DRUG TREATMENT OF HEART FAILURE

DRUG TREATMENT OF HEART FAILURE

Second Edition

Jay N. Cohn, MD
Editor

Advanced Therapeutics Communications International

SECAUCUS, NEW JERSEY • TOKYO • WORTHING, ENGLAND • MEXICO CITY

Before prescribing any medication, review the complete prescribing
information, including indications, contraindications, warnings,
precautions, and adverse effects.

Advanced Therapeutics Communications International
400 Plaza Drive
Secaucus, NJ 07096-1505

First edition published 1983. Second edition 1988
Printed in the United States of America

Library of Congress Cataloging-in-Publication Data

Drug treatment of heart failure.

   Includes bibliographies and index.
   1. Congestive heart failure—Chemotherapy.
I. Cohn, Jay N. [DNLM: 1. Heart Failure, Congestive
—drug therapy. 2. Heart Failure, Congestive
—physiopathology. WG 370 D794]
RC685.C53D78   1988   616.1′29061   88-22203
ISBN 0-911741-43-7

CONTENTS

Preface

In the past few years we have witnessed a remarkable growth of interest in the management of heart failure. Concern for this syndrome has intensified because of both its prevalence and lethality. As the population ages and as acute ischemic syndromes yield to aggressive interventional reperfusion efforts, pump dysfunction and accompanying heart failure become the most common problem facing the cardiologist. Furthermore, the now-recognized high mortality in the setting of severe left ventricular dysfunction has radically changed the perception of this disease from a chronic process of long duration to a high-risk process with a short life expectancy.

The second edition of this book represents an attempt to bring up to date the new concepts of this syndrome and, particularly, the newer approaches to its management. The available drug groups have not changed as much in the past few years as have the views regarding their use. Since many critical clinical trials utilizing some of these agents are still in progress, the views expressed by the authors of this book may change as new data become available. But the principles that must be applied to our evaluation of therapeutic agents should be constant. Since the pharmaceutical industry has supplied much of the innovation and, along with the government, most of the financial support for the drug development and clinical trials, they must be viewed as collaborators in the continuing investigative effort.

Our growing experience in the pharmacologic and physiologic management of heart failure has convinced us that precision in the use of available drugs can greatly enhance both the quality of life and its duration in patients with heart failure. To impart the principles of this precision to the practicing physician is one of the most important goals of this book.

I express my appreciation to the authors of chapters in the first edition who have revised and updated their contributions for the second edition. My special thanks to those who have prepared new chapters that have allowed us to expand this new edition into a more comprehensive treatise on the treatment of heart failure. The efforts of Randy Steer and John Russo of Advanced Therapeutics Communications and of Cheryl Yano in my office at the University of Minnesota have been critical to the success of this project.

Jay N. Cohn, MD

Contributors

Kanu Chatterjee, MB, FRCP
Professor of Medicine
Lucie Stern Professor of Cardiology
University of California, San Francisco
Associate Chief, Division of Cardiology
Director, Coronary Care Unit
H.M. Moffitt Hospital
San Francisco, California

Robert J. Cody, MD
Professor of Medicine
The Ohio State University Medical School
Research Director, Division of Cardiology
The Ohio State University Hospital
Columbus, Ohio

Jay N. Cohn, MD
Professor of Medicine
Head, Cardiovascular Division
University of Minnesota Medical School
Minneapolis, Minnesota

James E. Doherty, MD
Professor of Medicine and Pharmacology
University of Arkansas for Medical Sciences
Director of Cardiovascular Research
Veterans Administration Medical Center
Little Rock, Arkansas

Gary S. Francis, MD
Professor of Medicine
University of Minnesota Medical School
Director of Cardiovascular Research
Veterans Administration Medical Center
Minneapolis, Minnesota

Steven R. Goldsmith, MD
Associate Professor of Medicine
University of Minnesota Medical School
Director, Cardiology Clinics
Hennepin County Medical Center
Minneapolis, Minnesota

Norman K. Hollenberg, MD, PhD
Director and Professor of Physiologic
  Research
Departments of Medicine and Radiology
Brigham and Women's Hospital and Harvard
  Medical School
Boston, Massachusetts

Spencer H. Kubo, MD
Assistant Professor of Medicine
Director, Heart Failure Program
University of Minnesota Medical School
Minneapolis, Minnesota

John H. Laragh, MD
Professor of Medicine
Cornell University Medical College
Director, Cardiovascular and Hypertension
  Centers
The New York Hospital–Cornell University
  Medical Center
New York, New York

Milton Packer, MD
Associate Professor of Medicine
Mt. Sinai School of Medicine
City University of New York
Director, Cardiovascular Training Program
Director, Coronary Care Unit
Mt. Sinai Hospital
New York, New York

William W. Parmley, MD
Professor of Medicine
Chief, Division of Cardiology
University of California, San Francisco
San Francisco, California

Bertram Pitt, MD
Professor of Internal Medicine
Director, Division of Cardiology
University of Michigan Medical Center
Ann Arbor, Michigan

Elliot Rapaport, MD
Professor of Medicine
School of Medicine
University of California, San Francisco
Chief, Cardiology Division
San Francisco General Hospital
San Francisco, California

Edmund H. Sonnenblick, MD
Olson Professor of Medicine
Chief of the Division of Cardiology
Director of Cardiovascular Center
Albert Einstein College of Medicine
New York, New York

John E. Strobeck, MD, PhD
Clinical Assistant Professor of Medicine
Albert Einstein College of Medicine
Director, Coronary Care Unit
The Valley Hospital
Ridgewood, New Jersey

JAY N. COHN, MD

1

Heart Failure: An Overview

Congestive heart failure is so well recognized clinically that physicians have been lulled into a false confidence that they understand this syndrome. But as sophisticated techniques for measuring cardiac performance, neurohormonal activity, circulatory function, and exercise tolerance have become more readily available, the complexities of this disease process have become increasingly apparent. The most useful definition of congestive heart failure is that it represents a condition of impaired cardiac pumping ability that during exercise results in an attenuated rise in cardiac output and/or an exaggerated increase in cardiac filling pressure, which limits exercise capacity because of breathlessness or fatigue. Heart failure may develop as a major sign of progressively impaired cardiac pumping ability in all forms of heart disease.

If we accept this simple definition of heart failure, there still remain a vast number of unresolved questions relating to the etiology, pathophysiology, clinical recognition, treatment, and prognosis of this syndrome. Because an understanding of the present state of knowledge of these various aspects of heart failure may be vital in gaining insight into appropriate preventive and therapeutic measures, we shall briefly examine in this overview current concepts of this abnormal cardiac and systemic state. Details will then be provided in the chapters that follow.

ETIOLOGY Any disorder that produces primary damage to the myocardium or places the heart under chronically increased pressure or volume load may eventuate in the syndrome of heart failure. The deleterious effect of an increased pressure load was emphasized by data collected during the long-term Framingham study.[1] The vast majority of patients who developed heart failure in this study had, as an important factor, systemic hypertension. Even when rheumatic heart disease or coronary heart disease was present, the coexistence of hypertension was suggested by the Framingham data to be an important factor in the development of heart failure.[2] This experience not only provided a rational basis for understanding the development of heart failure but also implied that control of hypertension might be successful in eliminating most cases of heart failure observed in our society. It appears, however, that considerable change in the demographics of heart failure has taken place over the two decades since most of the Framingham data were collected. Treatment of hypertension has markedly improved and in most medical centers overt systemic hypertension as a direct etiologic factor in the development of heart failure is now much less common.

In most contemporary series, significant coronary artery disease is a likely etiologic factor in about 40% to 75% of patients presenting with signs and symptoms of congestive heart failure.[3] Even if hypertension had been a risk factor for the development of coronary artery disease at the time of the clinical appearance of heart failure, only a minority of these patients still manifest hypertensive blood pressure readings. Coronary disease appears capable of precipitating chronic heart failure in at least two different ways: (1) by an infarct or recurring ischemia that impairs the contractile performance of a sufficiently large area of the left ventricular myocardium so that overall pump performance is impaired, and (2) by a generalized hypokinesis of the entire left ventricle even in areas of the myocardium served by relatively normal coronary vessels. This latter syndrome is sometimes referred to as ischemic cardiomyopathy.[4]

The remaining 25% to 60% of patients with congestive heart failure do not have a history or findings compatible with significant coronary artery disease. Their heart muscle disease, therefore, may be viewed as probably nonischemic, although in some of these patients the possibility of a small vessel process leading to ischemia cannot be entirely excluded.[5] The exact mechanism of this muscle disease is not understood and probably involves a number of other possible etiologies. In a certain percentage of these patients with so-called nonischemic cardiomyopathy, the possibility of direct toxic damage to the myocardium, as from alcohol, nutritional deficiencies, viral infections, etc, can be identified. In others the absence of a known etiology dictates the use of the term *idiopathic*. Of particular interest in situations such as mitral regurgitation or aortic insufficiency is the progressive heart muscle disease that appears to accompany long-standing left ventricular volume overload. In these structural diseases the development of heart failure appears to represent a progressive deterioration of heart muscle function as a consequence of this long-standing overload. Nonetheless, if one views cardiac volume overload and the accompanying increase in wall stress as a stimulus to a progressive impairment of muscle function, then the pump dysfunction of congestive heart failure may represent, at least in part, the consequence of a self-perpetuated process initiated by cardiac dilatation.

CLINICAL RECOGNITION It is not a challenge for physicians to recognize congestive heart failure in patients with severe decompensation manifested by elevated central venous pressure, pulmonary rales, peripheral edema, small peripheral pulses, cardiac enlargement, and an S_3 gallop. More subtle and more important is the diagnosis of earlier stages of heart failure before these overt manifestations of decompensation become obvious.

2

Stress Testing   At earlier stages of heart failure it is usually mandatory to utilize some form of exercise stress in order to elicit the underlying functional cardiac deficiency. A bicycle ergometer or a treadmill can be used to quantitate impaired exercise capacity. Measurement of oxygen consumption by collecting expired gas during a progressive exercise test allows calculation of the peak oxygen consumption that the patient can achieve. Peak oxygen consumption less than 25 mL/kg/min measured at the time that dyspnea or fatigue prevents further exercise may be assumed to represent a limited oxygen consumption. If this limitation is related to cardiac dysfunction then cessation of exercise will be accompanied by a rising of respiratory quotient and a rising expired air oxygen content indicative of anaerobic metabolism and a peak cardiac output response. Use of these metabolic measurements to augment the more traditional exercise test provides more precise criteria for documentation of the presence and severity of exercise incapacity. Because heart failure is characterized by an exaggerated rise in cardiac filling pressure and an attenuated rise in cardiac output during stress, the invasive and noninvasive measurement of filling pressure and cardiac output provide physiologic evidence of the presence of pump failure.[6] These measurements are frequently conducted during heart catheterization in patients with suspected heart failure. However, it is now also possible to measure cardiac output during exercise by using noninvasive techniques, such as CO_2 rebreathing,[7] and to measure left heart filling pressure with the use of bedside balloon flotation catheterization or right atrial pressure by careful visual inspection of the jugular venous pulse.

The hepatojugular reflux test, conducted at the bedside, is a simple means of challenging the heart to detect early signs of heart failure. A sustained increase in jugular venous pressure during right upper quadrant abdominal compression has long been used by clinicians as a guide to the presence of cardiac decompensation. In normal individuals the jugular venous pressure is unaffected by this maneuver or, at most, shows a transient rise in venous pressure, which promptly falls to its previous level. If the head and neck are properly positioned for optimal utilization of the neck as a manometer, abdominal compression in patients with congestive heart failure usually reveals a prompt rise in the venous pressure, which remains elevated as long as abdominal compression is maintained. The pressure promptly falls to the previous level when abdominal compression is removed.

The mechanism of the positive hepatojugular reflux test has been controversial for many years.[8] We have demonstrated development of a positive hepatojugular reflux test in a dog model of heart failure that was, to some extent, independent of the mobilization of venous blood by abdominal compression. A large component of the rise of right atrial pressure during abdominal compression in the dog when the heart is enlarged could be explained by the mechanical effects of the rising diaphragm as it impinges upon cardiac filling.[9] It is therefore likely that the positive hepatojugular reflux test represents the summation of two phenomena: (1) a heart that cannot easily respond to the augmented venous return induced by blood mobilized from the abdominal viscera, and (2) a rising diaphragm that produces a form of tamponade that impedes cardiac filling and augments atrial pressure in the presence of the increased venous return. Regardless of the mechanism mediating this positive test, it has served as a useful clinical guide to early stages of heart failure that may not always be manifested by overt signs. Because this test can only assess the filling characteristics of the right heart, isolated left ventricular failure may not be recognized. Fortunately, even in predominantly left-sided heart failure, the hepatojugular reflux test is often positive. Nonetheless, the inability at the bedside to assess left-sided filling pressures does impair the precision of the clinical diagnosis of heart failure, which most commonly begins as a syndrome affecting the left ventricle.

The demonstration of abnormal cardiac findings at rest documents the presence of heart disease even if it does not in itself confirm the diagnosis of heart failure. Enlargement of the heart, a prominent apical impulse, an S_3 heart sound, an apical systolic murmur indicative of mitral regurgitation, left ventricular dilation (as demonstrated on a chest x-ray or echocardiography), or reduced ejection fraction (as shown with ventriculography or radionuclide scanning) may all be present in patients who manifest impaired functional capacity during exercise as a result of cardiac disease.

Classification of Severity of Heart Failure   Heart failure may be defined clinically either by the severity of cardiac dysfunction or by the severity of impaired exercise performance. The New York Heart Association classification, which is widely used to assess the severity of heart failure on clinical grounds, relies heavily upon the occurrence of symptoms during exertion. The goal of this classification is to provide a simple means of categorizing patients on the basis of severity of impairment of their life-style. The shortcoming of this assessment is that it depends entirely on subjective historical data. The degree of exercise impairment reported by the patient may bear surprisingly little relationship to the true limitation of exercise capacity. Patients who lead sedentary lives may report no symptoms despite considerable impairment of exercise performance; the history described by other patients may include marked limitations in exercise capacity, yet they perform remarkably well during quantitative exercise testing. Replacing the historical New York Heart Association classification with a classification based on objective measurements of exercise capacity (preferably supplemented by measurement of oxygen consumption) is a far more precise way to assess the limitations imposed by impaired cardiac performance. Such classifications have recently been reported from two different laboratories and appear to provide an objective measurement that is often at considerable variance from the New York Heart Association classification.[10,11]

An entirely independent method of assessing severity of heart failure is to quantitate the degree of cardiac dysfunction. This may be done by measuring heart size (by radiographic or echocardiographic techniques), by evaluating left ventricular ejection fraction (on the basis of ventriculography or radionuclide techniques), by quantitating heart muscle function by means of assessment of contractility (using invasive or noninvasive techniques), or by quantitating pump function (on the basis of the cardiac filling pressure and the stroke volume, cardiac output, or cardiac work). While intuitively it might be expected that the severity of resting pump dysfunction assessed by these invasive or noninvasive techniques would bear a close relationship to the impairment of exercise performance assessed by quantitative exercise testing, it appears that the correlation is surprisingly poor.[12] In some patients with relatively well-preserved resting ventricular function, severe symptoms develop during exertion, whereas in other individuals severe resting impairment of pump function may be associated with little or no symptoms of congestive heart failure. Therefore, it is likely that measurements of resting cardiac performance and functional capacity are independent phenomena.

Recently obtained data from the Veterans Administration Cooperative Study of Vasodilator Therapy of Heart Failure (V-HeFT) indicate that both ejection fraction and exercise tolerance are independent predictors of survival in heart failure. When both ejection fraction and peak O_2 consumption were below the median for the group, the subsequent mortality rate was at least twice that observed when only one of the measurements was below the median and nearly four times as great as when both measurements were above the median.[13]

PATHO-PHYSIOLOGY If heart failure were a direct consequence of damage to heart muscle, then it would be relatively simple to induce heart failure in an animal model by damaging the myocardium, and it could be expected that diseases such as acute myocardial infarction would precipitate the full-blown stable state of heart failure at the time of the initial event. Quite to the contrary, however, chronic heart failure is extremely difficult to produce in experimental animals despite the use of a variety of techniques to damage the myocardium.[14-16] Furthermore, patients who experience acute myocardial infarcts involving large areas of the left ventricle may spontaneously recover from acute left ventricular decompensation, yet they may present months later with signs and symptoms of congestive heart failure despite the fact that no further damage has apparently occurred to the myocardium.

In recent years, we have been able to develop a satisfactory dog model for heart failure that requires several months to develop after acute production of a fairly large area of myocardial damage by repetitive DC shock. These observations tend to confirm the impression that the syndrome of congestive heart failure that we recognize so well in the clinical setting represents the combined effects of a number of positive feedback mechanisms involving the heart, the peripheral circulation, and a number of vital organ systems. Although the complexity of this multisystem involvement makes it far more difficult to understand this disease, it also provides some basis for the thesis that the heart muscle disease itself may not be the limiting factor in satisfactory treatment of this disease state. Rather, positive feedback mechanisms may contribute to the syndrome to an extent that their interruption can produce a favorable clinical response. These positive feedback mechanisms may involve (1) aortic impedance; (2) ventricular preload; (3) myocardial hypertrophy; (4) sodium retention; (5) peripheral edema; (6) myocardial ischemia; and (7) neurohormonal responses, including the sympathetic nervous system, the renin-angiotensin-aldosterone system, the antidiuretic hormone-vasopressin system, and atrial natriuretic peptide.

Aortic Impedance Left ventricular emptying during systole is dependent, in part, upon the impedance the left ventricle confronts during ejection. This impedance includes a resistance component that resides largely in the small arteries and arterioles and a compliance component that resides in the larger arteries. The normal left ventricle is able to adjust to rather large changes in impedance with very small changes in emptying, in part by calling upon its Frank-Starling mechanism and perhaps in part by augmentation of contractile force as an intrinsic property of the normal myocardium (Fig. 1-1). In contrast, the damaged left ventricle loses this compensatory ability and becomes sensitive to even small changes in impedance.[17] Because vasoconstrictor mechanisms could be expected to reduce the caliber of the small arteries and arterioles and reduce the compliance of the large arteries, increased activity of the sympathetic nervous system, the renin-angiotensin-aldosterone system, or the vasopressin-antidiuretic hormone system could decrease stroke volume and cardiac output by imposing increased impedance on left ventricular emptying.[18] Because congestive heart failure is characterized by heightened activity of these neurohumoral vasoconstrictor systems, a positive feedback loop could be generated in which impaired pump performance increases impedance to left ventricular ejection, which further impairs the pump performance and sets in motion a vicious circle (Fig. 1-2).

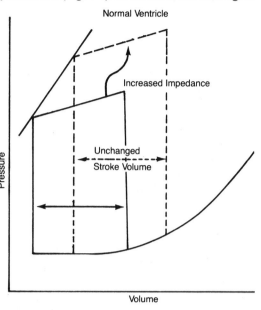

Fig. 1-1. Pressure-volume loop. In the normal heart, an increase in impedance (dashed line) may be counterbalanced by an increase in end-diastolic volume that maintains stroke volume constant. The diseased ventricle may lose this compensatory mechanism.

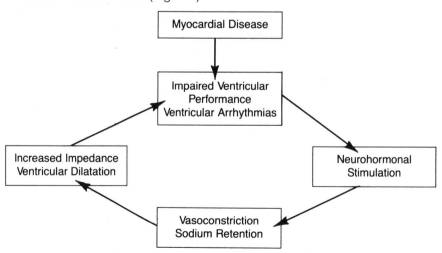

Fig. 1-2. Vicious circle of heart failure. As cardiac output falls, compensatory responses produce vasoconstriction and elevate systemic vascular resistance, which perpetuates myocardial failure.

Ventricular Preload   A high left ventricular filling pressure contributes to the pulmonary venous congestion of heart failure and probably plays an important role in precipitating the breathlessness that limits exercise tolerance. The elevated left ventricular filling pressure also contributes to the development of the elevated right ventricular filling pressure and peripheral edema that are also manifestations of chronic heart failure. The elevated cardiac filling pressure in heart failure probably is multifactorial. Impaired emptying of the left ventricle leaves a larger end-diastolic volume and pressure. Sodium retention caused by hormonal or renal perfusion abnormalities characterizes heart failure and leads to expansion of plasma volume. Decreased venous compliance reduces the capacitance of the venous system and could contribute to the rise in venous pressure even if the intravascular volume were normal.[19] Increased activity of the sympathetic nervous system probably plays a role in decreasing venous compliance, and the peripheral edema may further compress veins and contribute to this reduced venous capacitance. The elevated cardiac filling pressure also may reflect an abnormality in diastolic compliance of the ventricle.

Myocardial Hypertrophy   Protein synthesis and myocardial hypertrophy appear to be almost inevitable components of congestive heart failure. The pressure-overloaded and volume-overloaded ventricle responds to these abnormal loads by generating an increase in muscle mass, which initially appears as an appropriate response to maintain cardiac performance.[20] With time, however, this hypertrophic process may lead to further impairment of pump performance due to changes in either diastolic compliance as a result of a thickened ventricular wall, or impaired systolic pump performance due to impaired muscle function and/or the growth of collagen as well as muscle fibers during hypertrophy. Because failure induces hypertrophy and hypertrophy may thus induce failure, another positive feedback mechanism may have been identified.

Sodium Retention   Both hemodynamic and hormonal factors appear to contribute to the sodium retention that characterizes congestive heart failure. Abnormalities of renal perfusion appear to play a critical role in the abnormalities of sodium excretion.[21] A number of hormonal factors including the sympathetic nervous system, the renin-angiotensin-aldosterone system, and the vasopressin-antidiuretic hormone system, all of which are activated in heart failure,[22] probably contribute somewhat to the functional abnormality of the kidney. Thus, the kidney is integrally involved in the positive feedback loops contributing to the development of heart failure.

A new hormone, atrial natriuretic peptide, has recently been identified and characterized.[23] Studies suggest that levels of this hormone, which is thought to serve a regulatory role in the control of sodium excretion, are increased in patients with congestive heart failure. Although these elevated levels might be expected to produce a natriuresis, it is known that sodium excretion is markedly inhibited in congestive heart failure. One explanation for this paradox is that the sodium-retentive mechanisms in heart failure overwhelm the effect of the peptide; another is that the natriuretic effect is down regulated because of the chronically increased circulating levels of the hormone (see Chap. 3).

Peripheral Edema

A prerequisite for the development of peripheral edema on the basis of congestive heart failure is an elevated jugular venous pressure either at rest or during exercise. A number of factors, in addition to the elevated venous pressure, may contribute to the development of edema. The elevated venous pressure must be transmitted back to the capillary bed as an elevated capillary pressure in order to account for increased transudation out of capillaries in dependent portions of the body. Sodium and water retention and a decrease in plasma oncotic pressure may contribute to this transudation, as well as abnormalities of lymphatic drainage related in part to an elevated central venous pressure and resultant inhibition of thoracic duct drainage. In addition, the development of some edema may encourage further development of edema; edema may also influence venous compliance and thereby have an indirect effect on venous pressure itself, thus further perpetuating a vicious circle.

Myocardial Ischemia

It is well known that the subendocardial region of the myocardium must be perfused during diastole with a fairly low effective perfusion pressure. The maintenance of subendocardial perfusion is partially dependent on a low ventricular diastolic pressure that does not compress the subendocardial vessels directly adjacent to the ventricular chamber. If ventricular diastolic pressure rises to abnormal levels, the increased diastolic pressure will be transmitted into the subendocardial region and compress the subendocardial vessels. This abnormality may be a particularly important mechanism of ischemia in patients with proximal coronary artery stenosis in whom the distal coronary artery pressure is already strikingly reduced, and thus unable to maintain subendocardial perfusion in the presence of an elevated intracardiac pressure during diastole. Even in the presence of normal coronary arteries, however, subendocardial ischemia can be induced by experimental elevation of the left ventricular diastolic pressure.[24] Because myocardial ischemia can induce a rise in cardiac filling pressure by virtue of a decrease in compliance of the ventricle, and an elevated ventricular filling pressure can induce ischemia by virtue of subendocardial underperfusion, it is clear that potential for perpetuating a vicious circle may be generated by the coexistence of both ischemia and poor ventricular function.

Neurohormonal Responses in Heart Failure

Elevated plasma norepinephrine levels are a common finding in patients with congestive heart failure and suggest that the sympathetic nervous system is activated.[25] The systemic vasoconstriction and tachycardia that accompany heart failure provide further evidence for the involvement of the sympathetic nervous system in this process. Plasma renin activity often is elevated to very high levels in heart failure, whereas in some patients plasma renin activity is normal or even low.[26] Therefore, it is likely that in at least some patients with congestive heart failure, activation of the renin-angiotensin-aldosterone system represents another compensatory mechanism used by the body to adjust to an abnormality of pump performance.

Recent studies demonstrate that plasma arginine vasopressin levels are also increased in patients with congestive heart failure.[27] Because vasopressin is a potent vasoconstrictor as well as an antidiuretic hormone, it may well be that participation of this system in the neurohormonal response to heart failure further represents the body's efforts to constrict the peripheral vessels in an effort to support blood pressure. Activation of all these systems may be somewhat inappropriate on the basis of previous comments regarding aortic impedance. The interrelationship of these three endogenous vasoconstrictor systems and the precise mechanisms for their activation in congestive heart failure remain speculative (see Chap. 3).

PROGNOSIS In recent years it has become apparent that the functional state of the left ventricle is an important determinant of prognosis in patients with heart disease. In coronary disease, for instance, the severity of symptoms of heart failure and the ejection fraction as an index of ventricular function appear to be important independent predictors of survival above and beyond the severity of the coronary arterial lesions.[28] Similarly, in patients with acute myocardial infarction, mortality is directly related to the severity of ventricular dysfunction.[29,30] In addition, the syndrome of sudden death is relatively infrequent in the absence of considerable cardiac dysfunction,[31] and the risk of sudden death in patients with ventricular premature beats is directly related to the associated left ventricular dysfunction. From an epidemiologic standpoint, therefore, the majority of cardiovascular deaths in our society may be associated with or attributed to left ventricular dysfunction.

The etiology of heart failure appears to have less importance than might be suspected in the course of the disease. Thus, sudden death is an important terminal event in patients with idiopathic cardiomyopathy as well as in those with coronary artery disease. And the syndrome of heart failure appears to have a similarly poor prognosis in all subgroups of patients studied. Indeed, the poor prognosis in this syndrome has been newly emphasized in recent years by startlingly high mortality rates observed in patients followed after recognition of the presence of symptomatic heart failure.[3,32] Data from the V-HeFT trial as well as from other studies indicate that the mortality rate in congestive heart failure is related to the severity of left ventricular dysfunction, the degree of impairment of exercise tolerance, the presence of complex ventricular arrhythmias, and the level of plasma norepinephrine. All of these markers appear to reflect the severity of the myocardial disease or the magnitude of the compensatory response to that disease. The precise incidence of heart failure in our society is unknown. This dilemma is compounded by the likelihood that early stages of the disease are largely undiagnosed. If the early, presymptomatic phase of left ventricular dysfunction serves as a reservoir from which overt heart failure develops, then ventricular dysfunction should be considered to be "the disease." It would then be far more common than the current estimates of the incidence of overt heart failure.

THERAPY Major advances have been made during the past decade in drug therapy for congestive heart failure. The concept that the severely failing left ventricle is no longer capable of responding to pharmacologic intervention is no longer tenable. Even the most profoundly depressed left ventricular pump seems capable of augmenting its output in response to the appropriate vasodilator or inotropic stimulus. Therefore, one must conclude that the endogenous mechanisms that are supposedly available to improve the performance of the pump in response to disease or stress are not adequate to optimally maintain pump performance. These conceptual observations stress the potential for pharmacologic management in the restoration of cardiac performance even when all indices of cardiac function are severely impaired.

The quality of life, exercise capacity, and life expectancy of patients with heart failure may be alterable by the introduction of appropriate medical therapy at the appropriate time in the course of the patient's heart disease. In the chapters that follow, we shall explore in depth the various pharmacologic approaches available and the physiologic basis for their use in patients with failing hearts. This is a dynamic field in which new drugs that may be able to alter the performance of the heart are continually being synthesized and entered into clinical trials. Although many of these agents may utilize somewhat differing pharmacologic mechanisms, the overall theory behind these various approaches to heart failure probably will not change. Therefore, it is hoped that this volume will provide the framework upon which new drugs can be understood even if some newer agents that may soon become available are not specifically addressed.

Along with the rapid advances in drug therapy of heart failure have come new and aggressive approaches to life support of the patient whose clinical syndrome no longer appears to be responsive to pharmacologic intervention. Heart transplant has become a practical means of management for such patients, and the remarkable results with this procedure in selected institutions means that long-term survival and a productive life are the rule rather than the exception. The limitations of heart transplant as a practical mode of therapy for all patients with end-stage heart failure are, of course, obvious. Limited resources and limited donor hearts prevent this from becoming a solution to the problem. Development of an artificial heart to replace the human heart has been a high-priority research effort in several centers in the United States. A rational use of the present externally driven pumps can be seen in recent reports of limited success with the use of these mechanical devices as a bridge to heart transplants. Permanent implantation must await the development of a reliable, totally implantable device that can adjust its output to meet the changing needs of peripheral tissues.

In the long run, it appears that the goals of medicine should be to forestall the development of heart disease and, when this fails, to provide appropriate therapy for the earliest stages of heart muscle disease in order to prevent the development of end-stage heart failure. There is reason to suspect that both of these approaches may have long-term potential. Drug therapy may then have a place in the management of early stages of heart failure, which if left untreated might progress through activation of the positive feedback mechanisms outlined above to a later stage of the disease that eventually might become unresponsive to pharmacologic manipulation. Early intervention in such patients, if the proper time of intervention can be identified, might therefore have an important impact on the natural history of the disease. Such hopes for the future remain speculative, but it is clear that an understanding of the disturbed pathophysiology of heart failure is providing us with the necessary understanding with which these therapeutic attempts may be undertaken.

REFERENCES

1. McKee PA, Castelli WP, McNamara PM, et al: The natural history of congestive heart failure: The Framingham Study. *N Engl J Med* 1971;285:1441-1446.
2. Kannel WB, Castelli WP, McNamara PM: Role of blood pressure in the development of congestive heart failure: The Framingham Study. *N Engl J Med* 1972;287: 781-787.
3. Franciosa JA, Wilen M, Ziesche S, et al: Survival in men with severe chronic left ventricular failure due to either coronary heart disease or idiopathic dilated cardiomyopathy. *Am J Cardiol* 1983;51:831-836.
4. Burch GE, Giles TD, Colcolough HL: Ischemic cardiomyopathy. *Am Heart J* 1970;79:291-292.
5. Factor SM, Sonnenblick EH: Hypothesis: Is congestive cardiomyopathy caused by a hyperreactive myocardial microcirculation (microvascular spasm)? *Am J Cardiol* 1982;50:1149-1152.
6. Pierpont GL, Cohn JN, Franciosa JA: Congestive cardiomyopathy: Pathophysiology and response to therapy. *Arch Intern Med* 1978;138:1847-1850.
7. Franciosa JA, Ragan DO, Rubenstone SJ: Validation of the CO_2 rebreathing method for measuring cardiac output in patients with hypertension or heart failure. *J Lab Clin Med* 1976;88:672-682.
8. Burch GE, Ray CT: Mechanism of hepatojugular reflux test in congestive heart failure. *Am Heart J* 1954;48:373-382.
9. Cohn JN, Hamosh P: Experimental observations on pulsus paradoxus and hepatojugular reflux, in Reddy PS, Leon DF, Shaver JA (eds): *Pericardial Diseases.* New York, Raven Press, 1982, pp 249-258.
10. Franciosa JA, Park M, Levine TB: Lack of correlation between exercise capacity and indexes of resting left ventricular performance in heart failure. *Am J Cardiol* 1979;47:33-39.
11. Weber KT, Kinasewitz GT, Janicki JS, et al: Oxygen utilization and ventilation during exercise in patients with chronic cardiac failure. *Circulation* 1982;65:1213-1223.
12. Francis GS, Goldsmith SR, Cohn JN: The relationship of exercise capacity to resting left ventricular performance and basal plasma norepinephrine levels in patients with congestive heart failure. *Am Heart J* 1982;104:725-731.
13. Cohn JN, Ziesche SM, Archibald DG, et al: Quantitative exercise tolerance as a predictor of mortality in congestive heart failure: The V-HeFT Study. *Circulation* 1986;76(suppl 2):138.
14. Carlyle PF, Cohn JN: A non-surgical canine model of chronic left ventricular myocardial dysfunction. *Am J Physiol* 1983;244:H769-H774.
15. Franciosa JA, Heckel R, Limas C, et al: Progressive myocardial dysfunction associated with increased vascular resistance. *Am J Physiol* 1980;239:H477-H482.
16. Mehta J, Runge W, Cohn JN, et al: Myocardial damage after repetitive direct current shock in the dog: Correlation between left ventricular end-diastolic pressure and extent of myocardial necrosis. *J Lab Clin Med* 1978;91:272-279.
17. Cohn JN: Vasodilator therapy for heart failure: The influence of impedance on left ventricular performance. *Circulation* 1973;48:5-8.
18. Cohn JN, Mashiro I, Levine TB, et al: Role of vasoconstrictor mechanism in the control of left ventricular performance of the normal and damaged heart. *Am J Cardiol* 1979;44:1019-1022.
19. Wood JE: The mechanism of the increased venous pressure with exercise in congestive heart failure. *J Clin Invest* 1972;41:2020-2024.
20. Cohn JN, Limas CJ, Guiha N: Hypertension and the heart. *Arch Intern Med* 1974;133:969-979.
21. Barger AC: Renal hemodynamics in congestive heart failure. *Ann NY Acad Sci* 1973;139:786-797.

22. Cohn JN, Levine TB, Francis GS, et al: Neurohumoral control mechanisms in congestive heart failure. *Am Heart J* 1981;102:509-514.
23. deBold AJ, Borenstein HB, Veress AT, et al: A rapid and potent natriuretic response to intravenous injection of atrial myocardial extract in rats. *Life Sci* 1981;28:89-94.
24. Salisbury PF, Cross CE, Rieban PA: Acute ischemia of inner layers of ventricular wall. *Am Heart J* 1963;66:650-656.
25. Levine TB, Francis GS, Goldsmith SR, et al: Activity of the sympathetic nervous system and renin-angiotensin system assessed by plasma hormone levels and their relationship to hemodynamic abnormalities in congestive heart failure. *Am J Cardiol* 1982;49:1659-1666.
26. Curtiss C, Cohn JN, Vrobel T: Role of the renin-angiotensin system in the systemic vasoconstriction of chronic congestive heart failure. *Circulation* 1978;58:763-770.
27. Goldsmith SR, Francis GS, Cowley AW, et al: Increased plasma arginine vasopressin in patients with congestive heart failure. *J Am Coll Cardiol* 1983;1:1385-1390.
28. Califf RM, Bounous P, Harrell FE, et al: The prognosis in the presence of coronary artery disease, in Braunwald E, Mock MB, Watson J (eds): *Congestive Heart Failure.* New York, Grune and Stratton Inc, 1982, pp 31-40.
29. Cohn JN, Franciosa JA, Francis GS, et al: Effect of short-term infusion of sodium nitroprusside on mortality rate in acute myocardial infarction complicated by left ventricular failure. *N Engl J Med* 1982;306:1129-1135.
30. Sanz G, Castaner A, Betrui A, et al: Determinants of prognosis in survivors of myocardial infarction. *N Engl J Med* 1982;306:1065-1070.
31. Schultze RA, Strauss HW, Pitt BL: Sudden death in the year following myocardial infarction. *Am J Med* 1977;62:192-199.
32. Cohn JN: Part II: Clinical definitions and studies, in Braunwald E, Mock MB, Watson J (eds): *Congestive Heart Failure.* New York, Grune and Stratton Inc, 1982. pp 11-13.

JOHN E. STROBECK, MD, PhD, and
EDMUND H. SONNENBLICK, MD

2

Pathophysiology of Heart Failure: Deficiency in Cardiac Contraction

Congestive heart failure has traditionally been looked upon as a syndrome characterized by pulmonary and/or systemic venous congestion accompanied by a low cardiac output. Over the past 15 years, however, it has become clear that this broad definition has caused confusion in understanding this syndrome. While the term *congestive* acknowledges that venous congestion is present, we now know that severe heart failure may exist in the presence of normal or even low ventricular filling pressures. Also, some patients may have severe pulmonary or systemic venous congestion, while systolic ventricular performance is normal. Thus, in order for there to be a clear understanding of this syndrome, a distinction must be drawn between myocardial failure due to a defect in systolic performance, and congestive failure that results from a defect in diastolic function.

In this discussion of the pathophysiology of heart failure, the primary deficiencies of cardiac contraction that initiate compensatory mechanisms both in the heart and in the peripheral circulation of the patient with heart failure will be emphasized. These mechanisms result in cardiac chamber dilatation, myocardial hypertrophy, and activation of neural and humoral mechanisms that are designed to conserve body sodium and water, and maintain peripheral perfusion pressure. However, before theories or concepts of the pathogenesis of the deficiency of cardiac contraction leading to heart failure are presented, it is necessary to review the hemodynamic and muscular determinants of ventricular performance (ie, preload, afterload, contractility, and the interval between beats), as well as the neurohumoral factors affecting the interaction of the heart with the peripheral (arterial and venous) circulations. Consideration will also be given to how these factors are altered by disease.

**DETERMI-
NANTS OF
VENTRICULAR
PERFOR-
MANCE**

Preload

When isolated cardiac muscle is stimulated and held at a fixed length, the resultant contraction is termed isometric. In contrast to the situation with skeletal muscle, in which the force of contraction is nearly independent of muscle length over a wide range, and in which contraction is generally of a tetanic nature, the strength of individual isometric twitches in cardiac muscle is markedly length dependent. An increase in the initial muscle length, induced by a change in passive stretch of the muscle, produces a resting load that has been termed preload.

The effects of length on resting and developed force are established and expressed by the resting and active length-tension curves.[1] For reasons that remain incompletely understood, heart muscle is less compliant than skeletal muscle at rest,[2] so that resting tension rises more rapidly as heart muscle is stretched. It is also not known to what extent resting force is borne by passive elastic elements of the muscle, and to what extent it is maintained by active processes within the muscle. Regardless, the relatively high resting stiffness of cardiac muscle must be correlated with the inability to stretch the cardiac sarcomere beyond a length of about 2.2 μm.[1,2] At that sarcomere length the degree of overlap between actin and myosin filaments is optimal for contraction and muscle isometric force is maximal. This length is called L_{max}.

An increase in preload (eg, increased resting muscle length and sarcomere length) produces an increase in muscle force over the physiologic range and is responsible for the increase in stroke volume of the ventricle when end-diastolic volume is increased. The mechanisms of length-dependent muscle contractile behavior are not completely understood. Muscle force declines to zero between the optimum cardiac sarcomere length of 2.2 and 1.6 μm. Sarcomere length cannot be passively shortened below 2.0 μm.[3,4]

If a cardiac muscle cell is skinned of its sarcolemma, thus ensuring maximal activation and possibly removing internal loads, and the contractile apparatus is directly activated by Ca^{2+}, then the decline in force with shortening sarcomere length is less pronounced than in skeletal muscle (Fig. 2-1A).[5] In a skinned cardiac fiber, the relationship between muscle force and sarcomere length is shifted upward and to the left by increasing the extracellular Ca^{2+} concentration. When muscle force is corrected for passive resting force, borne presumably by noncontractile elements of the muscle, the relationship between muscle force and sarcomere length has a significantly steeper slope as calcium concentration is increased.[6,7] These data support the concept of a length-dependent activation process as the basis of the length-tension relation in cardiac muscle (Fig. 2-1B).

The exact nature of the length-dependent activation process is not known. It is unlikely that the length-tension relationship in cardiac muscle depends on length-dependent release of calcium to the myofilaments, because released calcium does not vary over a wide range of muscle and sarcomere lengths.[8] However, there is convincing evidence that, in cardiac muscle, myofilament sensitivity to calcium decreases with decreasing sarcomere length.[9,10] These data are not conclusive enough to rule out some effect of an internal load, because the nature of passive load-bearing structures

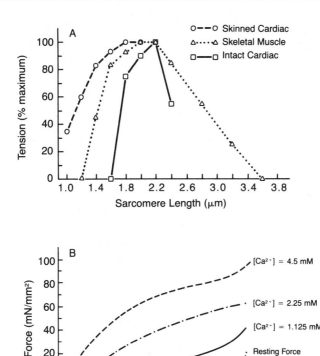

Fig. 2-1. A. Sarcomere length-tension relationships are depicted for skinned cardiac muscle, skeletal muscle, and intact cardiac muscle. Data from intact cardiac muscle[4] were obtained by fixing cat papillary muscles with glutaraldehyde at various diastolic lengths and recording the tension immediately before fixation. Average sarcomere length within tissue was determined electron microscopically. The relationship between tension development and sarcomere length obtained with skeletal fibers (Gordon et al, *J Physiol* 1966;184:170-192) is superimposed for comparison. Data from skinned cardiac muscle adapted from Fabiato and Fabiato[5] are also superimposed. In intact cardiac muscle, peak tension occurs with a diastolic sarcomere length of 2.2 μm,[4] whereas in skeletal muscle there is a plateau of developed tension between 2.2 and 2.0 μm. In intact cardiac muscle this is not the case, and developed tension falls as sarcomere length is decreased below 2.2 μm. There is a comparatively slower reduction in tension in skinned cardiac muscle that is maximally activated than in skeletal muscle. As intact cardiac muscle is stretched beyond 2.2 μm, resting tension rises substantially, while actively developed tension falls abruptly. In skeletal muscle, actively developed tension falls in a linear fashion between sarcomere lengths of. 2.2 and 3.6 μm. B. Relationships between force development and segment length (SL) at different calcium concentrations in mammalian cardiac muscle are shown. These curves are corrected for a segment-length-dependent passive force and show that the slope of the force–segment length relationship significantly increases as calcium concentration increases. This supports the existence of a length-dependent activation process that may reflect length-induced changes in calcium sensitivity of the myofilaments. (Adapted from DA Martyn, JF Rondinone, LL Huntsman, The dependence of force and velocity on calcium and length in cardiac muscle segments, *Adv Exp Med Biol* 1984;170:821-834, by permission of Plenum Publishing Corp.)

in cardiac muscle is not completely understood. Structures such as axially oriented collagen fibers[11] or surface fibers[12] might restrict shortening or elongation of sarcomeres and contribute to internal loads. However, the bulk of evidence suggests that, if present, the force of an internal load is small and will produce slight effects at physiologic lengths.[7]

Developed force, as noted earlier, is highly dependent on initial muscle length and hence sarcomere length; however, because of serial elasticities, peak muscle isometric force is obtained only with some obligatory sarcomere shortening during contraction. This shortening takes place at the expense of a series compliance, largely at the muscle ends.[4,13] Whether observed sarcomere shortening alters the isometric force that would have been generated at any myofilament overlap had no sarcomere shortening occurred has been determined.[9,14] Sarcomere length can be held reasonably constant by appropriate stretch of the muscle during the course of contraction. This method, which eliminates uncertainties due to series elasticity external to the sarcomere, proves that muscle force critically depends on a unique sarcomere length at the peak of contractile activity.[4]

The concept of isolated cardiac muscle mechanics takes on new dimensions when one considers the effect of muscle length on the mechanics of cardiac muscle in the ventricular wall. Increasing the length of ventricular muscle fibers is accomplished by a filling or distending pressure in the ventricular chamber created by inflow of blood during diastole. This pressure at end-diastole, termed ventricular preload, is a function of chamber shape and size, and the stiffness of the ventricular wall. The distending pressure in the ventricular chamber must be countered by an equal wall force that is generated by passive stretch of the muscle itself. The net wall force, which is the summated force from all the muscle fibers in the thickness of the wall, can be calculated for a spherical chamber as the product of intraventricular pressure and the cross-sectional area of the chamber at a given point along the long axis (net wall force $= P \times R_i^2$, where R_i is the internal radius of the spherical chamber). Wall stress (g/cm^2), the force borne by a unit-thickness area (cm^2) of myocardium is calculated by dividing wall force by $(R_o-R_i)^2$ where R_o is the outside radius of a spherical chamber, and R_i is the internal radius noted earlier. A midwall length of the "average" circumferential fiber is calculated as $2R_m$, where R_m is the midwall radius of the spherical chamber.

If ejection of blood from the ventricle during systole is prevented, an isovolumic contraction is generated. A series of isovolumic contractions from a variety of midwall circumferential lengths generates a pressure-length diagram that is analogous to the length-tension relationship in isolated cardiac muscle.

Starling's observations that "the mechanical energy set free on passage from the resting to the contracted state is a function of the muscle fibers' length (ie, the area of chemically active surfaces)"[15] underlie our current concepts of the relationship between the length-active tension curve in isolated muscle and the effect of end-diastolic pressure on stroke volume or stroke work in the intact ventricle (the Frank-Starling relationship). Shifts in the ventricular function curve, as shown in Figure 2-2, can also be used to demonstrate changes in contractility of the ventricle. Thus, the concept of ventricular function curves is useful in clinical settings to evaluate changes due to either load or contractility. In the heart, ventricular end-diastolic wall stress is analogous to the preload of an isolated muscle that, for physiologic loads, ultimately determines the resting length of sarcomeres in the ventricular wall. However, unlike the relation between muscle length and developed force in isolated muscle, where developed force reaches a maximum at a particular length (L_{max}) and then declines to form a "descending limb," in the normal ventricle an ascending limb of ventricular function (ie, the curve relating the increase in stroke volume with each increment in end-diastolic volume) continues above the range of normal end-diastolic pressures (ie, 12 to 14 mm Hg). Furthermore, at end-diastolic pressures greater than 20 mm Hg, or in certain disease states, the predicted relationship between midwall sarcomere lengths and diastolic wall stress is not always found.[1,16]

Fig. 2-2. Ventricular function curves expressed as the relationship between left ventricular end-diastolic pressure and stroke work. Increasing underlying myocardial contractility shifts the entire curve and changes its shape. Note that afterload, which can also change the shape and position of these curves, was constant during the experimental determination of these curves. (Adapted from JW Covell, J Ross, EH Sonnenblick, et al, Comparison of the force-velocity relation and the ventricular function curve as measures of the contractile state of the heart, *Circ Res* 1966;19:364-373, by permission of the American Heart Association, Inc.)

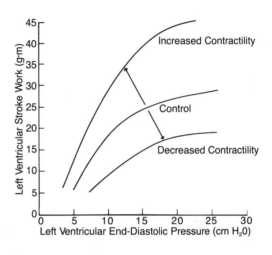

Sarcomere lengths vary considerably across the thickness of the ventricular wall. In the subendocardium, when studied at zero distending pressure, sarcomere lengths were longer than midwall or epicardial sarcomere lengths.[17,18] As distending pressure increased over the range of pressure defining the ascending limb of the length-tension curve in the intact left ventricle of open-chest dogs (2 to 20 mm Hg), sarcomere lengths approached their maximum (2.25 μm) at filling pressures of 10 to 12 mm Hg; however, shorter sarcomeres from both the inner and outer layers lengthened near 2.25 μm as filling pressure approached 20 mm Hg.[19] These findings may explain the apparent discrepancy between the observation that midwall sarcomere lengths in *in situ* hearts are near maximum when filling pressure is at the upper limit of normal (10 to 12 mm Hg), whereas an ascending limb of the ventricular isovolumic pressure-volume relationship is observed until even higher filling pressures are reached. Thus, at filling pressures above normal, recruitment of short sarcomeres from across the ventricular wall constitutes the functional reserve (preload reserve) of the Frank-Starling mechanism in the left ventricle.

The relative degree of sarcomere shortening during ejection in the left ventricle is also not the same in all layers of the ventricular wall (Fig. 2-3).[20] Thus, with 12% shortening in the midwall, epicardial fibers will shorten about 5% and endocardial layers will need to shorten approximately 20% of their initial lengths. Moreover, only the midwall fibers have been shown to shorten in a circumferential manner, whereas fibers in both the superficial and the endocardial layers shorten in an apex-to-base direction.[21] In angiographic studies circumferential shortening exceeds that of the apex-to-base direction, and large infoldings occur in the endocardial surfaces at end-systole. Thus, models directly relating fiber shortening in multiple layers of the heart to stroke volume are oversimplified.

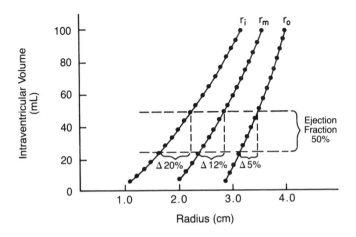

Fig. 2-3. Relationship between intraventricular volume and changes in circumference in the inner (i), middle (m), and outer (o) layers of the left ventricular wall. The dashed horizontal lines demark a change in volume from 50 to 25 mL, which represents a left ventricular ejection fraction of 50%. Such an ejection fraction would require a 5% change in the outer circumference of the heart, a 12% change in the midwall layers, and a 20% change in the inner circumference. (Adapted from EH Sonnenblick, Correlation of myocardial ultrastructure and function, *Circulation* 1968;38:29-44, by permission of the American Heart Association, Inc.)

Data obtained from fixed segments of cardiac muscle and from perfused intact heart,[22] in addition to the findings from recent studies of sarcomere motion,[2,7,12] permit construction of a diagram relating ventricular performance to sarcomere dimensions. Figure 2-4 represents the pressure-volume relationship of the intact heart, as well as the approximate length-tension relationship for the muscle composing the ventricular wall.[17,23,24] Moreover, because diastolic sarcomere length is determined by diastolic ventricular volume and hence diastolic muscle length, midwall diastolic sarcomere lengths measured at these volumes are shown below the pressure-volume curve.[12] These sarcomere lengths were obtained using rapid fixation methods that could produce as much as 5% shrinkage relative to the length occurring *in vivo*. Thus, a fixed sarcomere length of 2.0 μm might be 2.1 μm in living muscle.[25]

In Figure 2-4, hypothetical pressure-volume loops are portrayed on pressure-volume and pressure-sarcomere length axes. Loop ABCD represents contraction of the normal heart, loop EFGH shows a contraction potentiated by an inotropic stimulus, and loop IJKL illustrates a hypothetical loop for a failing ventricle.

Relative to the diastolic pressure-volume curve shown by connecting points I, L, A, E, D, and H, volume is not zero when filling pressure is zero.[17,26] Morever, to empty the ventricle completely, a substantial negative pressure (H) is required. In an intact heart at zero filling pressure, sarcomere lengths range from 1.90 to 2.00 μm, and sarcomere lengths shorter than 1.9 μm are not observed in the relaxed ventricular wall.[17] As noted earlier, diastolic sarcomere lengths in isolated cardiac muscle at slack muscle length also approximate 1.9 to 2.0 μm.[12] Shorter sarcomere lengths are attained during contraction, but sarcomeres reextend their lengths on relaxation. When contracting freely, with minimal or zero load, muscle cells in the ventricular wall will be expected to shorten to sarcomere lengths as short as 1.5 to 1.6 μm and then reextend to an equilibrium length of 2.0 μm on the basis of restoring forces alone.

Fig. 2-4. Relationship of ventricular performance, in terms of ventricular pressure-volume relationships, to average midwall sarcomere length is depicted under conditions of depressed, normal, and increased contractility. Intraventricular volume was obtained from dog left ventricle. These parameters can be translated into wall stress and circumferential fiber length, respectively, using formulas presented in this chapter. See text for further discussion. (Adapted from EH Sonnenblick, The structural basis and importance of restoring forces and elastic recoil for the filling of the heart, *Eur Heart J* 1980;1:107-110, with permission.)

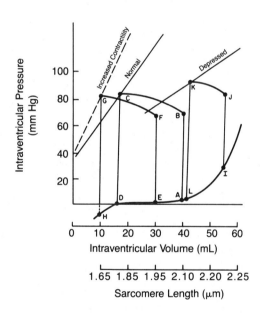

Returning to the pressure-volume (sarcomere) curve, a normal ventricle starts to contract from a sarcomere length of about 2.1μm. During isovolumic systole, sufficient force is generated to open the aortic valve (point B), followed by ventricular ejection (B to C). During ejection, the stress in the wall of the heart actually falls because of the progressive decline in ventricular volume, as predicted by the Laplace relation (tension = pressure × [R_i/2h], where R_i is the internal radius and h is wall thickness). Shortening continues until the end-systolic pressure (force)-volume (length) curve is reached. The position and slope of this curve are determined by the underlying contractility[27,28] and to a lesser degree by the afterload of the ventricle.[29,30] During systole, a normal heart ejects approximately two thirds of its initial volume; this corresponds to an end-systolic sarcomere length of approximately 1.8 to 1.9 μm. Thus, a normal heart begins its ejection from a sarcomere length that has a small but significant distending force and completes ejection at a sarcomere length at which elastic restoring forces will be relatively small. Accordingly, in a normally ejecting heart working at low heart rates, elastic recoil and early diastolic suction may make only a relatively small contribution to ventricular filling.[31]

In a heart in which contractility is increased, ventricular ejection begins at point E in Figure 2-4. The heart develops pressure and ejects volume to a midwall end-systolic sarcomere length of 1.65 μm.[23] At this sarcomere length, a substantial amount of elastic energy is stored during the process of systolic shortening and provides a significant elastic recoil during early diastole. It is clear that ventricular "suction" in early diastole should be most apparent and effective in augmenting early ventricular filling during periods when contractility is augmented and heart rate is increased (eg, during physical exercise). In a failing heart, the advantage of elastic recoil is diminished because of relatively long end-systolic sarcomere lengths. This may contribute to the inordinately elevated diastolic filling pressures seen in heart failure, especially during periods of demand for increased cardiac output. The loss of this elastic recoil also makes the failing heart more dependent on the contribution of atrial contraction to ventricular filling.

Afterload   Afterload, simply defined, is the load that the ventricular muscle senses and works against after it begins to contract. In experimental systems in which the load placed on an isolated muscle, or against which an isolated ventricle contracts, is controlled, the effects on systolic performance of varying afterload are clearly seen. However, when the intact circulation is considered as a ventricular pump that is coupled to a peripheral circulation with a characteristic input impedance, delineation of the factors contributing to the afterload on ventricular muscle becomes more complex. It has been argued that arterial input impedance best represents ventricular afterload,[32] but others consider systolic ventricular pressure[33] or wall tension[34] as more appropriate indices of afterload. It is clear that in a coupled cardiocirculatory system, a combination of cardiac and vascular factors, some of which are independent, contribute to the generation of ventricular afterload. Figure 2-5 illustrates some of the more important factors affecting ventricular afterload. It shows that cardiac-dependent ventriculoarterial coupling factors are independent of the vascular-dependent arterial afterload system. However, despite this theoretical independence, changes in arterial resistance and characteristic impedance have been shown to alter factors in the ventriculoarterial coupling system, such as wall stress and ventricular volume during systole.[30] The degree of independence also lessens significantly in disease states with myocardial failure.

Wall stress (force per unit area) is the most important afterload determinant of ventricular muscle. The ventricular wall stress during ejection (ventricular muscle afterload) significantly influences the quantity of blood ejected by the ventricles. For example, abrupt increases or decreases in ejection pressure inversely alter stroke volume. This occurs even when

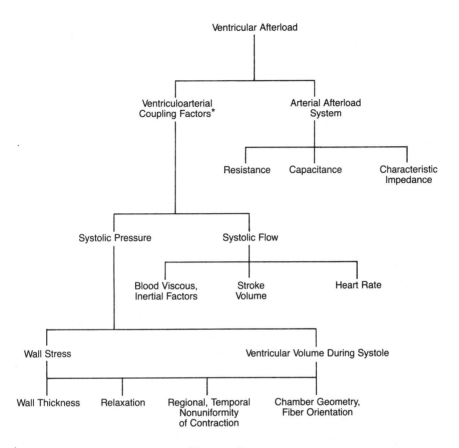

Ventricular Afterload

Ventriculoarterial Coupling Factors*   Arterial Afterload System

Resistance   Capacitance   Characteristic Impedance

Systolic Pressure   Systolic Flow

Blood Viscous, Inertial Factors   Stroke Volume   Heart Rate

Wall Stress   Ventricular Volume During Systole

Wall Thickness   Relaxation   Regional, Temporal Nonuniformity of Contraction   Chamber Geometry, Fiber Orientation

*This listing assumes a constant myocardial contractility.

Fig. 2-5. Factors affecting ventricular afterload.

end-diastolic volume is independently controlled.[10] Afterload is never constant during ventricular ejection. It continually declines as ventricular volume and midwall radius decrease, as predicted by the Laplace relation [wall stress $= Px(R_i/2h)$]. This type of contraction with continuously varying load is termed auxotonic contraction. Increasing afterload reduces stroke volume, as well as the extent and velocity of wall shortening, as shown in the end-systolic pressure-volume diagram (Fig. 2-6). If afterload is rapidly varied during the course of a single ejection, an instantaneous force-velocity-length relationship can be determined. Decreasing or increasing afterload causes immediate inverse changes in the velocity and extent of midwall shortening as well as the ejected volume. Also, analogous to what occurs in isolated muscle, the intact left ventricle reaches a point at end-systole that is near the isovolumetric length-active tension curve, regardless of the imposed afterload or the time course of its application (Fig. 2-6).[27] This relationship has recently been refined and discussed as a specific index of ventricular contractility.[29,30]

21

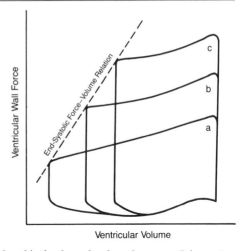

Fig. 2-6. Effects of changes in afterload, created by increasing the impedance to ejection, on the ventricular wall force–volume relationship during normal contraction with preload held constant. Contractions a, b, and c show decreasing end-systolic volume and wall force during the ejection of three levels of afterload. There is an inverse relationship between wall force during ejection and the extent of ventricular emptying. Not shown, but occurring simultaneously, were reciprocal changes in the rate of midwall ventricular shortening with load (force-velocity relationship). Note that at end-ejection, wall force and volume coincide with the isovolumic volume–wall force line describing underlying myocardial contractility.

Low impedance to ventricular ejection, as is produced by mitral regurgitation, patent ductus arteriosus, ventricular septal defect, or arteriovenous shunt, can increase ejection fraction in patients with normal ventricular contractility through a reduction in ventricular afterload. Increases in afterload, as when an infusion of angiotensin elevates systemic blood pressure, lead to compensatory alterations in preload, early diastolic ventricular function, and the contribution of ventricular volume to afterload,[32] which allow maintenance of stroke volume in the normal heart (Fig. 2-7).[33] When these compensatory mechanisms are impaired in diseased hearts, however, stroke volume and stroke work fall, with similar elevations in afterload. This response of the diseased heart depends on the extent of the reduction in ventricular contractility, as well as the capability for making adjustments in preload (Fig. 2-8). Thus, in the intact circulation, when there is relative hypovolemia and/or depressed ventricular contractility, a given increase in afterload will reduce stroke volume. This does not occur when contractility is higher or when preload can increase adequately.[33]

An understanding of the effects of afterload on ventricular muscle and ventriculoarterial coupling is crucial for an appreciation of the effects of chronic systemic pulmonary arterial hypertension, the consequences of obstructed ventricular ejection by valvular disease (eg, aortic or pulmonic stenosis), and the effects on hemodynamics of mitral or aortic regurgitation. For these conditions pharmacologic or surgical manipulation of afterload constitutes the primary mode of therapy.

Contractility　　Contractility is a concept, derived from isolated cardiac muscle studies,[35,36] that defines the intensity of activation of the myofibrils during contraction (ie, the processes leading to formation of force-generating sites and attachment of cross-bridges). Contractility can be influenced by membrane excitation, myoplasmic Ca^{2+}, interaction of Ca^{2+} with contractile proteins, and other properties of the contractile apparatus. Further, contractility represents the integrated effects of various cellular mechanisms involved in

Fig. 2-7. Response of the normal heart to increases in ventricular afterload that occur during functioning in the physiologic portion of the wall force–volume relationship. Loop 1, originating from a normal end-diastolic volume, ejects a normal quantity of blood (SV$_1$) for the basal level of contractility. With an increase in afterload, the initial result is loop 2, and a diminshed stroke volume. However, through the redistribution of total load and a slight increase in end-systolic volume, the heart uses its preload reserve and moves its functioning to loop 3. This beat originates from a slightly larger end-diastolic volume and contracts with slightly less afterload

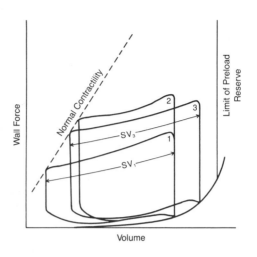

than loop 2, but ejects the same or nearly the same quantity of blood (SV$_3$) as loop 1. This sequence of events describes the process of afterload matching that is within the capability of the normal heart. The relationship between end-systolic wall force and volume is unique in describing underlying myocardial contractility. (Adapted from JE Strobeck, J Ross Jr, Afterload mismatch in the failing heart, *Heart Failure* 1985;1:84-92, with permission.)

Fig. 2-8. Result of increased afterload in a dilated, failing ventricle operating at a point in the wall force–volume plane that is very near the limit of preload reserve (loop 1). With an increase in afterload, a significant reduction in stroke volume (SV) occurs. The heart attempts to compensate by using preload reserve, but quickly reaches the limit without a significant increment in diastolic volume. Only a small increment in diastolic volume contributes further to the added afterload (loop 3) and produces a further decline in stroke volume. Thus, the failing heart, operating at the limit of preload reserve, is severely afterload de-

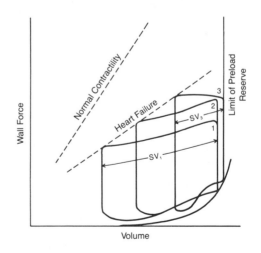

pendent for its stroke volume. At this level of functioning, very small reductions in ventricular afterload will produce a significant increase in stroke volume because of the relatively flat relationship between wall force and volume in the failing ventricle. (Adapted from JE Strobeck, J Ross Jr, Afterload mismatch in the failing heart, *Heart Failure* 1985;1:84-92, with permission.)

the initiation and regulation of contractile activity, such as processes that change intracellular Ca^{2+} concentration, change the sensitivity of myofilaments to Ca^{2+}, or produce shifts in the myosin ATPase isoenzyme population. Contractility has been defined in a variety of ways, most of which are specific to a given experimental preparation and experimental purpose.

In mechanical terms, contractility can be described in isolated heart muscle as a unique surface that is generated during the first two thirds of the contraction phase, as defined by the interrelated variables of muscle force, velocity, and length. Thus, for any instantaneous fiber length and total load on the muscle during the first two thirds of contraction, there is a unique velocity of shortening; the greater the contractility, the greater this velocity will be. From another point of view, at a given level of contractility and total load, the muscle will shorten to a particular end-systolic length, which can be predicted by the interrelationship. When load is changed, velocity and extent of shortening change, but the maximum rate of shortening at the lowest load is set by the level of contractility. Thus, the term *ventricular contractility* has a different connotation than the term *ventricular performance*. The former defines the properties of the muscle; the latter their expression as cardiac work. It is useful from a practical point of view to identify a change in contractility as an alteration in cardiac function that is independent of changes in ventricular performance, which, in general, are changes produced by alterations in either preload or afterload or both.

Calcium ions play a central role in the excitation-contraction coupling sequence of cardiac muscle cells, and calcium homeostasis in muscle cells involves a large number of separate processes. The individual parts involved in cellular Ca^{2+} homeostasis include the contractile proteins, intracellular Ca^{2+} levels, sarcolemmal processes, and intracellular organelles involved in calcium turnover. The binding of Ca^{2+} to troponin C on the thin filaments causes the activation of contraction. Troponin C interacts with troponin I and T and tropomyosin to uncover actin sites on the thin filament to which the myosin heads of the thick filaments can bind and perform work. The amount of Ca^{2+} required to activate contraction depends on that bound to calcium-specific sites on troponin C, but because other structures in muscle cells also bind Ca^{2+}, it is generally assumed that for troponin C to be fully saturated, a total rise in intracellular calcium of 100 μm/L is required.[25,34] The maximal activation of intact mammalian heart cells measured as force generation is less than 50% of that which can be achieved by direct activation of mechanically skinned preparations, suggesting that only 25 to 50 μm/L of calcium may be made available during each heart beat.[25] Measurements of intracellular calcium activity at rest and during contraction have been accomplished with ion-sensitive intracellular microelectrodes,[37] as well as by using the light-emitting Ca^{2+}-sensitive protein aequorin, injected into cells of mammalian cardiac muscle.[28,38] Experiments using aequorin as a Ca^{2+} indicator in mammalian ventricular muscle[28,39] confirm that most inotropic interventions increase the amplitude or duration of the accompanying Ca^{2+} transients (Fig. 2-9). These interventions include elevations of the external Ca^{2+} concentration, increasing heart rate, and exposure of the muscle to cardiac glycosides.[40] A second class of interventions leads to changes in developed tension that are not accompanied by proportional changes in the aequorin light transient. Thus, in addition to any changes in the Ca^{2+} transient that may occur, these interventions lead to changes in the sensitivity of the contractile proteins to Ca^{2+} and therefore exert their effects on contractility through a different mechanism. Examples of this type of intervention are the actions of catecholamines, caffeine, and hypoxia with acidosis.[28,41]

Quantitative consideration of all available information suggests that in the mammalian heart, most of the activating Ca^{2+} will cycle between the sarcoplasmic reticulum and the contractile proteins of the cell. As part of this cycle, a sarcolemmal calcium pump and sodium-calcium exchange transport out of the cell the Ca^{2+} that entered via the slow inward (Ca^{2+}) current and other sarcolemmal Ca^{2+} fluxes. Uptake of Ca^{2+} by mitochondria, which is of low capacity, may become important only when there is intracellular Ca^{2+} overload.[42]

Fig. 2-9. Effects of strophanthidin on calcium transients and developed tension from an aequorin-injected ferret papillary muscle. Aequorin light current measured by a photomultiplier tube is shown. The current output is a nonlinear function of the intracellular calcium concentration. The two superimposed contractions represent the average aequorin light (upper panel) and tension (lower panel) before and in the presence of 10 μM strophanthidin. (Adapted from DG Allen, CH Orchard, Measurements of intracellular calcium concentration in heart muscle: The effects of inotropic interventions and hypoxia, *J Mol Cell Cardiol* 1984;16:117-128, with permission.)

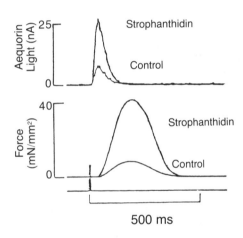

It is well known that changes in the contractile state of cardiac muscle are of physiologic and pathologic significance. Although the concept of contractile state is not difficult, important difficulties have developed in attempts to define it and measure it. This is because the contractile state is not a single measured variable. Instead, it is a description of the muscle's overall mechanical capabilities at that level. These capabilities encompass the capacity of the muscle to both develop force and to shorten. The extent to which the muscle will shorten is inversely related to the force it must develop in order to shorten. Similarly, the speed with which the muscle shortens is inversely related to the load against which it shortens. This inverse relationship between velocity of shortening and load is defined by the classic force-velocity curve, which can be seen as a way of relating the force-generating and shortening capabilities of the muscle at any given level of contractile state.

The mechanical behavior of heart muscle can be understood more simply with isolated muscle preparations in which force generation and shortening are unidirectional and can readily be normalized for differences in muscle thickness and length. The force-velocity curve of an isolated muscle preparation is generally constructed using peak velocity values measured in a series of contractions in which shortening occurs at different loads. When considered in terms of the simple Hill analog model of muscle in which the contractile element is in series with an elastic element, the course of isotonic shortening solely reflects the characteristics of the contractile element, because the length of the series elastic element is constant at any level of afterload.[43] As the afterload is increased, the peak velocity of isotonic shortening is reduced. Peak isometric force is produced when the load is so great that no contractile-element shortening occurs. When the curve that relates load and velocity is extrapolated to zero load, the maximum velocity of shortening (V_{max}) is obtained.[36]

The force-velocity relationship obtained from afterload isotonic contractions is of interest because it helps distinguish between two major ways in which cardiac performance can be altered, that is, changing the initial muscle length (the basis of the Frank-Starling phenomenon) and changing the contractile state through inotropic intervention. When the initial muscle length is increased, increases in the rate of force development (dF/dt) and peak isometric force (P_o) are noted, with slight but significant increases in the time to peak tension (Fig. 2-10). The force-peak velocity curves are shifted to the right, so that both P_o and the velocity of shortening with a given load are augmented. However, when the force-velocity curves have been extrapolated to zero load, V_{max} varies little with changes in initial muscle length over a physiologic range, although at shorter initial lengths V_{max} will fall.[44]

In Figure 2-11, the force-velocity-length relationship was plotted using data derived from recordings of shortening relative to muscle length in a series of afterload contractions. The base of this diagram shows a length-tension relationship; the projection to the rear illustrates the length-velocity relationship for the unloaded muscle; the projection to the left shows the force-velocity relationship. Point A on the base corresponds to the preload starting point. With activation, the contractile elements develop force along a hypothetical force-velocity curve, with force increasing until afterload is reached at point B, after which shortening proceeds across the surface until point C is reached. In any given contraction, the muscle moves in a predictable manner across the surface describing this relationship among force, length, and velocity.

Although the midportion of the force-velocity-length relationship characterizes the range of normal physiologic performance, analysis of this portion of the surface is complex.[45,46] Thus, the mechanical limits to both shortening and force development, representing either extreme of the surface, are of both theoretical and practical interest. Because measurements of velocity during a series of afterloaded isotonic contractions are, of necessity, made later during contraction and at progressively shorter contractile-element lengths as afterload is increased, an extrapolated V_{max} might be misleading. Unloading the muscle to near zero external load shortly after contraction begins has largely overcome this difficulty in determining V_{max} (Fig. 2-12).[47] In this manner, it has been suggested that V_{max} can be measured directly in isolated muscle.

Utilizing these concepts, left ventricular chamber mechanics have been further investigated using isolated canine hearts studied in a servo-controlled apparatus in which ventricular volume and pressure are completely controlled.[27,48] Using assumptions from either a spherical or

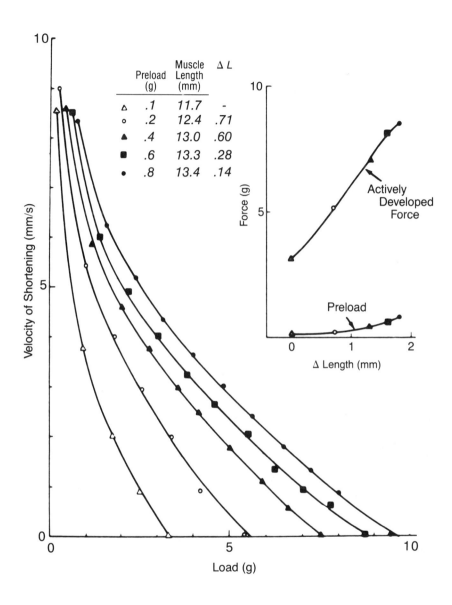

Fig. 2-10. Effects of increased initial muscle length on the force-velocity relationship and the length-tension relationship (inset). The relationship between peak velocity of afterloaded isotonic shortening and total load is shown for several initial muscle lengths of a cat papillary muscle. The inset shows the resting and developed active forces at these various lengths. When initial muscle length is increased, the actively developed force is augmented, as is the velocity of shortening with any individual load. Nevertheless, the maximum velocity of shortening is little altered with changes in preload alone. Moreover, extrapolation of these curves to zero load (V_{max}) would show little, if any, change. (Adapted from Braunwald et al[44] with permission.)

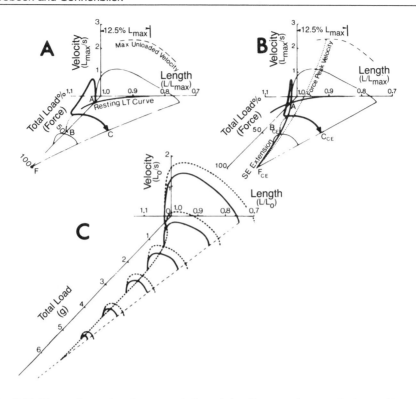

Fig. 2-11. Three-dimensional representation of simultaneous force, velocity, and length during contraction of papillary muscle. A. Velocity-length relationships of isotonic contractions obtained at L_{max} have been replotted as a function of total load (thin-line curves). Such a reconstruction can be obtained by plotting the velocity-length relationships at various loads. As the load increases, velocity and change in length decrease. The course of velocity of a hypothetical afterloaded isotonic contraction is superimposed (thick line). The velocity of shortening during the isometric phase of the contraction has been theoretically derived from a two-component muscle model. Velocity rises rapidly from point A to the appropriate level for the plane of this three-dimensional diagram. This plane also described the entire surface relating the three mechanical variables (length, load, and velocity) that define the contractility of the muscle. During isometric contraction, the contractile-element velocity falls as force rises. This velocity is not observed, but is expressed in terms of the rate of force development (ie, dP/dt). At level B, the force development equals the load; the external shortening can then proceed between point B and C. Velocity of shortening between B and C depends on the level of the force-velocity-length plane. The two-dimensional velocity-length relationship is projected to the right (A-1), and the maximum unloaded velocity of shortening (V_{max}) is also shown (dashed line). B. The curve is moved to the right in the force-velocity-length relationship of the same muscle as shown in panel A after correction for extension of the series elastic component. The dotted line shown on the plane created by the force-velocity-length relationship represents the force-velocity curve as obtained from afterloaded contraction. CE reflects the limits of contractile element shortening. C. The effect of a positive inotropic intervention (dotted lines) on the force-velocity-length relationship. The velocity of shortening at any given muscle length is augmented so that the entire surface relating force, velocity, and length is increased, and the extent of shortening is augmented. The projection of this surface to the right would be characterized by an increased V_{max}. (Adapted from Braunwald et al[44] with permission.)

ellipsoidal model of the ventricle, ventricular force-midwall length-circumferential velocity relationships were determined that agreed qualitatively with previously determined results in isolated ventricular muscle (see Figs. 2-8 to 2-10).[48] Analyzing the three-dimensional surface created by the interrelation of these variables in the ventricle produced a clear mechanical description of ventricular contractility that was very sensitive to changes in underlying contractile state.[49] However, most of the key measurements required mathematical derivation from pressure and volume data only after a multitude of assumptions were made, careful measurements were taken of wall thickness, and independent control of preload and afterload was accomplished. An easier, phenomenologic method was sought to measure alterations in ventricular contractility that reflected underlying myocardial strength, yet took into account the measured ventricular volume and the ventriculoarterial coupling factors outlined earlier. This process has led to examination of chamber elastance, the ratio of ventricular pressure to volume during contraction.[50] In analyzing the systolic pressure-volume relationship, end-systole can easily

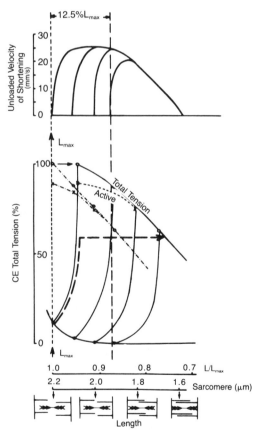

Fig. 2-12. The upper panel shows the velocity-length relationships of unloaded muscle, and the lower panel shows the length–active tension relationships of the contractile element (CE) in the papillary muscle of the cat. These are shown for contractions beginning from four different initial muscle lengths from L_{max} to 12.5% of L_{max}. At the bottom are shown the approximate sarcomere lengths related to the diastolic muscle lengths shown on the resting tension curve. When a contraction is initiated and then the preload removed (quick release), velocity rapidly rises to its peak level and then shows a constant velocity (upper panel). As shortening progresses, velocity of shortening decreases. When initial muscle length is decreased, velocity rises onto the same plateau and follows the same pathway, with velocity ultimately declining. Only with the shortest initial muscle length does the velocity fail to rise onto the same plateau of velocity of shortening. When the load is zero, the plateau approximates V_{max}. In the lower panel the contractile-element length–active tension curve shows a shift to the right with diminishing initial length. The heavy dashed line shows a hypothetical afterloaded isotonic contraction. Clearly, unloaded velocity of shortening, shown in the upper panel, occurs at longer contractile-element length than does the ultimate isometric force development, shown in the lower panel. This is due to the shortening of the contractile element when isometric force is generated. (Adapted from Braunwald et al[44] with permission.)

be determined as the point of maximum elastance (E_{max} equals the maximum P/V),[50,51] and if two contractions at different preloads or different afterloads are studied, the volume intercept (V_0) at zero pressure can be determined (Fig. 2-13). When elastance (P/V) is analyzed with respect to time, the curves in Figure 2-13 are obtained,[52] which show that changes in afterload do not affect the time course or the peak elastance measured. Changes in contractility, however, produce a shorter time course and higher peak elastance, making E_{max} a useful indicator of alterations in contractility.[27,52]

Although a linear relationship exists between points of peak elastance in a series of contractions at a given contractility that originates from different preloads,[27] it is debatable whether the slope of this line or the volume intercept (V_0) is altered independently by changes in afterload.[53,54] Recent evidence in isolated hearts and conscious animals[29,30] indicates that although the slope of the end-systolic pressure-volume relationship is unchanged by varying preload, higher levels of afterload produced a leftward, parallel shift in the relationship and lowered the volume intercept (V_0),[29,55] without an increase in contractility. Also, different slopes and intercepts may result when end-systolic pressure-volume relationships are constructed by varying venous return as opposed to changing arterial resistance or afterload.[46] The reason elevations in afterload exert a response that effectively increases the end-systolic pressure at a given end-systolic volume may relate to ventricular resistance during ejection.[56,57] In this model, end-systolic pressure is a function of end-systolic flow and end-systolic volume. At lower afterloads and higher flows, end-systolic pressure is lower than that predicted by a pure elastance model. At higher afterloads, end-systolic flow is lower, resulting in a higher peak end-systolic pressure-volume ratio. Thus, end-systolic pressure is not only a function of end-systolic volume and inotropic state but is also influenced by the resistance, capacitance, and characteristic impedance of the arterial circulation.[30] Although the end-systolic pressure-volume relationship will reliably detect acute changes in contractility in intact animals and humans, it is not clear that, as a clinical tool, it is superior to the conventional isovolumic indices such as peak dP/dt or dP/dt/P at 40 mm Hg developed pressure (DP). Ejection-phase indices such as the mean or maximum circumferential shortening velocity or ejection fraction are relatively insensitive to preload but are affected by changes in afterload.[58,59] Table 2-1 lists the published measures of contractility according to the portion of systole from which they are derived. All of the listed measures are sensitive to variations in contractility, but each has certain limitations that will be described later in this chapter.

In defining means to evaluate acute changes in ventricular contractility, isovolumic indices should be considered first. The value of dP/dt/DP at a developed pressure of 40 mm Hg is simple to obtain, and unlike maximum dP/dt, its peak occurs before aortic valve opening.[60,61] Both the maximum dP/dt and dP/dt/DP are insensitive to steady-state changes in afterload, but increase somewhat with large changes in preload. Both V_{max} calculated with total pressure and the more easily calculated point of maximum (dP/dt)/P (V_{pm}) fall with increasing end-diastolic pressure due to increased preload or afterload.[62] The use of V_{max} calculated with developed pressure obviates this problem, but appears to have little advantage over dP/dt/DP (40) or maximum dP/dt.[63] In addition, there are serious problems in extrapolating to zero pressure with these techniques. The ratio dP/dt/IIT (IIT = integrated ventricular pressure from the peak of the R wave to maximum dP/dt) was

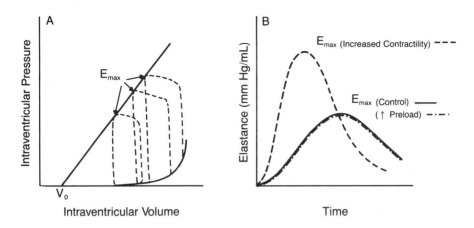

Fig. 2-13. A. Relationship between intraventricular pressure and volume during left ventricular contraction. Contractions in this figure originated at three different preloads with a constant afterload. End-systole is defined as the point at which the ratio of pressure to volume is maximal in each of the contractions. These points are illustrated at points of E_{max}. The end-systolic pressure–volume points are linearly related by a line that describes underlying myocardial contractility. The slope of this line and the volume intercept (V_o) are used to detect changes in underlying contractility. B. Plot of the ratio of pressure to volume (elastance) in a series of contractions that demonstrate the sensitivity of this index to increases in contractility (dashed lines) and insensitivity of the index to increases of preload (dot-dash line). Notice that the amplitude of peak elastance in a given contraction increases with increases in contractility, and the time to peak elastance is also shortened.

developed for completely isovolumic contractions, and derivatives of it have not been validated in the intact circulation.[64] A number of the ejection-phase indices of contractility listed in Table 2-1 are useful for detecting acute changes in contractility; these include stroke volume and stroke work, which are valid if they can be related to directional changes in ventricular end-diastolic volume or pressure in the form of a ventricular function curve.[1] All other ejection-phase indices are responsive to acute changes in contractility; they are relatively insensitive to acute changes in preload, but are influenced by acute alterations in afterload. Therefore, measures such as mean velocity of circumferential fiber shortening (V_{cf}) cannot be used to assess variations in contractility when substantial changes in ejection pressure occur.[54]

In assessing basal levels of contractility, a number of invasive and noninvasive approaches appear useful for separating groups of patients with normal left ventricular function from those with abnormal function. Of the isovolumic phase indices, V_{pm} and V_{max} based on total pressure appear to be most reliable, although considerable overlap exists between individuals in normal and abnormal groups.[65,66] V_{pm} correlates well with V_{max}, is more easily obtained, and avoids the problems inherent in extrapolation to zero pressure.

Maximum dP/dt exhibits a great deal more overlap between normal and abnormal groups than does V_{pm} or V_{max}, and the indices derived from developed pressure are not useful.[62] Ejection-phase indices corrected for end-diastolic volume or end-diastolic dimensions appear capable of detecting depressed contractility in the basal state of an individual patient and therefore seem preferable to the isovolumic indices for the purpose.[58] Mean V_{cf} and mean normalized systolic ejection rate may be more sensitive than the ejection fraction, particularly in assessing patients with mechanical overload such as mitral regurgitation. Ejection-phase measures, including E_{max}, offer the potential advantage of reliable determination, in many patients, by noninvasive echocardiographic techniques.[67,68]

Table 2-1. Measurements of myocardial contractility

Isovolumic phase indices (IPI)

(dP/dt)/developed pressure at 40 mm Hg (DP)
    Useful in acute changes of contractility
    Not useful in evaluating basal contractility

Maximum dP/dt
    Dependent on timing of aortic valve opening
    Useful in acute changes of contractility

V_{max} (based on total pressure)
    Will decrease with increased preload, afterload
    Not as useful as (dP/dt)/DP (40) in acute changes
    Useful in evaluating basal contractility

V_{pm} [point of maximum (dP/dt)/P]
    Most reliable IPI for evaluating basal contractility
    Dependent on preload and afterload at high levels of either

V_{max} (based on developed pressure)
    Useful in acute changes but little advantage over (dP/dt)/DP (40) or max dP/dt
    Not useful in evaluating basal contractility

(dP/dt)/IIT*
    Useful only in completely isovolumic contractions

Ejection-phase indices (EPI)

Stroke volume or stroke work related to diastolic volume or pressure
    Useful in acute changes of contractility if ventricular function curve obtained
    Not useful in evaluating basal contractility

Maximum acceleration of aortic blood flow

Ejection fraction
    Dependent on afterload
    Useful in evaluating basal contracility if corrected for diastolic volume

Mean velocity of circumferential fiber shortening (V_{cf})
    Dependent on afterload
    More sensitive than ejection fraction in evaluating basal contractility

Mean normalized systolic ejection rate
    Afterload dependent
    Less useful than mean V_{cf}

Maximum chamber elastance (E_{max})
    Useful in acute changes
    Not completely useful in evaluating basal contractility

---

*IIT = integrated ventricular pressure from the peak of the R wave to maximum dP/dt.

Premature depolarization of the intact ventricle, whether by atrial or ventricular extrasystole, results in a contraction whose strength decreases with increasing prematurity of the extrasystole. The contraction following the extrasystole is more forceful than normal because of an increase in the level of contractility. This phenomenon, post-extrasystolic potentiation, is independent of variations in diastolic filling of the ventricle,[69] and has been used in the cardiac catheterization laboratory, where application of timed premature beats demonstrates motion in previously motionless areas of the ventricular wall, where contractility is reduced but not absent. This technique provides a reliable estimate of myocardial contractility reserve and provides useful prognostic information in conditions associated with regional abnormalities of myocardial contractility, such as ischemic heart disease.

Heart Rate   Heart rate is the the fourth major determinant of cardiac performance. Increasing the frequency of contraction exerts a positive inotropic effect through the interval-strength relationship, although this effect is less prominent in intact conscious animals than in anesthetized animals or depressed heart. In a normal subject, pacing the heart rate between 60 and 160 beats per minute has little effect on cardiac output, despite increased contractility. Tachycardia reduces the duration of diastolic filling, but increased contractility, induced by the change in frequency, tends to restore normal filling dynamics through contractility-mediated reductions in the duration of systole.

DIASTOLIC PROPERTIES OF THE LEFT VENTRICLE   Before considering the diastolic properties of the intact ventricle it is important to differentiate the factors responsible for alterations in chamber stiffness, as derived from left ventricular diastolic pressure-volume data, from the factors affecting myocardial stiffness, as derived from the stress-strain characteristics of the left ventricular wall.

The intrinsic physical properties of cardiac muscle are described by calculating myocardial stiffness constants from muscle stress-strain data. Stress is the force per unit cross-sectional area; strain results from the application of the stress and is the fractional or percent change in dimension or size from the unstressed dimension. Elasticity is a property of recovery of a deformed material after removal of a stress. Use of the terms *stress* and *strain* allows normalization of values so that the properties of tissues obtained from organs of different sizes and shapes can be compared. Isolated cardiac muscle, like most biologic materials, exhibits a curvilinear relationship between diastolic stress and strain and is responsible for the nonlinear pressure-volume curve of the intact ventricle. Stiffness is defined by the instantaneous ratio of stress to strain at any given point on the curve relating stress to strain. The stiffness constant is the slope of the straight line relating these stress-strain ratios to the corresponding stress. The term *stiffness* has also been used when referring to the stiffness of the whole ventricular chamber and may be expressed in its simplified form as the ratio of change in pressure (dP) to a change in volume (dV).

Chamber stiffness is characterized by analyzing the curvilinear diastolic pressure-volume relationship. The normal ventricle typically has a small slope at low ventricular end-diastolic pressures, and this slope becomes steeper at the upper limit of normal end-diastolic pressure and above (10 to 20 mm Hg). The diastolic pressure-volume relation approximates an exponential curve. Thus as the chamber becomes progressively filled during each diastole, instantaneous ventricular compliance (dV/dP) decreases. The slope of the line relating dV/dP to P represents the elastic stiffness constant of the whole chamber and, while it does not exactly represent the stiffness constant of the ventricular wall muscle, its slope is relatively independent of ventricular shape and therefore may be useful for detecting changes in wall stiffness.

Although instantaneous compliance of the ventricular chamber varies as the heart fills, an alteration in the compliance of the whole chamber can be identified by a change in the shape and position of the entire curve relating ventricular diastolic volume to pressure (see Fig. 2-13). When incomplete relaxation due to tachycardia is excluded, acute interventions that alter myocardial contractility (other than myocardial ischemia) do not significantly shift the pressure-volume relationship of the left ventricle. Volume loading and elevation of arterial pressure cause no apparent shift in the ventricular diastolic pressure-diameter relationship during the slow phase of ventricular filling. However, during the rapid phases of ventricular filling, under some circumstances, inertial and viscous properties appear to influence the resulting shape of the curve, and therefore compliance.

In the intact heart, alterations in the filling of one ventricle can substantially alter the diastolic pressure-volume relationship of the opposite ventricle.[16,70,71] Therefore, when there are significant changes in right ventricular volume, changes in left ventricular end-diastolic pressure may not be a reliable guide even to directional changes of the diastolic pressure-volume curve of the ventricle.[70] Studies in which the pericardium is left intact show that end-diastolic pressure and the shape of the left ventricle are altered by increased right ventricular filling, with encroachment of the interventricular septum on the left ventricular cavity.[16,70,71]

THE FAILING HEART   A distinction between myocardial failure and congestive heart failure has provided a clearer understanding of the latter syndrome and has aided in the development of rational therapeutic modalities. In this discussion, heart failure is considered to be the pathophysiologic state in which an abnormality of myocardial function is responsible for the failure of the heart to pump blood at a rate commensurate with the body's metabolic requirements during exercise. Reduction in myocardial function leading to depressed cardiac output may result from a primary abnormality in the heart muscle (ie, cardiomyopathy), or it may be secondary to ischemia produced by obstructive coronary artery disease. Also, myocardial failure may result secondarily from anatomic lesions of the cardiac valves or pericardium that interfere with cardiac filling or emptying, or from severe or prolonged disorders of cardiac rate or rhythm.

In the presence of a defect in myocardial contraction induced by one or more of the factors outlined in Table 2-2, the heart is dependent on three principle compensatory mechanisms to maintain its normal function as a pump (Table 2-3). First, the Frank-Starling phenomenon is activated, and an increased preload (ie, elevated end-diastolic volume) sustains cardiac stroke volume. Second, myocardial hypertrophy occurs, which increases the mass of contractile tissue. Third, increased catecholamine release by adrenergic cardiac nerves and the adrenal medulla augment myocardial contractility. Initially these compensatory mechanisms have limited potential, and they ultimately fail. Thus, development of the syndrome of heart failure is a direct consequence of the limited ability and ultimate failure of these compensatory mechanisms.[15]

Contractility of Hypertrophied and Failing Myocardium When an excessive load (either a volume or a pressure load) is imposed on the ventricle, the development of myocardial hypertrophy reduces the stress per unit area of muscle toward normal values through an increase in myocardial mass, which permits the ventricle to sustain this burden. However, with prolonged overloads and greater degrees of hypertrophy, the ventricle ultimately fails. Results of early studies of myocardial contractility in patients and experimental animals with various forms of ventricular overload were variable and inconclusive because of limitations inherent in assessing the intrinsic contractility of the intact heart.[72-77] For this reason, there has been interest in the analysis of isolated muscle behavior in experimental models of pressure or volume overload.

Pulmonary artery banding in a variety of mammalian species, producing right ventricular pressure overload and hypertrophy with progression to overt ventricular failure, has been studied extensively.[78,79] Right ventricular hypertrophy and failure reduced the maximum velocity of shortening (V_{max}) below values obtained in muscles from normal animals. The changes were more marked in muscles from animals with heart failure than in those with hypertrophy alone (Fig. 2-14). Heart failure depressed maximum isometric tension, but hypertrophy without failure produced only mild depressions of peak force. Thus, ventricular hypertrophy in the absence of failure in this experimental model was associated with depressed contractility per unit area of myocardium. Ventricular compensation preventing development of signs of heart failure was maintained by an increase in muscle mass. The precise alterations in subcellular function regulating myocardial contraction during the development of hypertrophy and failure have been studied in

---

Table 2-2. Primary etiology of myocardial failure

Work overloads
Increased pressure load
   High "central" resistance, eg, valvular stenosis
   High "peripheral" resistance, eg, hypertension
Increased volume load
   Valvular regurgitation
   High output, eg, A-V shunt, thyrotoxic

Oxygen deprivation
Hypoxia and ischemia { Akinesis
                         Asynergy
                         Dyssynergy
Infarction and/or fibrosis

Myocardiopathy
Idiopathic, hereditary, or acquired
Viral
Metabolic, eg, ethanol, cobalt

detail.[80-84] Multiple defects occur, including defects in energy production, calcium metabolism, and membrane function.[85]

Table 2-3. Secondary compensations of myocardial failure

Compensation	Mechanism	Limit
↑ Volume	Length-tension	Structure of sarcomere
	Sarcomere	"Fibril slippage" Laplace relation $(T = P \times r)^*$
↑ Hypertrophy	↑ Muscle mass	↑ Total force, but ↓ force/unit mass, ↓ actomyosin ATPase
↑ Sympathetic drive	Norepinephrine release	Norepinephrine depletion ↓ Tyrosine hydroxylase

$^*T$ = wall tension; P = pressure; r = radius of the ventricle.

The contractile performance of the intact right ventricle of the same animals revealed depressed function that paralleled the muscle function studies.[79] Wall force developed by the right ventricle at equivalent end-diastolic fiber lengths was significantly lower than normal in animals with heart failure. Reducing or augmenting the end-diastolic volume in the heart failure group demonstrated that the relationship between end-diastolic volume and stroke volume or stroke work was shifted downward and to the right of the normal curves, indicating depressed performance. Thus, during the development of heart failure, ventricular volume increases and the performance of the ventricle returns to near-normal values through movement to the right and upward along a depressed ventricular function curve. Ventricular performance is thus preserved in the face of a reduction in overall contractility at the expense of an increased end-diastolic pressure, volume, and fiber length.

More recently, experimental models of pressure overload hypertrophy and failure have been reexamined in order to understand the results of muscle studies and relate them to the type, duration, and severity of the overload, as well as to the abruptness with which it was applied to the ventricle. Newer models, such as renal vascular hypertension in rats, provide more clinically relevant temporal relationships between the application of the overload and the development of myocardial hypertrophy, consequent alterations in ventricular function, and their reversibility upon relief of the overload.[86,87]

When muscle was removed from animals with chronic volume overload (atrial septal defect), contractility was normal and exhibited none of the changes in the force-velocity or length-tension curves noted in muscles obtained from animals with pressure overload hypertrophy.[88] Thus, the nature of the stress responsible for inciting the hypertrophy appears to play a critical role in determining whether or not hypertrophy is detrimental to myocardial contractility. Following the development of an arteriovenous fistula, the left ventricular end-diastolic pressure rises and stabilizes, while the left ventricular end-diastolic diameter progressively increases and the wall becomes thicker. With chronic adjustments to the shunt and to elevated

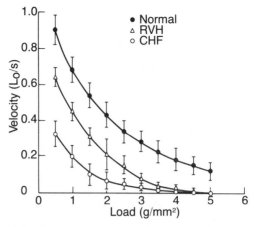

Fig. 2-14. Force-velocity relations in three groups of cat papillary muscles: normal; right ventricular hypertrophy without failure (RVH); and right ventricular hypertrophy with congestive heart failure (CHF). Velocity is expressed in muscle lengths per second (L_o/s). Note the parallel depression of the lower load velocity with the development of hypertrophy and failure. (Adapted from JF Spann Jr, RA Buccino, EH Sonnenblick, et al, Contractile state of cardiac muscle obtained from cats with experimentally produced ventricular hypertrophy and heart failure, *Circ Res* 1967;21:341-354, by permission of the American Heart Association, Inc.)

diastolic filling, myocardial function, as reflected in measurements of mean velocity of circumferential fiber shortening, remains normal. However, worsening of the shunt and, hence, development of signs of congestive failure are uniformly associated with depressions of myocardial contractility. Thus, the development of hypertrophy with primary chamber enlargement in volume overload alters ventricular geometric relationships in a way that allows maintenance of normal wall stress as well as optimal sarcomere length. This permits an enhancement of overall myocardial performance while contractility remains normal.[89-91] With further overload, however, these mechanisms of compensation are inadequate.[91]

As a result of the compensatory mechanisms serving the heart, ventricular performance is usually not markedly affected until the signs and symptoms of congestive heart failure develop. Therefore, indices of ventricular contractility, reflecting the intrinsic state of the myocardium itself, have been sought to more precisely define the course of myocardial deterioration in various myocardial diseases, as well as provide an early indication of the need for either pharmacologic or surgical therapy. The search for the ideal index of ventricular contractility, defined in mechanical terms, has been hampered by both incomplete understanding of ventricular contraction and significant assumptions required before analysis of ventricular function can be undertaken in terms of isolated muscle mechanics.[92,93]

Nearly all indices of ventricular contractility are performance dependent, which means their sensitivity in detecting a change in contractility is diminished to the extent they are influenced by preload, afterload, and heart rate, important determinants of ventricular performance. However, despite these obstacles, ejection-phase indices such as the ejection fraction (ratio of stroke volume to end-diastolic volume) and the velocity of circumferential fiber shortening have clinical usefulness.[94] By definition, these indices remain incomplete, and their limitations must be considered when they are applied to a clinical problem. With more precise information on ventricular contraction dynamics, it is hoped that more sensitive indices will emerge to permit early detection of myocardial failure and allow therapy to begin before compensatory mechanisms are exhausted.

Adrenergic Nervous System in Heart Failure The third form of compensation for failure of myocardial contraction is augmented sympathetic nervous system activity with increased release of norepinephrine into the myocardium. Increased release of norepinephrine in the normal state augments myocardial contractility and participates in the regulation of cardiac performance during acute stress or exercise. During early stages of heart failure, urinary excretion of catecholamines is elevated.[95] However, during sustained loads with developing myocardial failure, the myocardium becomes depleted of its catecholamine stores. This depletion is related to failure of the adrenergic nerves of the heart.

Thus, with chronic failure, the myocardium may become effectively denervated by progressive failure of the sympathetic nerve endings of the heart to synthesize, store, and release catecholamines. The myocardial catecholamines appear to be most depleted in situations in which the myocardium is most depressed. This does not mean, however, that a loss of myocardial catecholamine stores per se directly leads to heart failure, because pharmacologic depletion of myocardial catecholamine stores in the normal state does not alter basal contractility.[96]

However, in heart failure with depressed myocardial contractility, the ability to augment contractility through localized catecholamine release may be lost even though the responsiveness of the myocardium is normally sustained. While there is an augmentation of the circulating catecholamines in the presence of heart failure, the degree to which these circulating catecholamines serve to support contractility of the heart is unknown. Since use of β-adrenergic blockade in severe myocardial failure may be limited by further depression of the heart, it is apparent that myocardial contractility may still be dependent on adrenergic mechanisms.[87]

Chronic elevations of circulating catecholamines also affect peripheral vascular resistance in patients with congestive heart failure, often producing a significant increase in order to maintain blood pressure.[97] This results in increased impedance to ventricular ejection, which, in combination with a dilated heart, leads to significant elevations of afterload and decreasing ventricular performance (see Chap. 3).

Pathophysiology of Heart Failure Myocardial failure resulting in ventricular dysfunction and ultimate depression of cardiac pump performance remains a fundamental, unsolved clinical problem. It invariably leads to a limitation of normal activities and early death of the patient. Indeed, the presence of myocardial failure appears to be the primary determinant of short- or long-term patient survival, independent of etiology or whether treatment is medical or surgical.[94]

The syndrome of heart failure may be considered in relation to two conditions (Table 2-4). The first is diffuse or segmental myocardial failure characterized by a decrease in speed and force of muscle contraction. When myocardial depression is great enough, it is manifested as a decrease in the reserve of pump function and ultimately pump failure. Pump failure is then defined as the inability to provide adequate cardiac output, on demand, to meet the peripheral needs during exercise. The second condition is congestive heart failure, which reflects systemic responses to an inadequate pump. It is characterized by augmented sympathetic nervous system activity, renal vasoconstriction, and activation of the renin-angiotensin system with peripheral congestion and edema.

Experimental heart failure has been studied in several animal models, all of which are characterized by hemodynamic pressure or volume overload. In these models, the time between the creation of the hemodynamic overload and the appearance of myocardial failure depends on the type of overload created (pressure or volume), the abruptness with which it is applied, and the severity of the overload created. Whereas initial hypertrophy in response to the hemodynamic overload tends to normalize the load per unit of myocardium and maintain pump performance early in the course, myocardial failure ultimately develops in most, but not all, instances. Whether or not depression of myocardial function ensues has correlated with the severity of the overload and the extent of resultant myocardial hypertrophy.[98] The contribution of other factors, such as age of the host when the overload occurs and concurrent vascular disease, is not clear.

From early studies of the mechanical correlates of acute pulmonary artery banding in the cat,[78] it is clear that moderate degrees of obstruction of the pulmonary artery lead to right ventricular hypertrophy but not ventricular failure. With more severe obstruction, a greater systolic pressure overload is produced and more severe hypertrophy occurs, as well as right ventricular failure. Studies of papillary muscles removed from hypertrophied heart without congestive failure showed decrements in the maximum velocity of shortening of unloaded myocardium (V_{max}), but not in peak force development (P_o). Ultrastructural and biochemical studies done in the same preparation showed little histologic change aside from cell enlargement, little or no change in mitochondrial function, an increase in connective tissue,[99] and a significant decrease in the rate-limiting enzymatic step for muscle shortening, namely actomyosin ATPase.[100] A slowing of calcium binding by the sarcoplasmic reticulum from such preparations has also been found.[93] As the systolic overload was increased further, additional myocardial failure as well as ventricular failure occurred, characterized by a fall in force production as well as a further decrease in velocity of the isolated papillary muscle.[79] In addition to a further decline in actomyosin ATPase, catecholamine depletion occurred in the heart with failure of cardiac nerves to synthesize, store, or release norepinephrine.[101,102]

Table 2-4. The myocardial and systemic components of heart failure

Myocardial failure

Decrease in force development and shortening secondary to myocyte loss and hypertrophy → pump failure (↓ CO on demand)

Congestive failure

Peripheral effects of failure of pump to meet peripheral needs
　↑ Sympathetic tone and renin-angiotensin activity
　↑ Peripheral congestion, edema, and/or fatigue

Not all experimental systolic overloads result in a clear-cut depression of myocardial function. This may be explained, at least in part, by variations in the severity and duration of the overload. Moreover, most studies of hypertrophy have involved acute imposition of the load. This may produce initial pump failure with focal myocardial damage and subsequent recovery with residual scarring and hypertrophy. In studies of a more physiologic model of systolic pressure overload (eg, renal vascular hypertension), V_{max} falls as a function of hypertrophy, yet force development is maintained.[98,103] Thus, systolic (renal) hypertension in the rat, which mimics hypertensive hypertrophy of humans, is associated with changes in contractile properties of the myocardium characterized by a decrease in relaxation rate.[98,103] Actomyosin ATPase rates fall *para passu* with these mechanical events.[103] Of greater importance is the fact that all of these contractile changes are reversible when the hypertension is corrected.[103]

Experimental diabetes mellitus in the rat was recently shown to lead to contractile changes characterized by a decrease in V_{max} and slowed relaxation.[104] Once again, this was associated with a decrease in actomyosin ATPase[105] and reduced rates of calcium binding by isolated sarcoplasmic reticulum.[106] These alterations are reversed by treatment of a diabetic rat with insulin.[107]

Diastolic overloads (volume overload) impose a change in diastolic volume without an increase in the systolic load on the myocardium. An increase in ventricular mass occurs but does not produce the same fall in contractility observed following systolic overloads.[88,108] The reason for this discrepancy is not known; one potential explanation is that diastolic overload may not lead to the same degree of cell enlargement during hypertrophy. However, with substantial volume overloads, sarcomeres in the wall of the heart are stretched to the limit of their length-tension curve and "plastic" alterations occur, leading to further dilatation.[109] Further, when volume is increased, without unloading of tension in the wall by increased ventricular emptying, the tension in the wall rises as a result of the Laplace relationship and hypertrophy ensues. This may then lead to late declines in contractility from this secondary tension overload. All of the changes in mechanics described are subject to reversal upon removal of the overload.[110-112]

Understanding what factors lead to irreversible depression of myocardial function and ultimate pump failure in the face of a compensatory hypertrophic response to various pump overloads is of essential pathophysiologic importance to the problem of myocardial failure. Recent studies in four different forms of cardiomyopathy have produced some insight into this question. These forms of cardiomyopathy include the hereditary cardiomyopathy that occurs in the Syrian hamster[113] and the cardiomyopathy that develops in rat hypertensive diabetic hearts,[114] human diabetic hearts,[115] and rat renal vascular hypertension.[86,98] Histologic studies in each type of myopathy have all shown regions of fibrosis, myocytolysis, and even calcification adjacent to regions of severely hypertrophied but normal-appearing muscle.[113]

The hereditary cardiomyopathic Syrian hamster develops focal myocardial necrosis beginning as early as one month of age, which leads to eventual myocardial failure within a year. Studies of isolated muscle from such hearts demonstrate substantial decrements in force development as early as 50 days after birth, with subsequent restoration of total force development as compensatory hypertrophy develops.[114] In contrast, V_{max} is preserved early on but falls as the hypertrophic process progresses. Such findings are consistent with an early loss of myocytes that produces a fall in force with V_{max} unchanged, followed by later changes reflecting progressive hypertrophy of the remaining cells that is characterized by a decline in V_{max}.

Continued progression of the latter process leads to congestive cardiomyopathy and death of the animal. Treatment of young Syrian hamsters with the calcium channel blocker verapamil, during the period when the animals normally develop focal myocardial necrosis (30 to 44 days of age), prevented the myocytolytic lesions and abolished the microvascular hyperreactivity.[116] Thus, in this case, a drug was capable of preventing the development of cardiomyopathy.

Vascular hyperreactivity provides a rational explanation for the early pathologic lesions in the Syrian hamster, and it is believed that these microcirculatory lesions are not limited to this model. Similar abnormalities have been demonstrated in the hypertensive diabetic rat, an experimental model of human disease.[117,118] The animals in this model develop focal, discrete areas of fibrosis in the myocardium, similar to those seen in the Syrian hamster. In vivo perfusion of these hypertensive diabetic rats with silicone rubber solutions also reveals a multiplicity of constrictions, tortuosities, and true microaneurysms.[117,118] Whether these lesions can be prevented with a calcium channel blocker such as verapamil is currently under study. Microvascular constriction is demonstrable with postmortem perfusions of human diabetic hearts.[115] In this investigation, typical microaneurysms similar to those seen in diabetic retinas were observed, but in addition, focal vascular constrictions identical to those reported in the Syrian hamster studies were also seen. Constricted lesions following Microfill injection have also been demonstrated in renal hypertensive rats.[118]

Because microvascular hyperreactivity is present in all models and leads to focal cell necrosis and subsequent fibrosis, it has been speculated whether such circulatory lesions are a feature of congestive cardiomyopathy in general. Most human forms of cardiomyopathy have focal myocardial fibrosis as their most significant pathologic feature.[119,120] Because adult myocardial cells do not proliferate, microvascular spasm with focal myocytolytic necrosis will result in decreased numbers of ventricular myocytes. This increases the load borne by the remaining myocytes, leading to their compensatory hypertrophy. Subsequently, in later stages of the cardiomyopathy, one would expect to find areas of focal necrosis and fibrosis intermingled with hypertrophied myocardium. Severe hypertrophy that results from this underlying microvascular process and the persistent hemodynamic overload results in extremely large cells in which activation is impaired and actomyosin ATPase activity is reduced. Widespread fibrosis also has substantial effects on overall ventricular compliance. Dilatation of the heart may then be superimposed in an attempt to compensate for decreased myocardial function. Thus, what began as widespread focal and even unrecognized myocyte necrosis, secondary to microvascular hyperreactivity and spasm, may terminate as hypertrophic myopathy characterized by large ventricular myocytes with impaired contractility, ultimately producing myocardial failure.

CONCLUSION The current concept of the systemic response to myocardial failure is summarized in Figure 1-2. Myocardial failure eventually ensues after cardiac compensatory mechanisms are exhausted. An essential consideration relative to therapy and outcome of the process leading to myocardial failure depends on what is reversible (Table 2-5). Reversible factors include hypertrophy when the load is removed prior to substantial cell loss. Ischemia is reversible until necrosis and cell loss occur, whether the result of large vessel obstruction or spasm. Once myocyte loss occurs, an irreversible process develops that depends on the extent of further cell loss for its progression.[121]

Current therapy for the treatment of myocardial failure, as well as the systemic response to myocardial failure (congestive heart failure), has traditionally involved medication aimed at improving the contractile function of myocardial cells, as well as relieving the hemodynamic effects of the systemic response to myocardial failure. However, these medications provide palliative relief and in no way reverse the abnormality of the activating system or contractile proteins of the myocardium that is observed in the presence of severe hypertrophy. Moreover, the process of microvascular spasm and loss of cardiac cells with further fibrosis may proceed and even be worsened by inotropic therapy. Although the need for palliative therapy in heart failure is not questioned, physicians must remain critically aware that the initial lesion, namely myocyte loss, causing an ultimate downhill course for the myocardium, is not being approached directly by these medications. Alternatively, it is possible that agents that affect microvascular spasm and perhaps other yet unknown factors may ultimately improve myocardial performance by preventing progression of the primary disease. These considerations strongly suggest that interest should shift from continued therapeutic attempts to bolster the already irreversibly damaged heart to attempts to identify patients with certain forms of cardiomyopathy at an earlier stage of the disease, when an opportunity to truly affect the long-term outcome exists.

Table 2-5. Reversible and irreversible factors in heart failure

Reversible

Hypertrophy
Volume increase—elastic
Ischemia*
  Large vessel (coronary artery disease)
  Small vessel (spasm)

Irreversible

Myocardial cell loss and fibrosis
  Segmental
  Diffuse focal
Volume increase—dilatation with "plastic" changes ("fiber slippage")
Catecholamine depletion (?)

---

*Ischemia includes both large vessel obstructive disease and microvascular spasm prior to myocardial necrosis.

REFERENCES

1. Sonnenblick EH, Skelton CL: Reconsideration of the ultrastructural basis of cardiac length-tension relations. *Circ Res* 1974;35:517.
2. Spiro D, Sonnenblick EH: Comparison of the ultrastructural basis of the contractile process in heart and skeletal muscle. *Circ Res* 1964;15(suppl 2):14-37.
3. Julian FJ, Sollins MR: Sarcomere length-tension relations in living rat papillary muscle. *Circ Res* 1975;37:299-308.
4. Pollack GH, Krueger JW: Sarcomere dynamics of intact cardiac muscle. *Eur J Cardiol* 1976;(suppl 4):53-65.
5. Fabiato A, Fabiato F: Dependence of contractile activation of skinned cardiac cells on the sarcomere length. *Nature* 1975;256:54-56.
6. Jewel BR: A re-examination of the influence of muscle length on myocardial performance. *Circ Res* 1977;40:221-230.
7. Martyn DA, Rondinone JF, Huntsman LL: The dependence of force and velocity on calcium and length in cardiac muscle segments. *Adv Exp Med Biol* 1984;170:821-834.
8. Allen DG, Kurihara S: Calcium transients at different muscle lengths in rat ventricular muscle. *J Physiol* 1979;292:680-692.
9. Fabiato A, Fabiato F: Myofilament tension oscillations during partial calcium activation and activation dependence of the sarcomere length-tension relation of skinned cardiac cells. *J Gen Physiol* 1978;72:667-699.
10. Hibbert MG, Jewell BR: Length dependence of the sensitivity of the contractile system to calcium in rat ventricular muscle. *J Physiol* 1979;290:30-41.
11. Caulfeld JB, Bony TK: Collagen network of myocardium. *Circulation* 1978;58:240-255.
12. Ohrenstein J, Hogan D, Bloom S: Surface cables of cardiac myocytes. *J Mol Cell Cardiol* 1980;12:771-780.
13. Krueger JW, Pollack GH: Myocardial sarcomere dynamics during isometric contraction. *J Physiol* 1975;251:627-643.
14. Strobeck JE, Krueger JW, Sonnenblick EH: Load and time considerations in the force-length relation of cardiac muscle. *Fed Proc* 1980;39:175-182.
15. Patterson SW, Piper H, Starling EH: The regulation of the heart beat. *J Physiol* 1914;48:465-513.
16. Tyberg JV, Misbach GA, Glantz SA, et al: A mechanism for shifts in diastolic, left ventricular pressure-volume curve: The role of the pericardium. *Eur J Cardiol* 1978;7(suppl 6):163-173.
17. Spotnitz HM, Sonnenblick EH, Spiro D: Relation of ultrastructure to function in the intact heart: Sarcomere structure relative to pressure-volume curves of the intact left ventricles of the dog and cat. *Circ Res* 1966;18:49-66.
18. Grimm AF, Lin HL, Grimm BR: The pattern of sarcomere lengths through the left ventricular free wall: Difference between open- and closed-chest rats. *Basic Res Cardiol* 1983;78:560-570.
19. Yoran C, Covell JW, Ross J Jr: Structural basis for the ascending limb of left ventricular function. *Circ Res* 1973;32:297-303.
20. Sonnenblick EH: Correlation of myocardial ultrastructure and function. *Circulation* 1968;38:29-44.
21. Streeter DD Jr, Vaishnav RN, Patel DJ, et al: Stress distribution in the canine left ventricle during diastole and systole. *Biophys J* 1970;10:345-363.
22. Ross J Jr, Sonnenblick EH, Covell JW, et al: Architecture of the heart in systole and diastole: Technique of rapid fixation and analysis of left ventricular geometry. *Circ Res* 1967;21:409-421.
23. Sonnenblick EH, Ross J Jr, Covell JW, et al: The ultrastructure of the heart in systole and diastole. *Circ Res* 1967;21:423-431.
24. Sonnenblick EH: The structural basis and importance of restoring forces and elastic recoil for the filling of the heart. *Eur Heart J* 1980;1:107-110.

25. Robertson SP, Johnson JD, Potter JD: The time course of Ca^{++} exchange with calmodulin, troponin, parvalbumin, and myosin in response to transient increase in Ca^{++}. *Biophys J* 1981;34:559-569.
26. Tyberg JV, Keon WJ, Sonnenblick EH, et al: Mechanics of ventricular diastole. *Cardiovasc Res* 1970;4:423-428.
27. Suga H, Sagawa K: Instantaneous pressure-volume relationships and their ratio in the excised, supported canine left ventricle. *Circ Res* 1974;35:117.
28. Allen DG, Kurihara S: Calcium transients in mammalian ventricular muscle. *Am Heart J* 1980;1:5-15.
29. Sodums MT, Badke FR, Starling MR, et al: Evaluation of left ventricular contractile performance utilizing end-systolic pressure-volume relationships in conscious dogs. *Circ Res* 1984;54:731-739.
30. Maughan WL, Sunagawa K, Burkoff D, et al: Effect of arterial impedance changes on the end-systolic pressure-volume relation. *Circ Res* 1984;54:595-602.
31. Brecher GA, Kissen AT: Relation of negative intra-ventricular pressure to ventricular volume. *Circ Res* 1958;6:554-566.
32. Colan SD, Borow KM, Neumann A: Effects of loading conditions and contractile state (methoxamine and dobutamine) on left ventricular early diastolic function in normal subjects. *Am J Cardiol* 1985;55:790-796.
33. Ross J Jr: Afterload mismatch and preload reserve: A conceptual framework for analysis of ventricular function. *Prog Cardiovasc Dis* 1976;18:255-264.
34. Chapman RA, Coray A, McGuigan JAS: Sodium-calcium exchange in mammalian heart: The maintenance of a low intracellular calcium concentration, in Drake A, Noble MIM (eds): *Cardiac Metabolism*. London, Wiley, 1984.
35. Abbott BC, Mommaerts WFHM: A study of inotropic mechanisms in the papillary muscle preparation. *J Gen Physiol* 1959;42:533-551.
36. Sonnenblick EH: Instantaneous force-velocity-length determinants in the contraction of heart muscle. *Circ Res* 1965;16:441-451.
37. Coray A, McGuigan JAS: Measurement of intracellular ionic calcium in guinea pig papillary muscle, in Sykova E, Hnik P, Vylickyl L (eds): *Ionselective Microelectrodes and Their Use in Excitable Tissues*. New York, Plenum, 1981, pp 299-301.
38. Allen DG, Blinks JR: Calcium transients in aequorin-injected frog cardiac muscle. *Nature* 1978;273:509-513.
39. Blinks JR, Rudel R, Taylor SR: Calcium transients in isolated amphibian skeletal muscle fibres: Detection with aequorin. *J Physiol* 1978;277:291-323.
40. Blinks JR, Wier WG, Morgan JP, et al: Regulation of intracellular (Ca^{++}) by cardiotonic drugs, in *Advances in Pharmacology and Experimental Therapeutics II: Cardiorenal and Cell Pharmacology, Proceedings of the 3rd International Congress of Pharmacology*. Oxford, England, Pergamon Press, 1981, pp 205-216.
41. Allen DG, Orchard CH: Measurements of intracellular calcium concentration in heart muscle: The effects of inotropic interventions and hypoxia. *J Mol Cell Cardiol* 1984;16:117-128.
42. Becker GL: Regulation of free Ca^{++} by cardiac mitochondria in skinned myocytes, in Bronner F, Peterlik M (eds): *Calcium and Phosphate Transport Across Biomembranes*. New York, Academic, 1981, pp 79-82.
43. Sonnenblick EH: Implications of muscle mechanics in the heart. *Fed Proc* 1962;21:975-990.
44. Braunwald E, Ross J Jr, Sonnenblick EH: *Mechanisms of Contraction in the Normal and Failing Heart*, ed 2. Boston, Little, Brown, 1976.
45. Covell JW, Ross J, Sonnenblick EH, et al: Comparison of the force-velocity relation and the ventricular function curve as measures of the contractile state of the heart. *Circ Res* 1966;19:364-373.
46. Sodums MT, Badke FR, O'Rourke RA: Differing effects of venous and arterial loading on end-systolic pressure-volume relations. *Circulation* 1982;66(suppl 2):347.

47. Brutsaert DL, Claes VA, Sonnenblick EH: Effects of abrupt load alterations on force-velocity-length and time relations during isotonic contractions of heart muscle: Load clamping. *J Physiol* 1971;216:319-326.

48. Weber KT, Janicki JS: Instantaneous force-velocity-length relations in isolated dog heart. *Am J Physiol* 1977;232:H241-H249.

49. Peterson KL, Uther JB, Shabetai R, et al: Assessment of left ventricular performance in man: Instantaneous tension-velocity-length relation obtained with the aid of an electromagnetic velocity catheter in the ascending aorta. *Circulation* 1973;47: 924-935.

50. Suga H, Sagawa K, Shoukas AA: Load independence of instantaneous pressure-volume ratio of the canine left ventricle and effects of epinephrine and heart rate on the ratio. *Circ Res* 1973;32:314-322.

51. Sagawa K, Suga H, Shoukas AA, et al: End-systolic pressure/volume ratio: A new index of ventricular contractility. *Am J Cardiol* 1977;40:748-753.

52. Suga H, Sagawa K, Kostuik DP: Controls of ventricular contractility assessed by the pressure-volume ratio, Emax. *Cardiovasc Res* 1976;10:582-592.

53. Grossman W, Braunwald E, Mann T, et al: Contractile state of the left ventricle in man as evaluated from end-systolic pressure-volume relations. *Circulation* 1977;56:845-852.

54. Mahler F, Covell JW, Ross J Jr: Systolic pressure-diameter relations in the normal conscious dog. *Cardiovasc Res* 1975;9:447-455.

55. Sungawa K, Maughan WL, Burkhoff D, et al: The effect of arterial impedance changes on the end-systolic pressure-volume relation. *Circulation* 1981;84(suppl 4):209-221.

56. Shroff SG, Janicki JS, Weber KT: Left ventricular systolic dynamics in terms of its chamber mechanical properties. *Am J Physiol* 1983;245:H110-H124.

57. Hunter WC, Janicki JS, Weber KT, et al: Systolic mechanical properties of the left ventricle. *Circ Res* 1983;52:319-327.

58. Gault JH, Ross J, Braunwald E: Contractile state of the left ventricle in man: Instantaneous tension-velocity-length relations in patients with and without disease of left ventricular myocardium. *Circ Res* 1968;22:45-56.

59. Ross J Jr, McCullough WH: The nature of enhanced performance of the dilated left ventricle during chronic volume overloading. *Circ Res* 1972;30:549-556.

60. Mason DT, Braunwald E, Covell JW, et al: Assessment of cardiac contractility: The relation between the rate of pressure rise and ventricular pressure during isovolumic systole. *Circulation* 1971;44:47-58.

61. Davidson DM, Covell JW, Malloch CI, et al: Factors influencing indices of left ventricular contractility in the conscious dog. *Cardiovasc Res* 1974;8:299-312.

62. Peterson KC, Sklovan D, Ludbrook P, et al: Comparison of isovolumetric and ejection phase indices of myocardial performance in man. *Circulation* 1974;49: 1088-1101.

63. Grossman W, Haynes F, Paraskos JA, et al: Alterations in preload and myocardial mechanics in the dog and man. *Circ Res* 1972;31:83-94.

64. Hisada S: Myocardial contractility and pumping function of the ventricle. *Jpn Circ J* 1969;33:1557-1563.

65. Nejad NS, Klein MD, Mirsky I, et al: Assessment of myocardial contractility from ventricular pressure recordings. *Cardiovasc Res* 1971;5:15-23.

66. Mehmel H, Krayenbuehl HP, Rutishauser W: Peak measured velocity of shortening in the canine left ventricle. *J Appl Physiol* 1970;29:637-645.

67. Marsh JD, Green LH, Wynne J, et al: Left ventricular end-systolic pressure-dimension and stress-length relations in normal human subjects. *Am J Cardiol* 1979;44:1311-1317.

68. Borow KM, Neumann A, Wynne J: Sensitivity of end-systolic pressure-dimension and pressure-volume relations to the inotropic state in humans. *Circulation* 1982;65:988-997.

69. Lendrum B, Feinberg H, Boyd E, et al: Rhythm effects on contractility of beating isovolumic left ventricles. *Am J Physiol* 1960;199:115-126.

70. Glantz SA: Ventricular pressure-volume indices change with end-diastolic pressure. *Circ Res* 1976;39:772-785.

71. Ross J Jr: Acute displacement of the diastolic pressure-volume curve of the left ventricle: Role of the pericardium and the right ventricle. *Circulation* 1979;59:32.

72. Braunwald E, Welch GH Jr, Sarnoff SJ: Hemodynamic effects of qualitatively varied experimental mitral regurgitation. *Circ Res* 1957;5:539-555.

73. Grant C, Greene DG, Bunnell IL: Left ventricular enlargement and hypertrophy: A clinical angiocardiographic study. *Am J Med* 1965;39:895.

74. Hood WP Jr, Rackley CE, Rolett EL: Wall stress in the normal and hypertrophied human left ventricle. *Am J Cardiol* 1968;22:550.

75. Urschel CW, Covell JW, Sonnenblick EH, et al: Myocardial mechanics in aortic and mitral valvular regurgitation: The concept of instantaneous impedance as a determinant of the performance of the intact heart. *J Clin Invest* 1968;47:867.

76. Urschel CW, Covell JW, Graham TP, et al: Effects of acute valvular regurgitation on the oxygen consumption of the canine heart. *Circ Res* 1968;23:33.

77. Welch GH Jr, Braunwald E, Sarnoff SJ: Hemodynamic effects of quantitatively varied experimental aortic regurgitation. *Circ Res* 1957;5:546.

78. Spann JF Jr, Buccino RA, Sonnenblick EH, et al: Contractile state of cardiac muscle obtained from cats with experimentally produced ventricular hypertrophy and heart failure. *Circ Res* 1967;21:341-354.

79. Spann JF Jr, Covell JW, Eckberg DL, et al: Contractile performance of the hypertrophied and chronically failing cat ventricle. *Am J Physiol* 1972;223:1150.

80. Alpert NR, Gordon MS: Myofibrillar adenosinetriphosphate activity in congestive failure. *Am J Physiol* 1962;202:940-952.

81. Chidsey CA, Weinbach EC, Pool PE, et al: Biochemical studies of energy production in the failing human heart. *J Clin Invest* 1966;45:40.

82. Conway GF, Roberts JL: Comparison of molecular weight of myosin from normal and failing dog hearts. *Am J Physiol* 1965;208:342.

83. Katz AM: Biochemical "defect" in the hypertrophied and failing heart. *Circulation* 1973;47:1076.

84. Olson RE, Ellenbogen E, Lyengar R: Cardiac myosin and congestive heart failure in dog. *Circulation* 1961;24:471.

85. Entman ML, Van Winkle B, Tate CA, et al: Pitfalls in biochemical studies of hypertrophied and failing myocardium, in Braunwald E (ed): *Congestive Heart Failure: Current Research and Clinical Applications*. New York, Grune & Stratton, 1982, pp 51-64.

86. Capasso J, Strobeck JE, Sonnenblick EH: Myocardial mechanical alterations during gradual onset of long-term hypertension in rats. *Am J Physiol* 1981;241: H435-H441.

87. Epstein SE, Braunwald E: The effect of β-adrenergic blockade on patterns of urinary sodium excretion: Studies in normal subjects and in patients with heart disease. *Ann Intern Med* 1966;75:20.

88. Cooper G IV, Puga F, Zujko KJ, et al: Normal myocardial function and energetics in volume-overload hypertrophy in the cat. *Circ Res* 1973;32:140.

89. Grossman W, Jones D, McLaurin LP: Wall stress and patterns of hypertrophy in the human left ventricle. *J Clin Invest* 1975;56:56.

90. McCullagh WH, Covell JW, Ross J Jr: Left ventricular dilatation and diastolic compliance changes during chronic volume overloading. *Circulation* 1972;45:943.

91. Ross J Jr: Adaptations of the left ventricle to chronic volume overload. *Circ Res* 1974;35(suppl 11):64.

92. Gunther S, Grossman W: Determinants of ventricular function in pressure overload hypertrophy in man. *Circulation* 1979;59:679.

93. Sordahl LA, McCollum WB, Wood WB, et al: Mitochondrial and sarcoplasmic reticulum function in cardiac hypertrophy and failure. *Am J Physiol* 1973;224: 497-502.

94. Cohen PF, Gorlin R, Cohn LH, et al: Left ventricular ejection fraction as a prognostic guide in surgical treatment of coronary and valvular heart disease. *Am J Cardiol* 1974;34:136-141.

95. Chidsey CA, Braunwald E, Morrow AG: Catecholamine excretion and cardiac stores of norepinephrine in congestive heart failure. *Am J Med* 1965;39:442.

96. Spann JF Jr, Sonnenblick EH, Cooper T, et al: Cardiac norepinephrine stores and the contractile state of heart muscle. *Circ Res* 1966;19:317.

97. Higgins CB, Vatner SF, Franklin D, et al: Effects of experimentally produced heart failure on the peripheral vascular response to severe exercise in conscious dogs. *Circ Res* 1972;31:186.

98. Strobeck JE, Aronson RS, Capasso JM, et al: Hypertensive hypertrophy effects on cardiac contractile and electrophysiological behavior. Proceedings of the Second US-USSR Joint Symposium of Hypertension. Dept HEW, NIH 80-2016, 1980, pp 107-123.

99. Buccino RA, Harris E, Spann JR Jr, et al: Response of myocardial connective tissue to development of experimental hypertrophy. *Am J Physiol* 1969;216:425-428.

100. Chandler BM, Sonnenblick EH, Spann JR, et al: Association of depressed myofibrillar adenosine triphosphatase and reduced contractility in experimental heart failure. *Circ Res* 1967;21:717-725.

101. Chidsey CA, Kaiser GA, Sonnenblick EH, et al: Cardiac norepinephrine stores in experimental heart failure in the dog. *J Clin Invest* 1964;43:2386-2393.

102. Spann JF Jr, Chidsey CA, Pool PE, et al: Mechanism of norepinephrine depletion in experimental heart failure produced by aortic constriction in the guinea pig. *Circ Res* 1965;17:312-321.

103. Capasso J, Strobeck JE, Malholtra A, et al: Contractile behavior of rat myocardium after reversal of hypertension. *Am J Physiol* 1982;242:H882-H889.

104. Fein F, Kornstein L, Strobeck JE, et al: Altered myocardial mechanics in diabetic rats. *Circ Res* 1980;47:922-933.

105. Malholtra A, Penpargkul S, Fein FS, et al: Effect of streptozotocin-induced diabetes in rats on cardiac contractile proteins. *Circ Res* 1981;49:1243-1250.

106. Penpargkul S, Fein F, Sonnenblick EH, et al: Depressed cardiac sarcoplasmic reticular function from diabetic rats. *J Mol Cell Cardiol* 1981;13:303-309.

107. Fein FS, Strobeck JE, Malholtra A, et al: Reversibility of diabetic cardiomyopathy with insulin in rats. *Circ Res* 1981;49:1251-1261.

108. Mehmel HC, Mazzoni S, Krayenbuchl HP: Contractility of the hypertrophied human left ventricle in chronic pressure and volume overload. *Am Heart J* 1975;90:236-240.

109. Bishop SP: Structural alterations of the myocardium induced by chronic work overload, in Bloor CM (ed): *Comparative Pathophysiology of Circulatory Disturbances*. New York, Plenum, 1972, pp 289-314.

110. Coulson RL, Yazdanfar S, Rubio E, et al: Recuperative potential of cardiac muscle following relief of pressure overload hypertrophy and right ventricular failure in the cat. *Circ Res* 1977;40:41-49.

111. Jouannot P, Hatt PY: Rat myocardial mechanics during pressure-induced hypertrophy development and reversal. *Am J Physiol* 1975;229:355-364.

112. Sasayama S, Ross J, Franklin D, et al: Adaptations of the left ventricle to chronic pressure overload. *Circ Res* 1977;38:172-178.

113. Strobeck JE, Factor SM, Bhan A, et al: Hereditary and acquired cardiomyopathies in experimental animals: Mechanical, biochemical, and structural features. *Ann NY Acad Sci* 1979;317:59-88.

114. Factor SM, Minase T, Sonnenblick EH: Microvascular abnormalities in the hypertensive-diabetic rat heart. *Circulation* 1980;62(suppl 3):247.

115. Factor SM, Okun EM, Minase T: Capillary microaneurysms in the human diabetic heart. *N Engl J Med* 1980;320:384-388.

116. Factor SM, Cho S, Sonnenblick EH: Verapamil treatment of cardiomyopathic Syrian hamster: Effects on the microcirculation and the extent of myocardial necrosis. *Fed Proc* 1981;40:758.

117. Factor SM, Minase T, Sonnenblick EH: Clinical and morphological features of human hypertensive-diabetic cardiomyopathy. *Am Heart J* 1980;99:446-458.

118. Factor SM, Bhan R, Minase T, et al: Hypertensive-diabetic cardiomyopathy in the rat: An experimental model of human disease. *Am J Pathol* 1981;102:219-228.
119. Olsen EGJ: The pathology of cardiomyopathies: A critical analysis. *Am Heart J* 1979;98:385-392.
120. Roberts WC, Ferrans VJ: Pathologic anatomy of the cardiomyopathies: Idiopathic dilated and hypertrophic types, infiltrative types, and endomyocardial disease with and without eosinophilia. *Hum Pathol* 1975;6:287-342.
121. Sonnenblick EH, Factor SM, Strobeck JE, et al: The pathophysiology of heart failure: The primary role of microvascular hyperreactivity and spasm in the development of congestive cardiomyopathies, in Braunwald E (ed): *Congestive Heart Failure: Current Research and Clinical Applications*. New York, Grune & Stratton, 1982, pp 87-97.

STEVEN R. GOLDSMITH, MD, and
SPENCER H. KUBO, MD

3

Pathophysiology of Heart Failure: Peripheral Vascular Factors and Neurohormonal Mechanisms

It is now clear that congestive heart failure due to congestive cardiomyopathy is a syndrome that must be viewed in terms of an interaction between a diseased left ventricle and numerous factors involving the peripheral circulation. The syndrome begins with impaired left ventricular function, but its full expression depends, to a large degree, on the overall circulatory consequences of this impairment. These consequences are responsible for many of the clinical aspects of the syndrome and also lead in a vicious circle to further reductions in left ventricular function (Fig. 3-1). Recognition of the complexity of the syndrome of heart failure has led to significant advances in therapy for this illness because it has proved much easier to design safe and effective therapy directed at the peripheral circulation than it has to favorably influence ventricular function directly.

Understanding congestive heart failure requires an appreciation of the different relationships among contractility, preload, and afterload in this condition as compared with normal physiology. The function of the normal left ventricle is quite dependent upon preload, but in congestive heart failure, the relationship between contractility and preload, as defined by the Frank-Starling curve, is both depressed and flattened. The result is that increases in preload do not result in improved stroke volume over the usual range of pressures observed in this condition, but rather produce pulmonary and systemic venous congestion. Furthermore, overfilling of the ventricle contributes to increased wall stress and subendocardial underperfusion that may have additional adverse effects on myocardial function.

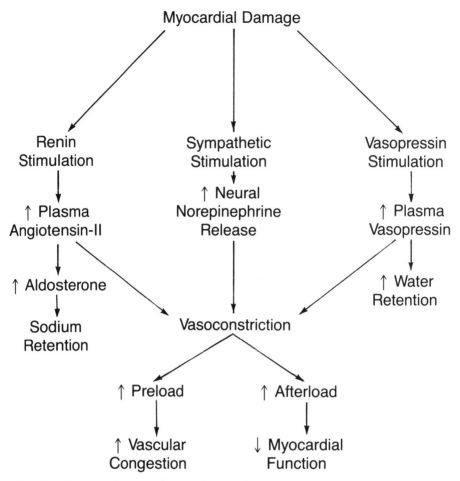

Fig. 3-1. Neurohumoral response in heart failure.

In contrast to the relative independence of the failing left ventricle from changes in preload, the abnormal heart is exquisitely sensitive to alterations in afterload. Very small increases in afterload may significantly worsen ventricular function, while very small decreases in afterload may significantly improve ventricular function in heart failure.[1] Because decreased afterload is therefore theoretically desirable, it may be somewhat paradoxical, from a teleological standpoint, that impaired left ventricular function leads to a rise in afterload as a result of reflex responses to diminished cardiac output, which are designed to maintain perfusion to vital organs. But while such circulatory adjustments undoubtedly occur in response to acute, severe heart failure (as they would to a fall in cardiac output from whatever cause), it is by no means clear that such a process occurs in the insidious development of chronic congestive heart failure. Vasoconstriction may never be "desirable" in chronic congestive heart failure—and if not, the search for the mechanisms that lead to abnormal loading conditions in chronic heart failure may need to consider factors other than those known to be associated with vasoconstriction in response to severe acute circulatory derangement.

The importance of afterload in the regulation of left ventricular function in congestive heart failure was not appreciated until comparatively recently. As a result, until the early 1970s therapy for congestive heart failure was limited either to mild inotropic support with digitalis or treatment with diuretics, which, while relieving symptoms due to pulmonary and venous congestion, did little to alter the fundamental pathophysiology of the syndrome. Since the advent of vasodilator therapy for congestive heart failure, however, dramatic improvements have been made in both the relief of symptoms and even improved survival. Indeed, two recent studies, the V-HeFT trial[2] and the CONSENSUS Trial[3] have demonstrated that the use of two different types of vasodilator therapy can reduce mortality in patients with moderate and severe congestive heart failure. The importance of vasoconstriction in the overall pathophysiology of congestive heart failure is therefore securely established. Interruption of vasoconstriction should clearly be a goal of therapy, certainly in the later and possibly even at very early stages of the disease. No data yet exist for such an approach at the earliest stages, but clinical trials are under way, and at least one study in an animal model suggests that early treatment with a vasodilator may actually retard the development of the full syndrome.[4]

The mechanisms by which left ventricular dysfunction leads to vasoconstriction have been and continue to be the focus of intense study. Increased preload results initially from decreased left ventricular contractile function because end-diastolic volume increases to allow maintenance of stroke volume via the Frank-Starling mechanism. However, impaired cardiac output and/or regional maldistribution of cardiac output (due in part to neurohumoral activation as discussed below) soon leads to sodium and water retention by the kidney. This process expands intravascular volume and further increases preload. Increases in preload lead directly to some increase in afterload. This occurs because salt- and water-engorged blood vessels may not respond normally to physiologic regulation[5] and because one component of afterload is wall tension, which is influenced by left ventricular end-diastolic size and pressure. Afterload is otherwise composed of additional factors that include aortic and large artery impedance, and the resistance produced by arteriolar constriction. Recent studies based on pulse contour analysis and Fourier analysis of simultaneous recordings of pressure and flow in the aorta make it clear that even this last statement is an oversimplification, because many elements including the compliance of muscular arteries, elasticity factors in the large central arteries, and the caliber and tone of small resistance arteries and arterioles must all be accounted for in an overall assessment of impedance.[6,7] These observations may have consequences for therapy because various classes of vasodilating drugs may not affect the different components of impedance to the same degree.

Perhaps the largest body of research data accumulated in recent years regarding the mechanisms of vasoconstriction in heart failure is that dealing with the role of neurohumoral pathways in mediating vasoconstriction in this syndrome.[8] It is now well recognized that there is increased activity of the sympathetic nervous system and the renin-angiotensin system as well as high circulating levels of the potent vasoconstrictor arginine vasopressin. In addition, there may also be deficiencies or deficient activities of endogenous vasodilator systems such as the prostaglandin E series, atrial natriuretic factor, and dopamine. The importance of investigating these neurohumoral pathways as mediators of vascular abnormalities in congestive heart failure lies in the likelihood of being able to modulate either the control or the effects of these neurohumoral systems and so provide targeted, rational therapy for the vasoconstriction of congestive heart failure beyond that which is available from nonspecific vasodilating agents. Thus far, the most dramatic evidence of the success of such an approach has come from the renin-angiotensin system and the development of the angiotensin converting-enzyme inhibiting agents. Indeed, the importance of the renin-angiotensin system is such that a separate chapter within this text is devoted specifically to a discussion of this system and the consequences of modifying it in congestive heart failure. The remaining part of this chapter, therefore, will focus on reviewing the available information dealing with the other neuroendocrine pathways associated with vasoconstriction and vasodilation in heart failure. Specifically, the roles of increased activity of the sympathetic nervous system and high circulating levels of arginine vasopressin, as well as the possible contribution of deficiencies in vasodilator prostaglandins, atrial natriuretic factor, and endogenous dopamine, will be discussed.

THE SYMPATHETIC NERVOUS SYSTEM

Physiology of the Sympathetic Nervous System

The sympathetic nervous system forms one of the major branches of the autonomic nervous system. The afferent limb of the system consists of fibers carried into the central nervous system by the vagus, splanchnic, and other assorted autonomic nerves. In the brain stem and hypothalamus, numerous connections are made with efferent signals sent via preganglionic fibers that synapse at a variety of ganglions, giving rise in turn to postganglionic fibers, which travel to numerous widely distributed nerve terminals. Acetylcholine mediates the responses of preganglionic fibers; however, at the neuroeffector junction, the main neurotransmitter of the sympathetic system is norepinephrine. Norepinephrine interacts with several types of receptors, and it is the net result of multiple possible effects of this interaction that governs the hemodynamic response to a sympathetic stimulus.[9,10] The major receptor subtypes include the postsynaptic α_1- and α_2-receptors, which mediate vasoconstriction; the presynaptic α_2-receptor, which inhibits norepinephrine release; the β_1-receptor, which mediates inotropic and chronotropic responses in the myocardium; and the β_2-receptor, which mediates vaosdilation and, to an extent, chronotropic responses in the myocardium.[11] There may be presynaptic β-receptors as well, which enhance norepinephrine release.

An important concept for cardiovascular physiology, particularly as it relates to congestive heart failure, is the recognition that adrenergic receptors are capable of undergoing "down regulation."[12] As these receptors are exposed to high circulating concentrations of their respective agonists, diminished numbers of active receptors are available to implement their respective physiologic functions. Down regulation is a reversible process and may develop very quickly, within minutes, as in vitro studies have suggested. It is also reversible once high concentrations of agonist are removed.[13] An awareness of these functional characteristics of the sympathetic nervous system is essential for understanding the observations on sympathetic control and effects in disease states such as congestive heart failure, in which there are abnormalities both in the control of sympathetic nervous system activity and in sympathetic nervous system function.

Control of Sympathetic Nervous System Activity

Sympathetic nervous system activity is under a complex series of controls.[14] Most prominently, these involve central command, baroreceptor influences, and either chemo- or mechanoreceptor influences in the peripheral musculature. *Central command* refers to the observation that under conditions of stress or anticipated exercise, sympathetic nervous system activity increases in the resting state prior to activation of other reflex factors. Baroreceptor influences responsible for controlling sympathetic nervous system activity include the cardiopulmonary baroreceptors and the sinoaortic baroreceptors. There is tonic inhibition of sympathetic nervous system activity mediated by the resting level of stretch in both the "low-pressure" cardiopulmonary and "high-pressure" sinoaortic baroreceptors. When stretch is reduced by a fall in intracardiac volume or arterial pressure, the degree of inhibition is diminished and an increase in sympathetic nervous system activity results. Conversely, if cardiac volume expands or if blood pressure rises, enhanced inhibition of sympathetic nervous system activity results. It is important to realize that the efferent limb of the sympathetic nervous system is not an "all-or-nothing" response when exposed to these types of influences. There may be selective connections between the different baroreceptors and various circulatory beds with the cardiopulmonary reflexes linked to forearm vascular and renovascular control and the sinoaortic reflex to splanchnic and cardiac efferents.[14] Finally, sympathetic nervous system activity increases dramatically during physical exercise.[15] Part of this has been attributed to central command influences, but as baroreceptors tend to be "loaded" during exercise, other factors are clearly capable of overriding this baroreceptor inhibition and stimulating sympathetic activity. This phenomenon is not well understood, but it appears that receptors are located within the musculature that are sensitive either to the mechanical stretch of the muscle during activity or to local chemical imbalances produced during exercise, such as tissue acidosis, that may in turn lead to an increase in sympathetic activity. This sequence would promote further increases in cardiac output and vasoconstriction in the nonexercising muscle bed in order to maintain arterial pressure.

Sympathetic Nervous System in Congestive Heart Failure

Sympathetic nervous system activity is increased in patients with congestive heart failure, and the degree of increased activity roughly parallels the severity of the disease. Evidence for this comes both from measurements of plasma norepinephrine levels[16,17] and more recently from actual neural recordings.[18] The plasma norepinephrine level may be increased either by increased sympathetic activity or by diminished clearance of norepinephrine. Recent data suggest that both increased release and decreased clearance play a role in determining the plasma norepinephrine level in this condition.[19] Plasma norepinephrine may therefore be a crude index of overall sympathetic nervous system activity, but the actual level of nerve traffic recorded from peroneal nerves in patients with this condition correlates with the plasma norepinephrine level, at least at rest.[18] It therefore seems reasonable to use plasma norepinephrine as a guide to sympathetic activity in this condition. The mechanism by which sympathetic nervous system activity is enhanced in congestive heart failure is not known. It has been speculated that baroreceptor influences may play a role. If, for example, a patient is hypotensive, has a narrow pulse pressure, or has a diminished cardiac output, relative unloading of the sinoaortic baroreceptors that could lead to increased sympathetic nervous system activity may be present. Most patients with congestive heart failure have increased cardiac filling pressures, however, which should decrease sympathetic nervous system activity. But since it has been reported in animal models that structural abnormalities develop in these receptors during the development of chronic congestive heart failure,[20] perhaps some degree of tonic inhibition of sympathetic nervous system activity is lost. In opposition to the baroreceptor theory for either the low- or high-pressure system, however, is the phenomenon of adaptation.[21] While acute changes in activity of these reflexes may stimulate or inhibit sympathetic nervous system activity, once a steady state is reached, the receptors tend to regain function at a higher or lower level. This observation diminishes the likelihood that these reflex networks would be involved in the long-term stimulation or suppression of sympathetic activity.

Down regulation of myocardial β-receptors occurs in congestive heart failure,[22] and it has been generally assumed that the down regulation results from high concentrations of synaptic cleft norepinephrine. However, it is at least theoretically possible that as congestive heart failure progresses and as abnormalities progressively develop within the myocardium, functional β-adrenergic receptors are lost. Hearts from patients with congestive failure do exhibit reduced norepinephrine content. If there were a primary problem with receptors in cardiomyopathic ventricles, then it is possible that increased sympathetic activity could develop as a compensatory response to diminished cardiac output due, in part, to abnormal sympathetic responsiveness. This concept is only speculative, however, and most authorities favor the alternative theory that elevated levels of norepinephrine in the synaptic cleft lead to down regulation in the myocardium.

While the mechanism by which sympathetic nervous system activity is increased in heart failure is not known, much is known about the responsiveness of the sympathetic nervous system to its known modulating influences in congestive heart failure. In general, the pattern is one of blunted responsiveness. Normal individuals, when subjected to passive upright tilt or lower body negative pressure (which creates relative venous pooling in the lower extremities), respond rapidly by increasing plasma norepinephrine levels and exhibit accompanying vasoconstriction in the forearm, renal, and hepatic beds. When patients with congestive heart failure are subjected to lower body negative pressure or upright tilt, however, plasma norepinephrine levels tend not to increase and there is either no decrease or even, at times, paradoxical increase in peripheral blood flows.[23-25] This abnormal response is not uniform in congestive heart failure and there seems to be a correlation between the severity of the disease and the degree to which the reflex responsiveness is blunted.[26] The mechanism by which this blunting comes about is unknown. It seems that the afferent signal, in terms of a reduction in cardiac filling pressures, is present in the sense that significant reductions in atrial pressure have been recorded during these stimuli, although inadequate afferent stimulation is still a possible factor because the absolute pressure at the nadir is rarely as low as in a normal person. Other explanations may include abnormal central integration of the efferent signal or a blunting of the efferent component of the reflex arc.

Similar findings have been observed with the high-pressure baroreceptors. A normal subject given sodium nitroprusside to the point that the arterial pressure declines will respond rapidly with an increase in plasma norepinephrine. Patients with congestive heart failure given sodium nitro-prusside tend to respond with either no change or only a small increase in plasma norepinephrine.[27] This observation suggests blunting of the responsiveness to the high-pressure baroreceptor in analogous fashion to that of the low-pressure or cardiopulmonary baroreceptor network. Again, the reason for this abnormality is not clear. It is of interest to note that as a normal subject becomes hypotensive, the cardiac output is apt to decrease; whereas in a patient with congestive heart failure, cardiac output tends to rise as afterload is reduced.[1] To the limits of our understanding, the sinoaortic baroreceptor is sensitive to stretch, and it may be that although the mean arterial pressure or pulse pressure is decreasing, these receptors are somehow capable of sensing improved cardiac function and are responding in what is, in fact, an "appropriate" pattern for the overall circulatory effects of the intervention. While teleologically appealing, this concept has yet to be explained in specific terms. It should be noted, however, that the disturbances in the sinoaortic baroreceptor control of the sympathetic nervous system are not due to permanent structural damage, because the response to upright tilt largely normalizes following cardiac transplantation.[16] Mohanty et al[28] recently showed that the response to lower body negative pressure, dependent largely on the ventricular stretch receptors in the "low-pressure" network, does not normalize following transplantation because reinnervation of these receptors does not occur. Therefore, impaired response to orthostasis probably comes about from reversible physiologic dysfunction in the sinoaortic baroreceptor. This possibility is also suggested by studies demonstrating normalization of the response to tilt after pharmacologic treatment of heart failure.[29,30]

The response of the sympathetic nervous system to exercise has also been studied in congestive heart failure. If a normal individual exercises on a bicycle, plasma norepinephrine increases, but only to a significant degree as exercise becomes quite intense. It was observed long ago that in congestive heart failure there was a rather rapid early rise in plasma norepinephrine during exercise, and this observation led to the conclusion that there was heightened sympathetic activity for any given level of exercise in congestive heart failure.[31] As we have confirmed,[32] this is true in absolute terms, but if one examines the plasma norepinephrine level during exercise as a function of the peak exercise capability in patients with heart failure and normal subjects, one reaches exactly the opposite conclusion.[33] Plasma norepinephrine may be higher at 50 watts of bicycle exercise in a heart failure patient compared with a normal subject at that load, but if the patient can only achieve 75 watts with a limited peak norepinephrine response, whereas the normal subject may be able to achieve 275 watts with a very high final norepinephrine level, the proportional increase in plasma norepinephrine at 50 watts as a function of the maximum achievable exercise capacity is, in fact, reduced in the patient with heart failure. This analysis is therefore more consistent with the observations already discussed regarding baroreceptor control of sympathetic activity in congestive heart failure. It suggests that there may be some blunting of the exercise response as well. Whether or not this blunted sympathetic response to exercise is causally related to the blunted heart rate and blood pressure response to exercise in congestive heart failure is not known; but in the study in which it was observed that plasma norepinephrine response was blunted as a function of exercise level, heart rate and arterial pressure responses were significantly decreased as well.[33] At low levels of exercise, however, the degree of increased sympathetic nervous system activity may well be impeding further exercise capacity due to vasoconstriction in nonexercising muscle beds, but proof of this hypothesis with appropriate drug intervention is lacking.

Significance of the Abnormal Sympathetic Nervous System in Congestive Heart Failure

The data reviewed above suggest that there is enhanced sympathetic nervous system activity in congestive heart failure and that its response to various physiologic interventions that are designed to increase sympathetic activity is abnormal. What, therefore, is the pathophysiologic significance of these findings? Sympathetic nervous system activity, at least as reflected by plasma norepinephrine, correlates inversely with survival in heart failure (ie, higher plasma norepinephrine is associated with a poorer prognosis for an individual patient[34]; Fig. 3-2). This observation, however, does not distinguish between sympathetic nervous system activity as simply concomitant to worsening congestive heart failure, in which case it could be teleologically viewed as playing a supportive role in the circulation as it deteriorates (supporting inotropic responses in the myocardium as well as perfusion of vital organs), or as a contributor to the worsening of congestive heart failure. The latter possibility is intriguing, because it suggests that interventions designed to decrease sympathetic stimulation in heart failure would be of therapeutic value.

There are at least three mechanisms by which enhanced sympathetic activity may be deleterious to ventricular function in congestive heart failure. The first is the well-known toxic effects of plasma catecholamines on the myocardium. In experimental models of cardiomyopathy, high levels of sympathetic activity are toxic and may be involved in the progression of the disease.[35] It is possible that such a circumstance could exist in human heart failure as well. A precedent for this might be the cardiomyopathy that develops with very high levels of plasma norepinephrine in cases of pheochromocytoma but no other cause of heart failure.[36] A second mechanism would be the aforementioned down regulation of β-adrenergic responsiveness of the left ventricle. β-Receptors in the myocardium are down regulated in human congestive heart failure.[22] Recent studies have shown that the biochemical response characteristics of tissue from failing human hearts is normal once one moves distal to the β-receptor. Hence, abnormal β-receptor function may be a significant component of impaired left ventricular contractile

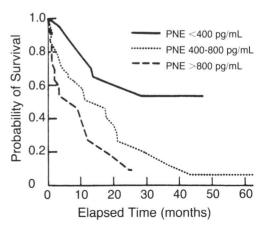

Fig. 3-2. Relationship of plasma norepinephrine (PNE) to prognosis of CHF. (Adapted from Cohn et al.[34] Reprinted, by permission of *The New England Journal of Medicine*, 311;819-823, 1984.)

responsiveness to stress. In this case, interfering with the down regulatory process either by decreasing plasma norepinephrine or antagonizing the β-adrenergic receptor in congestive heart failure could conceivably be of therapeutic value. There are few data concerning such approaches, but preliminary data with β-adrenergic blocking drugs in congestive heart failure suggest that the general effect of such interventions may be beneficial in terms of preservation of left ventricular function.[37]

The third mechanism by which sympathetic activity may be deleterious in heart failure would be from peripheral vasoconstriction mediated either by the α_1-receptor or, if we postulate possible down regulation of the α_1-receptor, even the postsynaptic α_2-receptor. The α_2-receptor may respond more to circulating norepinephrine than to that released locally at the sympathetic cleft,[10] making it also more likely to be active in a condition when plasma levels of norepinephrine are high. In support of this possibility is the observation that the acute administration of vasodilating drugs that act by inhibiting either or both the α_1- and α_2-receptors, such as phentolamine,[38] or selectively inhibiting the α_1-receptor with prazosin or trimazosin[39] produces striking acute vasodilatation with attendant improvements in left ventricular function. Chronic therapy directed at the α_1-receptor has been less successful, probably due to activation of opposing neurohumoral forces or to up regulation of the α_2-receptor blockade, but the principle has been demonstrated that vasoconstriction mediated via α-adrenergic receptors can be deleterious in congestive heart failure.

Finally, although not necessarily related to ventricular function per se, increased sympathetic activity in heart failure may also lead to inappropriate tachycardia, which may shorten filling times and worsen pulmonary congestion, and to arrhythmias, which may lead to diminished cardiac output, syncope, and death. Increased sympathetic activity may also contribute to salt and water retention by causing renal vasoconstriction, direct effects in the renal tubule, and stimulation of the renin-angiotensin system.

As with the phenomenon of vasoconstriction in heart failure, conventional wisdom suggests that increased sympathetic activity in this syndrome is a normal adaptive process gone awry. The range and seriousness of possible adverse influences from sympathetic activation in chronic failure suggest that this is incorrect. If there is no constructive role for enhanced sympathetic activity in chronic heart failure, then perhaps the mechanism by which such sympathetic activation occurs does not involve the reflexes that generate the teleologically desirable responses to hypovolemia and exercise stress. Attention may need to be refocused towards less understood phenomena including the functional characteristics of adrenergic receptors in abnormal myocardium and perhaps the central nervous system control of sympathetic activity. More importantly, if enhanced sympathetic activity is more of a liability than an asset in heart failure, therapeutic attempts to inhibit sympathetic activity may be useful from the earliest stages of the disease. Few data derived from such approaches are available because no long-term trials of centrally acting agents have been conducted, and, for reasons previously discussed, chronic α_1-antagonism has not proved efficacious. Early reports of a controlled trial with β-blockade, however, appear promising, and further attempts with such an approach may be worthwhile.[37]

ARGININE VASOPRESSIN IN CONGESTIVE HEART FAILURE

Vasopressin as Vasopressor

The antidiuretic hormone arginine vasopressin is perhaps the most potent circulating vasoconstrictor substance in the body.[40] In fact, it was the pressor activity of the antidiuretic hormone that led to its original name. It was only recently, however, that a significant physiologic role for the vasoconstrictor properties of arginine vasopressin was elucidated. Research in this area was hampered until the early 1970s by the absence of sensitive and specific radioimmunoassay techniques that allowed arginine vasopressin to be measured at low, and therefore physiologic, concentrations. Further, it has only recently been understood that arginine vasopressin interacts in a unique fashion with the sinoaortic baroreceptor such that when vasoconstriction is induced by arginine vasopressin, signficant potentiation of the baroreflex occurs as reflected in greater reductions in heart rate and cardiac output than are seen in response to comparable degrees of vasoconstriction induced by other agents.[41] As a result, if arterial pressure is the only variable measured in response to an increase in vasopressin, little change will be seen until comparatively high, and therefore pharmacologic, levels of vasopressin are achieved, because as systemic vascular resistance increases, cardiac output declines and arterial pressure remains unchanged. If, however, more thorough hemodynamic assessment is made during infusion of arginine vasopressin, significant vasoconstriction (as reflected both by increased peripheral resistance and redistribution of cardiac output) is observed at very low plasma levels of arginine vasopressin that are well within the usual physiologic range for this hormone.[41] These observations have led to a series of studies in experimental animals demonstrating that arginine vasopressin is an important homeostatic hormone in circulatory regulation (for a review, see Goldsmith[42]).

Arginine Vasopressin in Congestive Heart Failure

Investigation of a possible role for vasopressin in heart failure began with characterization of baseline levels of the hormone in this condition. Reports during the late 1960s using bioassay techniques suggested that arginine vasopressin levels were high in congestive heart failure.[43] Later reports using sensitive and specific radioimmunoassays confirmed that in patients with heart failure arginine vasopressin levels are two to three times those found in a normal control population.[44-47] The absolute level of arginine vasopressin varies somewhat due to methods of reporting the radioimmunoassay, but in our laboratory, the latest statistical comparison of 72 patients and 50 normal subjects gave a mean arginine vasopressin level of 9.8 ± 2.6 pg/mL, with a normal value of approximately 3.5 ± 0.5 pg/mL. Other laboratories, in which the normal value for arginine vasopressin is somewhat lower, report roughly the same proportional increase in congestive heart failure patients.

Arginine vasopressin levels, therefore, tend to be increased in patients with congestive heart failure, although obviously there is considerable heterogeneity and not every patient with congestive heart failure will have a high arginine vasopressin level. This is due to that fact that arginine vasopressin is under a complex series of control systems involving interaction between osmolality and various nonosmotic factors, both of a reflex and central neurohumoral character.[48,49]

The mechanism by which vasopressin levels are increased in heart failure is not yet known. Correlations have been sought between arginine vasopressin and hemodynamics in congestive heart failure, and none have been found in any series, thus diminishing the likelihood that a specific hemodynamic derangement accounts for nonosmotic stimulation of arginine vasopressin. Also, hemodynamic factors involving reflex control of vasopressin release may be comparatively unimportant modulators of arginine vasopressin secretion in humans as compared with experimental animals.[50-52] And as with the sympathetic nervous system, adaptation of the reflex control mechanisms of vasopressin secretion also militates against hemodynamic factors being responsible for chronic, as opposed to acute, stimulation of vasopressin.

The osmoreceptor has also been investigated in congestive heart failure.[53,54] The consensus from current studies is that osmoreceptor function is essentially intact. Vasopressin does decline normally after a given osmotic inhibitory stimulus; however, after such a stimulus, vasopressin levels remain above those levels found in normal subjects even prior to osmotic inhibition, suggesting that undefined factors are responsible for overriding what should be a more complete osmotic inhibition in relative if not absolute terms.

There was a significant correlation between arginine vasopressin and plasma renin activity in at least one series in which plasma vasopressin levels in heart failure were reported.[44] Arginine vasopressin inhibits renin secretion at the renal level, yet angiotensin-II is capable of stimulating arginine vasopressin if levels are high enough in the central nervous system.[55] In addition, furosemide stimulates arginine vasopressin release in heart failure, probably as a result of its effects on renin and angiotensin-II.[56] It is therefore possible that angiotensin-II, at least under some circumstances, may account for some stimulation of arginine vasopressin; but it cannot be the only determinant of a high level of arginine vasopressin in congestive heart failure, because acute administration of converting-enzyme inhibitors does not result in an acute fall in plasma arginine vasopressin levels.[44,57]

Numerous other central neurohumoral influences such as the α_2-receptor, dopaminergic mechanisms, opioid mechanisms, and various central prostaglandin pathways reportedly influence arginine vasopressin secretion either in the basal state or in response to osmotic manipulation.[49] These relationships have not been extensively investigated in humans, and not at all in congestive heart failure. An imbalance in such influences, particularly in a neurohumorally active state such as congestive heart failure, could also contribute to a high arginine vasopressin level for the prevailing osmolality on a nonosmotic basis.

Regardless of the mechanism by which arginine vasopressin levels are increased in congestive heart failure, two lines of evidence suggest that vasopressin is capable of adversely influencing hemodynamics in patients with this condition. Arginine vasopressin infusions have been given to a limited number of patients with congestive heart failure with the goal of determining whether small increases in plasma arginine vasopressin, within the basal range seen in the syndrome, are capable of influencing hemodynamics.[58] When such infusions were given, significant reductions in cardiac output with accompanying increases in systemic vascular resistance were found at levels of arginine vasopressin seen in the basal state in roughly one third of the population of congestive heart failure patients. The mechanism of the adverse hemodynamic effects is not clear, because there was a decrease in cardiac output due to a fall in stroke volume with no change in arterial pressure and an accompanying calculated increase in systemic resistance. The most likely explanation is that plasma arginine vasopressin induced peripheral vasoconstriction, which imposed an enhanced afterload stress on an already failing left ventricle and thus led to a reduction in stroke volume and cardiac output. The data are also consistent with a primary myocardial depressant effect of arginine vasopressin, and while most of the literature suggests that cardiodepression due to arginine vasopressin is related to reflex factors, some direct cardiodepression cannot be excluded. The nature of the hemodynamic response in congestive heart failure was, however, quite different from that seen in normal experimental animals or in normal humans in which a slight degree of cardiodepression, as already noted, occurs in response to increased systemic vascular resistance. In normal experimental animals and humans, cardiodepression occurs primarily as a result of a reflex reduction in heart rate, while no reduction in heart rate was found in the heart failure patients. The mechanism of cardiodepression in response to vasopressin in heart failure is, therefore, not a result of the normal observed physiologic response to the hormone.

A second line of evidence supporting a possible hemo-dynamic effect of arginine vasopressin in congestive heart failure comes from preliminary studies in which patients with congestive heart failure were given an experimental antagonist of the vascular receptor for vasopressin.[38,59] The renal and vascular receptors for vasopressin are pharmacologically distinct.[60] Selective antagonism of these receptors is therefore possible, and when patients with congestive heart failure were given an antagonist of the V_1-receptor, vasodilation and improved cardiac function were seen in patients with a high baseline arginine vasopressin level (Fig. 3-3). This has only been the case in a minority of the patients in whom the inhibitor has been studied to date, and the observations by Creager et al[38] suggest that if the arginine vasopressin level is low or normal, there may be some agonist effects from this compound. Further study is therefore necessary with this or other com-pounds to define the extent to which arginine vasopressin may contribute to vasoconstriction in a population of patients with severe congestive heart failure. Also unknown at the present time is the degree to which inhibiting the vascular receptor for arginine vasopressin may be enhanced by simul-taneous or combined inhibition of the adrenergic nervous system or the renin-angiotensin system. Vasopressin potentiates the pressor response to angiotensin-II and norepinephrine.[61] Further, there seems to be functional redundancy in these three systems in the degree to which they support arterial pressure in response to hypovolemia or hypotension. By analogy, combined inhibition of these networks in disease states may result in greater pharmacologic vasodilation than achieved by inhibiting individual systems alone. This has been shown in the laboratory,[62] but data on the inhibition of vasopressin along with the inhibition of other neurohumoral systems are not available in congestive heart failure. An interesting clinical precedent may exist in the hypertension literature,[63] however, in that patients with severe

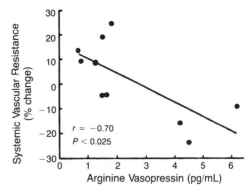

Fig. 3-3. Correlation of baseline arginine vasopressin with percent change in systemic vascular resistance after administration of the vasopressin antagonist. (Adapted from Creager et al.[38] Reprinted with permission from the American College of Cardiology [*Journal of the American College of Cardiology* 1986;7:758-765].)

hypertension already treated with converting-enzyme inhibitors and large doses of clonidine achieved significant further reductions in their arterial pressure when given an antagonist of the vascular receptor for arginine vasopressin.

For completeness, it should be mentioned that in preliminary studies of different animal models of congestive heart failure, vasopressin has been demonstrated to be of pathophysiologic importance. In dogs in which congestive heart failure is induced by a combination of pulmonic stenosis and tricuspid valve ablation, arginine vasopressin levels are increased and apparently associated with adverse hemodynamic effects as judged by the response to V_1-inhibitors.[64] And in rabbits with Adriamycin cardiomyopathy, vasopressin antagonists produce hemodynamic benefit even if the baseline arginine vasopressin level is normal.[65] Studies in these and other animal models may shed further light on the mechanisms by which arginine vasopressin levels are increased in congestive heart failure, as well as provide a more controlled environment in which to examine the possible interrelationships among vasopressin, norepinephrine, and angiotensin-II in this syndrome.

ATRIAL NATRIURETIC FACTOR

Intense interest in the pathophysiology of atrial natriuretic factor (ANF) has existed since the identification of secretory granules within mammalian atria by Jamieson and Palade[66] and the landmark experiments of deBold et al,[67] who demonstrated that atrial, but not ventricular, extracts produce a marked increase in sodium and water excretion in rats. This interest is related to the extraordinary number of physiologic actions of ANF (eg, natriuresis, diuresis, vasodilatation, and suppression of the renin-angiotensin system) and the mechanisms by which this hormone could contribute to blood pressure and body volume homeostasis.[68,69] In particular, it has been postulated that ANF may have a critical role in the pathophysiology of edema-forming states, including congestive heart failure. It is therefore timely to review some of the data on the multiple physiologic actions of ANF, as they specifically relate to human subjects and patients with congestive heart failure.

Structure

Atrial natriuretic factor has been purified, sequenced, and synthesized.[70-73] It appears that there is a precursor that contains 152 amino acids, including a signal peptide of 24 amino acids and a 126-amino-acid prohormone, which is the primary form in which the peptide is stored in atrial granules. Several circulating peptides have been described that contain an identical core sequence of 17 amino acids, but with some differences in overall length, leading to several different names including cardionatrin, atriopeptin I, II, and III, and auriculin A and B. These different peptides appear to be related to proteolysis during the isolation procedure, and the circulating form of human ANF appears to contain 28 amino acids.[73,74]

Physiologic Regulation of ANF

ANF can be detected in the plasma of normal human subjects. Under basal conditions, levels of ANF are usually very low. This is consistent with continuous release of ANF into the circulation. Although a number of stimuli will acutely increase ANF release into the systemic circulation, the most effective and important mechanism appears to be atrial distension. This was confirmed by a number of in vitro and in vivo experiments. Dietz,[75] using an isolated rat heart-lung preparation, demonstrated that increasing venous return to increase right atrial pressure resulted in the release of a potent natriuretic factor. These findings were confirmed by Lang et al[76] and Schwab et al,[77] who found that volume loading resulted in a marked increase in plasma levels of atrial natriuretic factor and natriuresis.

Significant correlations between atrial pressure and plasma levels of ANF in patients undergoing cardiac catheterization have been demonstrated in several laboratories.[78-80] These studies indicate that both right and left atrial pressures are important in the regulation of ANF release. In addition, maneuvers that increase central blood volume and/or atrial distension increase ANF levels. Thus, head-out water immersion,[81] head-down tilt,[82] rapid atrial pacing,[83] and high salt intake[84,85] all acutely increase ANF secretion into the circulation. Similarly, head-up tilt during sodium loading decreases ANF levels.[84] These data are consistent with the hypothesis that ANF secretion is an important effector mechanism by which the heart responds to changes in blood volume.

ANF granules have been identified in a number of tissues in the body, but the cardiac atria remain the primary source of circulating ANF. Although both right and left atria are capable of secreting ANF, the contribution is somewhat greater from the right atrium. In a cardiomyopathic hamster model, however, there are large quantities of ventricular ANF granules, suggesting that the decrease in ventricular function stimulates ANF production in ventricular myocytes and that the contribution of ventricular ANF may increase in congestive heart failure.[86] ANF appears to exit the heart via the coronary sinus,[83] as suggested by the "step-up" in ANF levels, with the highest levels found with atrial sampling, as compared with arterial and venous sites.

Patients with symptomatic congestive heart failure generally have higher levels of ANF than normal subjects, as suggested by the correlations between atrial pressure and ANF levels.[78,79,87] This suggests, therefore, that the avid sodium retentive state that is characteristic of many patients with congestive heart failure is not related to a deficiency of ANF but possibly to a diminished physiologic responsiveness to the hormone.[87]

Effects on Renal Hemodynamics and Excretory Function   One of the most prominent effects of ANF is an increase in glomerular filtration rate and a sustained natriuresis and diuresis. The increase in glomerular filtration rate has been demonstrated in the isolated perfused rat kidney[88] and in intact animals.[89-91] The mechanisms by which ANF leads to an increase in glomerular filtration rate are complex and multifactorial, but appear to be independent of changes in total renal blood flow. It is likely that efferent arteriolar constriction is an important mechanism, because the increase in glomerular filtration rate is accompanied by an increase in filtration fraction. However, dilatation of the afferent arteriole[90,92] and a direct effect on the glomerular membranes to alter the hydraulic permeability-filtration area coefficient[90] have also been proposed as potential mechanisms contributing to the increase in glomerular filtration rate.

As suggested by its trivial name, steady-state infusions of ANF cause a profound natriuresis and diuresis, associated with increases in calcium, magnesium, phosphate, and potassium excretion.[87,89,91] The mechanisms of the natriuretic effect have received intense scrutiny. Although the increase in glomerular filtration rate and increased filtered sodium load are undoubtedly important, they probably do not fully account for the observed natriuretic effect. There appears to be a complex interplay between the increase in glomerular filtration rate and peritubular physical factors that influence sodium excretion,[93] including a washout of the medullary interstitial gradient and an intrarenal shift of blood flow to the medulla.[94] In addition, direct tubular actions may also contribute.[95] That these nonglomerular factors are important for the natriuretic effect was underscored by a study by Burnett et al,[96] demonstrating that the natriuretic response to ANF was still present, although attenuated, when the increase in glomerular filtration was blocked.

These renal hemodynamic and excretory effects of ANF were recently evaluated in normal subjects and patients with congestive heart failure using steady-state intravenous infusions.[87] In normal subjects, ANF given at a dose of 0.10 μg/kg/min caused a marked increase of urinary sodium excretion from 160 $\pm$ 23 to 725 $\pm$ 198 μEq/min, an increase in urine flow from 10 $\pm$ 1.6 to 20 $\pm$ 2.6 mL/min, and an increase in fractional excretion of sodium from 1% to 4% (all $P < 0.05$). There were also significant increases in osmolar clearance from 3.2 $\pm$ 0.6 to 6.8 $\pm$ 1.2 mL/min and free water clearance from 6.8 $\pm$ 1.6 to 13.6 $\pm$ 1.6 mL/min. There were minor changes in glomerular filtration rate (117 $\pm$ 15 to 133 $\pm$ 10 mL/min) and renal blood flow (1,100 $\pm$ 125 vs 998 $\pm$ 77 mL/min) that were not statistically significant. Because of the tendency for an increase in glomerular filtration rate and a decrease in renal blood flow, there was a significant increase in filtration fraction from 20 $\pm$ 1% to 26 $\pm$ 2% ($P < 0.05$). Although glomerular filtration rate did not increase significantly in this study, it should be noted that there may be important species and dose-related differences that may affect the renal responses to ANF.[97]

In contrast to the responses in normal subjects, the identical administration of ANF in patients with congestive heart failure produced variable but generally smaller changes in renal hemodynamics and excretory function, consistent with an overall blunting of responsiveness. There was no change in mean glomerular filtration (93 $\pm$ 13 to 91 $\pm$ 10 mL/min), renal blood flow (542 $\pm$ 104 vs 527 $\pm$ 85 mL/min), or filtration fraction (33 $\pm$ 4%

vs 32 ± 5%). Furthermore, there were no significant changes in urinary sodium excretion (31 ± 22 vs 59 ± 39 μEq/min), or urinary flow rates (1.67 ± 0.38 vs 2.21 ± 0.59 mL/min), although there was some interpatient variability. The attenuated renal responses to ANF are summarized in Figure 3-4, which plots the net changes in urine volume and sodium excretion over the dose range of ANF given (0.01 to 0.10 μg/kg/min), as compared with placebo infusion, for both normal subjects and heart failure patients.[87] It is clear that the responses in patients with heart failure were considerably less than those of normal subjects, even when a substantially lower dose (0.03 μg/kg/min) was given to the normal subjects. Thus, the effects of ANF on renal excretory function are diminished in heart failure, consistent with the hypothesis that sodium and water retention in patients with heart failure may be related to diminished responsiveness rather than a deficiency of ANF. However, there may be considerable heterogeneity in ANF responsiveness among patients with heart failure, due to differences in the degree of avid sodium retention and activation of the renin-angiotensin system.

Vascular
Smooth Muscle
Several investigators have shown that ANF has potent direct relaxant effects on blood vessels.[98,99] In models using preconstricted aortic rings, ANF inhibited the contractions produced by angiotensin-II and norepinephrine, as well as non-receptor-mediated, potassium-induced vasoconstriction.[99] Of note, ANF was more effective in antagonizing contractions produced by angiotensin-II than norepinephrine, because sufficiently high concentrations of norepinephrine can overcome the ANF inhibitor effect. Thus, although ANF has general vasorelaxant properties, it may be particularly effective as a functional antagonist of angiotensin-II.[88,99]

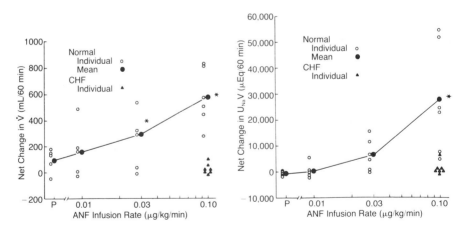

Fig. 3-4. Net changes in urine volume (V̇) and urinary sodium excretion (U_{Na}V) in response to placebo (P) and atrial natriuretic factor (ANF) infusions, in both normal subjects and heart failure patients (CHF). For normal subjects, there were significant ($P < 0.05$) increases (asterisks) in urine volume and urinary sodium excretion at the 0.10 μg/kg/min infusion rate. The net change in urine volume and urinary sodium excretion for patients with heart failure was markedly less than that observed for normal subjects, consistent with hyporesponsiveness to ANF administration. (Adapted from *The Journal of Clinical Investigation* 1986; 78:1362-1374 by copyright permission of the American Society for Clinical Investigation.)

The mechanism for ANF's vascular relaxant property is not known, but appears to be a direct effect on vascular smooth muscle, because the same effects can be seen when the endothelium is not present.[100] Since the renal hemodynamic effects of ANF are attenuated when isolated kidneys are perfused with low calcium concentrations or in the presence of the calcium channel blocker verapamil, it has been suggested that calcium fluxes are important.[88] Alternatively, the vasodilator action of ANF is associated with an increase in tissue cyclic guanosine monophosphate (cGMP), which may be an important second messenger for its vascular relaxant effect.[100]

This vasodilating capacity of ANF has been confirmed in human studies using an isolated forearm model and intra-arterial infusions.[101,102] In this model, the direct vasoactive properties of infused agents can be assessed *in vivo*, excluding the effects of autonomic reflexes that are potentially activated during systemic administration. Intra-arterial infusion of ANF in normal subjects caused dose-dependent increases in forearm blood flow and decreases in forearm vascular resistance.[101] The maximal effect of ANF was a 3.4-fold increase in forearm blood flow, which was approximately 60% of the maximal response to nitroprusside, but considerably less than the vasodilating responses observed with the calcium antagonist verapamil and with postocclusion reactive hyperemia.[103]

In similar experiments, Cody et al[102] compared vasodilating responses of ANF in normal subjects and patients with heart failure. Similar to the attenuated renal effects following intravenous administration, the identical intra-arterial doses of ANF did not produce as large an increase in forearm blood flow in patients with congestive heart failure as was observed in normal subjects. This apparent diminished potency, however, may be due to a decrease in overall vasodilating capacity seen in patients with heart failure.[5] Thus, when the ANF responses were compared as a fraction of the post-ischemic reactive hyperemia response, the relative increases in forearm blood flow were comparable between normal subjects and patients with heart failure.

Actions on the Blood Pressure and Circulation The exogenous administration of ANF in intact animals has generally resulted in a depressor response[104,105] that is even more marked in renin-dependent forms of hypertension.[91,106] Although it was originally thought that the reduction in blood pressure was secondary to its vasodilator properties, most studies show that systemic resistance is not decreased,[104,107] and that the reduction in blood pressure is related to a reduction in cardiac output. The most likely mechanism responsible for the decrease in cardiac output is a reduction in venous return, rather than a negative effect on contractility. The mechanisms contributing to the reduction in preload have not been identified, but may be related to an increase in venous capacitance, or a fluid shift from the intravascular compartment to the interstitium.

The depressor action of ANF has been confirmed in humans. In normal subjects in the seated position, ANF at a dose of 0.10 μg/kg/min caused a significant decrease in systolic blood pressure, but no change in diastolic blood pressure.[87] To further explore the hemodynamic action of ANF in human subjects, these same doses were given during an invasive hemodynamic study.[87] ANF administration was associated with a significant reduction in pulmonary wedge pressure from 11 ± 1 to 7 ± 1 mm

Hg ($P < 0.05$) and a smaller decrease in right atrial pressure from 4 ± 2 to 3 ± 1 mm Hg (NS), consistent with preload reduction (Fig. 3-5).[87] However, when these patients were studied in the supine position, there was no change in cardiac index or systemic vascular resistance. Furthermore, there was no change in systolic, diastolic, or mean arterial pressure. It can be expected, however, that a reduction in cardiac output and blood pressure due to preload reduction would be more prominent in the seated position, when compared with the supine position.

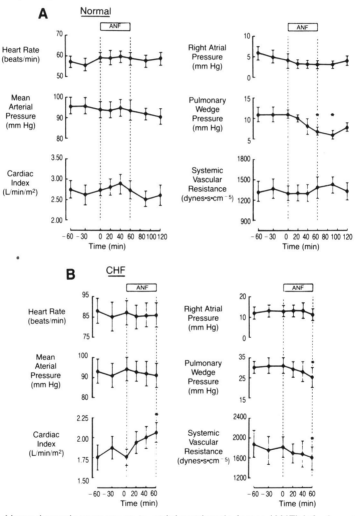

Fig. 3-5. Hemodynamic responses to atrial natriuretic factor (ANF) infusion at a rate of 0.10 μg/kg/min in (A) normal subjects and (B) heart failure patients. In normal subjects, ANF administration caused a significant reduction (asterisks indicate $P < 0.05$) in pulmonary wedge pressure and a trend toward a reduction in right atrial pressure. There were no significant changes in heart rate, mean arterial pressure, cardiac index, or systemic vascular resistance. In heart failure patients, there was also a reduction of pulmonary wedge pressure. However, there was a reduction in systemic vascular resistance and an increase in cardiac index with ANF administration. (Adapted from *The Journal of Clinical Investigation* 1986;78:1362-1374 by copyright permission of the American Society for Clinical Investigation.)

In patients with heart failure[87] ANF administration was also associated with a significant decrease in pulmonary wedge pressure from 31 ± 4 to 25 ± 5 mm Hg ($P < 0.05$; Fig. 3-5). In contrast to normal subjects, however, there was a significant reduction in systemic vascular resistance from $1,831 \pm 208$ to $1,597 \pm 243$ dynes·s·cm^{-5}, and an increase in cardiac index from 1.77 ± 0.6 to 2.07 ± 0.13 L/min/m^2 (both $P < 0.05$). Systolic, diastolic, and mean arterial pressure were unchanged. The explanation for these different hemodynamic responses may be related to the multiple physiologic actions of ANF and the differences in the hemodynamic profile of normal subjects and heart failure patients. The most consistent hemodynamic effect is a reduction in preload, as manifested by a reduction of pulmonary wedge pressure. In the seated position, this reduction in preload may reduce cardiac output and mean arterial pressure by a Starling mechanism. In heart failure, where vasoconstriction from activation of the sympathetic nervous system and renin-angiotensin system is prominent, the administration of ANF could lead to an important arterial dilator action, reducing impedance and leading to an increase in cardiac output. Thus, in many respects, the combined venous and arterial hemodynamic profile of ANF is similar to that of intravenous nitroglycerin.

Hormonal and Hemo-concentrating Effects

ANF has also been shown to have several effects on circulating hormone levels. Administration of ANF will promptly suppress renin secretion even in the setting of decreased mean arterial pressure. The mechanism of renin suppression is most likely related to an increase in distal sodium delivery to the macula densa.[91,108,109] This has also been shown in normal subjects[87] in whom plasma renin activity decreased 67% from 2.9 ± 0.4 to 1.9 ± 0.2 ng/mL/h ($P < 0.02$). In patients with heart failure, in whom basal levels of plasma renin activity are frequently elevated, ANF produced a small but nonsignificant decrease in plasma renin activity from 8.6 ± 5.2 to 6.1 ± 3.4 ng/mL/h. ANF has also been shown to decrease aldosterone secretion from the adrenal cortex,[87,91,110,111] without affecting secretion of cortisol.

Thus, ANF appears to be uniquely designed to counteract the effects of the renin-angiotensin system on multiple levels. It can suppress renin secretion, decrease aldosterone secretion, act as a vasodilator opposing the vasoconstrictor effects of angiotensin-II, and act as a natriuretic agent opposing the sodium-retaining action of aldosterone. This multiple level coordination with the renin-angiotensin system suggests that these dual pathways could be an important modulator of blood pressure and body volume regulation.[68]

Another intriguing effect of ANF is the finding of hemoconcentration and a contraction of the intravascular compartment. In normal subjects, ANF infusion at a rate of 0.10 μg/kg/min resulted in a significant and reversible increase of hematocrit from 45.7 ± 0.08 vol% to 48.6 ± 0.9 vol%, and total protein from 6.8 ± 0.1 to 7.3 ± 0.3 g/dL (both $P < 0.05$).[87] This hemoconcentrating effect could not be explained by a natriuretic effect and is most consistent with a fluid compartment shift from the intravascular space to the interstitial or intracellular compartments.[87,91] Although the mechanisms have not been clarified, these findings are consistent with an increase in capillary permeability, which may be an important factor contributing to the effect of ANF on preload reduction.

PROSTA-GLANDINS   Prostaglandins are a heterogeneous group of fatty acids resulting from the metabolism of arachidonic acid through a series of steps catalyzed by enzymes known collectively as cyclo-oxygenase.[112] There are several different types of prostaglandins, some with contrasting effects. For example, prostaglandin I_2 (PGI_2 or prostacyclin) and prostaglandin E_2 (PGE_2) have potent vasorelaxant activity, while thromboxane A_2 is a potent vasoconstrictor. There is a large data base demonstrating that prostaglandins have vasodilator actions that are important in maintaining vascular tone and circulatory homeostasis, particularly in counteracting the vasoconstrictor effects of norepinephrine and angiotensin-II. This has been demonstrated in dog models where cardiac output is acutely decreased by the inflation of a balloon in the thoracic inferior vena cava[113] and in other animal models following surgery,[114] hypotensive hemorrhage,[115] and sodium depletion.[116] These interventions share several common features, including simultaneous activation of the sympathetic nervous system and the renin-angiotensin system, as well as increased synthesis and release of renal prostaglandins.[117] It is hypothesized that the vasodilator actions of the renal prostaglandins are critical for the maintenance of renal blood flow by counteracting the vasoconstrictor actions of angiotensin-II and norepinephrine. This is further supported by the effects of the administration of an inhibitor of prostaglandin synthesis, which typically results in a decrease in renal blood flow and/or glomerular filtration rate,[113,114,116] probably secondary to unopposed vasoconstriction from angiotensin-II and norepinephrine. Furthermore, prostaglandin synthesis and release are increased in response to exogenous infusions of angiotensin-II and norepinephrine.[118-121] These cumulative data are consistent with the hypothesis that the maintenance of the renal circulation is dependent on the balance between the vasoconstrictors and vasodilators.[117]

Other data suggest that prostaglandins are important in maintaining circulatory homeostasis in patients with congestive heart failure. Dzau et al[122] studied 38 patients with evidence of severe left ventricular dysfunction and found that the average plasma levels of prostaglandin E_2 metabolite (843 ± 20 pg/mL) and 6-keto-prostaglandin $F_{1\alpha}$ (128 ± 31 pg/mL) were significantly increased when compared with normal subjects. The plasma concentration of PGE_2 metabolite varied directly and linearly with plasma renin activity ($r = 0.72$; $P < 0.005$) and with plasma angiotensin-II concentrations ($r = 0.84$; $P < 0.001$). When patients were grouped according to their serum sodium concentration, increased levels of PGE_2 metabolite, plasma 6-keto-$PGF_{1\alpha}$, and plasma renin activity were primarily observed in patients with a serum sodium less than 135 mmol/L. Similar findings were reported by Punzengruber et al.[123] The observation that a subgroup of patients with congestive heart failure can have increased levels of vasoconstrictor substances, while at the same time having increased levels of vasodilating substances, provides further evidence that peripheral vascular tone represents a balance between these competing systems. At this time, however, the explanation for this relationship is not clear, as it may reflect activation of prostaglandin synthesis by angiotensin-II, increased release of renin by prostaglandins, or possibly a common stimulus.

Dzau et al[122] also evaluated the hemodynamic effects of indomethacin, a prostaglandin synthetase inhibitor. After indomethacin, patients with low sodium concentrations showed a significant decrease in cardiac

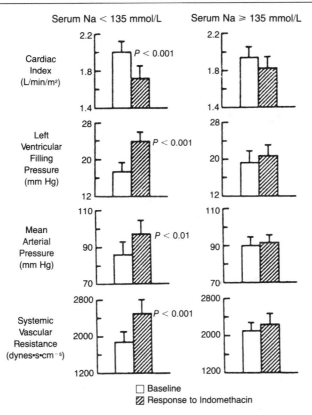

Serum Na < 135 mmol/L Serum Na ≥ 135 mmol/L

Cardiac Index (L/min/m²)

Left Ventricular Filling Pressure (mm Hg)

Mean Arterial Pressure (mm Hg)

Systemic Vascular Resistance (dynes•s•cm⁻⁵)

P < 0.001

P < 0.001

P < 0.01

P < 0.001

☐ Baseline
▨ Response to Indomethacin

Fig. 3-6. Hemodynamic changes following administration of indomethacin in patients with congestive heart failure. In those patients with hyponatremia, indomethacin caused an increase in left ventricular filling pressure, mean arterial pressure, and systemic vascular resistance, associated with a decrease in cardiac index. In contrast, there were no significant hemodynamic changes in those patients with normal serum sodium concentrations. (Adapted from Dzau et al.[122] Reprinted, by permission of *The New England Journal of Medicine*, 310;347-352, 1984.)

index from 1.99 ± 0.12 to 1.72 ± 0.13 L/min/m² associated with an increase in pulmonary capillary wedge pressure from 17.4 ± 2.0 to 24 ± 1.9 mm Hg, mean arterial pressure from 86 ± 6.7 to 96.9 ± 7.6 mm Hg, and systemic vascular resistance from $1,882 \pm 239$ to $2,488 \pm 315$ dynes•s•cm⁻⁵ (all $P < 0.01$; Fig. 3-6).[122] In contrast, there were no significant hemodynamic changes in patients with normal serum sodium concentrations. The hemodynamic deterioration from indomethacin in the patients with low serum sodium concentrations is likely to be secondary to the reduction in vasodilator tone from prostaglandins, and resultant unopposed vasoconstriction. That this hemodynamic deterioration could become clinically significant is supported by adverse clinical experiences with the nonsteroidal anti-inflammatory agents.[124]

The vasodilating actions of prostaglandins have been confirmed in studies evaluating the effects of an intravenous infusion of a PGE_2 analog, viprostol.[125] In both normal subjects and patients with congestive heart failure, viprostol produced a significant decrease in mean arterial pressure and systemic vascular resistance. Similar data were seen in two patients given another PGE_2 analog, CL 115,347.[126] Of note, it appears that heart failure patients, despite having elevated basal levels of PGE_2, remain responsive to the vasodilator actions of the exogenously administered prostaglandin analogs.

In addition, prostaglandin infusions had important effects on plasma renin activity and plasma norepinephrine. In normal subjects, PGE_2 analog infusion was associated with an increase in plasma norepinephrine from 268 ± 110 to 622 ± 110 pg/mL ($P < 0.01$) and in plasma renin activity from 1.6 ± 0.6 to 16.2 ± 13.5 ng/mL/h ($P < 0.05$).[125] In heart failure patients, viprostol caused a significant increase in plasma renin activity from 9.6 ± 6.4 to 46.5 ± 37.9 ng/mL/h ($P < 0.01$). The mechanism of stimulation of renin release was probably a secondary response to a direct effect of PGE_2 on the macula densa, as similar degrees of vasodilation produced by nitroprusside did not increase plasma renin activity. These findings are similar to data reported with PGE_2 in dogs[127] and prostacyclin in normal humans.[128] Thus, not only will the vasoconstrictor hormones increase prostaglandin release, but prostaglandins will increase the release of vasoconstrictor hormones.

In addition to their direct vasodilator actions, prostaglandins may mediate the effects of several vasodilating drugs, including captopril, hydralazine, nitrates, and nitroprusside.[129-132] Nitroglycerin added to cultured endothelial cells resulted in a dose-dependent increase in the synthesis of the potent vasodilator PGE_2, which could be inhibited by pretreatment with aspirin.[129] This mediation by prostaglandins is supported by the effects of indomethacin, which appears to partially mitigate the hemodynamic effects of these vasodilator drugs.[131,132]

The mechanism of the vasodilator effect of captopril has been of particular interest because converting enzyme is identical to one of the kinin-degrading enzymes, kininase-II. Bradykinin increases prostaglandin release; therefore, inhibition of kinin degradation may be an important component of the vasodilating action of the converting-enzyme inhibitors. Moore et al[130] measured prostaglandins and the effect of indomethacin on the antihypertensive effect of captopril in 31 patients with essential hypertension. After a single oral dose of captopril, blood pressure and angiotensin-II levels fell as anticipated. Kinin levels increased, as did the metabolite of prostaglandin E_2. After inhibition of prostaglandin synthesis with indomethacin, the increases in prostaglandin E metabolite following captopril were blocked. While indomethacin had no effect on the angiotensin-II responses to captopril, the depressor effect was significantly blunted. Thus, these data suggest that the antihypertensive effect of captopril may be mediated through prostaglandins. It has also been suggested that the increase in prostaglandins is important for the clinical efficacy of captopril in patients with congestive heart failure.[133]

DOPAMINE   Since the identification of the potent vasodilating action of dopamine, many investigators have suggested that endogenous dopamine may be another important vasodilating system in patients with congestive heart failure.
There appear to be two distinct dopamine receptors, DA_1 and DA_2.[134] DA_1-receptors are located postsynaptically and mediate vasodilatation in the renal, mesenteric, coronary, and cerebral circulations. DA_2-receptors are presynaptic, located on postganglionic sympathetic nerves and autonomic ganglia. They inhibit norepinephrine release from sympathetic

nerve endings. Therefore, stimulation of both DA_1- and DA_2-receptors produces vasodilation. The pharmacologic actions of exogenously administered dopamine are dependent on the infusion rate. DA_1- and DA_2-receptors are activated at the lowest infusion rates, producing vasodilatation and a reduction in the systemic vascular resistance. In addition, there is an increase in renal blood flow, due to a direct vasodilating effect on the renal vasculature, which generally increases urine flow rates and the excretion of sodium. At infusion rates above 2 µg/kg/min, β_1-adrenoreceptors are activated, with an increase in contractility and cardiac output.[135] At higher doses, above 5 to 10 µg/kg/min, there is further activation of α_1- and α_2-adrenoceptors, resulting in an overall increase in systemic vascular resistance.

Limited data are available to assess the status of endogenous dopamine in patients with congestive heart failure. Circulating levels of plasma dopamine are frequently increased in patients with heart failure.[136,137] It is not known if these high circulating levels reflect increased secretion of dopamine or the inability of the failing heart to metabolize norepinephrine. In addition, myocardial concentrations of dopamine are increased,[138,139] possibly reflecting a change in the rate-limiting step for myocardial norepinephrine synthesis. However, the precise stimulus for increased dopamine levels in patients with heart failure has not been identified. There was no correlation between dopamine levels and systemic hemodynamics, suggesting that the higher levels in patients with heart failure are not solely due to the reduction in cardiac output.[137] However, increases in plasma dopamine levels were more prominent in patients in whom there was an activated renin-angiotensin system.[136] Thus, similar to prostaglandins, patients with heart failure may simultaneously activate vasoconstrictor pathways and dopamine pathways, so that vascular tone represents a balance between these counterregulating systems.

Although patients with congestive heart failure frequently have elevated levels of dopamine, they remain responsive to exogenous infusions of dopamine.[135,140,141] The combined renal and systemic hemodynamic effects of intravenous infusions in nine patients with severe congestive heart failure were studied by Maskin et al in 1985.[141] At an infusion rate of 2 µg/kg/min, renal blood flow increased from 304 ± 120 to 604 ± 234 mL/min ($P < 0.01$), while the increase in cardiac index was smaller, from 1.96 ± 0.36 to 2.38 ± 0.35 L/min/m^2 ($P < 0.05$). These data are consistent with a selective renal vasodilating effect of dopamine, as the renal flow fraction, or the ratio of renal blood flow to cardiac output, increased from $17 \pm 7\%$ to $27 \pm 8\%$. At a higher dose of 4.0 µg/kg/min, there was no change in renal blood flow, but a further increase in cardiac index to 2.87 ± 0.46 L/min/m^2 ($P < 0.05$). Thus, these data suggest that the dose-response relationship of dopamine remains relatively intact in patients with congestive heart failure.

Other data have confirmed the vasodilating action of dopamine using orally active dopamine agonists. Thus, bromocriptine,[142] ibopamine,[143,144] fenoldopam,[145] and levodopa[146] have all been shown to acutely improve the hemodynamic profile of patients with congestive heart failure, with beneficial decreases in systemic vascular resistance and increases in cardiac output. These studies are consistent with a potential vasodilator effect of dopamine and suggest that there may be an important role for dopamine agonists in the treatment of patients with heart failure, although this evaluation still requires controlled trials.

REFERENCES

1. Cohn JN, Franciosa JA: Vasodilator therapy of cardiac failure. *N Engl J Med* 1977;297:27-31, 254-258.
2. Cohn JN, Archibald DG, Ziesche S, et al: Effect of vasodilator therapy on mortality in chronic congestive heart failure: Results of a Veterans Administration Cooperative Study. *N Engl J Med* 1986;314:1547-1552.
3. CONSENSUS Trial Study Group: Effects of enalapril on mortality in severe congestive heart failure: Results of the Cooperative North Scandinavian Enalapril Survival Study (CONSENSUS). *N Engl J Med* 1987;316:1429-1435.
4. Riegger GAJ, Liebau G, Holzschuh M, et al: Role of the renin-angiotensin system in the development of congestive heart failure in the dog as assessed by chronic converting enzyme blockade. *Am J Cardiol* 1984;53:614-618.
5. Zelis R, Nellis SH, Longhurst J, et al: Abnormalities in the regional circulations accompanying congestive heart failure. *Prog Cardiovasc Dis* 1975;18:181-199.
6. Finkelstein SM, Cohn JN, Collins RV, et al: Vascular hemodynamic impedance in congestive heart failure. *Am J Cardiol* 1985;55:423-427.
7. Gabe IT, Karnell J, Porje IG, et al: The measurement of input impedance and apparent phase velocity in the human aorta. *Acta Physiol Scand* 1984;61:73-84.
8. Francis GS, Goldsmith SR, Levine TB, et al: The neurohormonal axis in congestive heart failure. *Ann Intern Med* 1984;101:370-377.
9. Langer SZ: Presynaptic receptors and their role in the regulation of transmitter release. *Br J Pharmacol* 1977;60:481-497.
10. Langer SZ, Hicks PE: Alpha-adrenergic subtypes in blood vessels in physiology and pharmacology. *J Cardiovasc Pharmacol* 1984;6:S547-S558.
11. Ginsburg R, Bristow MR, Zera P: β_2-Receptors are coupled to muscle contraction in human ventricular myocardium (abstract). *Circulation* 1984;70:II-67.
12. Lefkowitz RJ: Direct binding studies of adrenergic receptors: Biochemical, physiologic and clinical implications. *Ann Intern Med* 1979;91:450-458.
13. Limas CJ, Limas C: Rapid recovery of cardiac β-adrenergic receptors after isoproterenol induced "down" regulation. *Circ Res* 1984;55:524-531.
14. Abboud FM, Heistad DD, Mark AL, et al: Reflex control of the peripheral circulation. *Prog Cardiovasc Dis* 1976;18:371-403.
15. Mitchell JH, Kaufman MP, Iwamoto GA: The exercise pressor reflex: Its cardiovascular effects, afferent mechanisms, and central pathways. *Annu Rev Physiol* 1983;45:229-242.
16. Levine TB, Olivari MT, Carlyle P, et al: Reversibility by heart transplantation of abnormal neurohormonal control mechanisms in chronic congestive heart failure. *Circulation* 1982:66:II-192.
17. Thomas JA, Marks BH: Plasma norepinephrine in congestive heart failure. *Am J Cardiol* 1978;41:233-243.
18. Leimbach WN, Wallin BG, Victor RG, et al: Direct evidence from intraneural recordings for increased central sympathetic outflow in patients with heart failure. *Circulation* 1986;73:913-919.
19. Hasking GJ, Esler MD, Jennings GL, et al: Norepinephrine spillover to plasma in patients with congestive heart failure: Evidence of increased overall and cardiorenal sympathetic nerve activity. *Circulation* 1986;73:615-621.
20. Zucker IH, Gilmore JP: Aspects of cardiovascular reflexes in pathologic states. *Fed Proc* 1985;44:2400-2407.
21. Kunze DL: Role of baroreceptor resetting in cardiovascular regulation: Acute resetting. *Fed Proc* 1985;44:2408-2411.
22. Bristow MR, Ginsburg R, Minobe W, et al: Decreased catecholamine sensitivity and beta-adrenergic receptor density in failing human hearts. *N Engl J Med* 1982;307:205-211.

23. Brigden W, Sharpey-Schafer EP: Postural changes in peripheral blood flow in heart failure. *Clin Sci* 1950;9:93-97.
24. Goldsmith SR, Francis GS, Levine TB, et al: Regional blood flow response to orthostasis in patients with congestive heart failure. *J Am Coll Cardiol* 1983;1:1391-1395.
25. Lilly L, Dzau VJ, Williams GH, et al: Hyponatremia in congestive heart failure—implications for neurohormonal activation and responses to orthostasis. *J Clin Endocrinol Metab* 1984;59:924-930.
26. Levine TB, Francis GS, Goldsmith SR, et al: Activity of the sympathetic nervous system and renin-angiotensin system assessed by plasma hormone levels and their relationship to hemodynamic abnormalities in congestive heart failure. *Am J Cardiol* 1983;49:1659-1666.
27. Olivari MT, Levine TB, Cohn JN: Abnormal neurohumoral response to nitroprusside infusion in congestive heart failure. *J Am Coll Cardiol* 1983;2:411-417.
28. Mohanty PK, Thames MD, Arrowood JA, et al: Impairment of cardiopulmonary baroreflex after cardiac transplantation in humans. *Circulation* 1987;75:914-921.
29. Cody RJ, Franklin KW, Kluger J, et al: Mechanisms governing the postural response and baroreceptor abnormalities in chronic congestive heart failure: Effects of acute and long-term converting enzyme inhibition. *Circulation* 1982;66:135-142.
30. Timmis AD, Kenny JF, Smyth P, et al: Restoration of normal reflex responses to orthostatic stress during felodipine therapy in heart failure. *Cardiovasc Res* 1984;18:613-619.
31. Chidsey CA, Harrison DC, Braunwald E: Augmentation of the plasma norepinephrine response to exercise in patients with congestive heart failure. *N Engl J Med* 1962;267:650-654.
32. Francis GS, Goldsmith SR, Ziesche SM, et al: Response of plasma norepinephrine and epinephrine to dynamic exercise in patients with congestive heart failure. *Am J Cardiol* 1982;49:1152-1156.
33. Francis GS, Goldsmith SR, Ziesche SM, et al: Relative attenuation of sympathetic drive during exercise in patients with congestive heart failure. *J Am Coll Cardiol* 1985;4:832-839.
34. Cohn JN, Levine TB, Olivari MT, et al: Plasma norepinephrine as a guide to prognosis in patients with chronic congestive heart failure. *N Engl J Med* 1984;311:819-823.
35. Eliot RS, Todd GL, Clayton FC, et al: Experimental catecholamine-induced acute myocardial necrosis. *Adv Cardiol* 1978;25:107-118.
36. Garcia R, Jennings JM: Pheochromocytoma masquerading as a cardiomyopathy. *Am J Cardiol* 1972;29:568-571.
37. Engelmeier RS, O'Connell JB, Walsh R, et al: Improvements in symptoms and exercise tolerance by metoprolol in patients with dilated cardiomyopathy: A double-blind, randomized, placebo controlled trial. *Circulation* 1985;72:536-546.
38. Creager MA, Faxon DP, Cutler SS, et al: Contribution of vasopressin to vasoconstriction in patients with congestive heart failure: Comparison with the renin-angiotensin system and the sympathetic nervous system. *J Am Coll Cardiol* 1986;7:758-765.
39. Miller RR, Awan NJ, Maxwell KS, et al: Sustained reduction of cardiac impedance and preload in congestive heart failure with prazosin. *N Engl J Med* 1977;297:303-307.
40. Monos E, Cox RH, Peterson CH: Direct effect of physiologic doses of arginine vasopressin on the arterial wall *in vivo*. *Am J Physiol* 1978;243:H167-H173.
41. Liard JF: Vasopressin in cardiovascular control: Role of circulating vasopressin. *Clin Sci* 1984;67:473-481.
42. Goldsmith SR: Vasopressin as vasopressor. *Am J Med* 1987;82:1213-1219.
43. Yamane Y: Plasma ADH level in patients with chronic congestive heart failure. *Jpn Circ J* 1968;32:745-759.

44. Goldsmith SR, Francis GS, Cowley AW, et al: Increased plasma arginine vasopressin levels in patients with congestive heart failure. *J Am Coll Cardiol* 1983;1:1385-1390.
45. Prebiscz J, Seasley J, Laragh J, et al: Platelet and plasma vasopressin in essential hypertension and congestive heart failure. *Hypertension* 1983;5(suppl 1):129-132.
46. Riegger GAJ, Liebau G, Kochsiek K: Antidiuretic hormone in congestive heart failure. *Am J Med* 1982;72:49-52.
47. Uretsky B, Verbalis J, Generalovitch T, et al: Plasma vasopressin response to osmotic and hemodynamic stimuli in congestive heart failure. *Am J Physiol* 1985;248:H396-H402.
48. Schrier RW, Berl T, Anderson RJ: Osmotic and non-osmotic control of vasopressin release. *Am J Physiol* 1979;236:F321-F332.
49. Sklar AH, Schrier RW: Central nervous system mediators of vasopressin release. *Physiol Rev* 1983;63:1243-1265.
50. Goldsmith SR, Francis GS, Cowley AW, et al: Reponse of vasopressin and norepinephrine to lower body negative pressure in humans. *Am J Physiol* 1982;272:H970-H973.
51. Goldsmith SR, Francis GS, Cowley AW, et al: Effects of increased central venous and aortic pressure on plasma vasopressin in man. *Am J Physiol* 1984;246:H647-H651.
52. Goldsmith SR, Dodge-Brown D, Pederson W: Arterial baroreceptor unloading and vasopressin secretion in humans. *Circulation* 1986;74:II-430.
53. Goldsmith SR, Cowley AW, Francis GS, et al: Arginine vasopressin and the renal response to water loading in congestive heart failure. *Am J Cardiol* 1986;58:295-299.
54. Pruszczynski W, Vahanian A, Ardaillou R: Role of antidiuretic hormone in impaired water excretion in patients with congestive heart failure. *J Clin Endocrinol Metab* 1984;58:599-605.
55. Share L: Interrelations between vasopressin and the renin-angiotensin system. *Fed Proc* 1979;38:2267-2271.
56. Francis GS, Siegel R, Goldsmith SR, et al: Acute vasoconstrictor response to furosemide in patients with chronic congestive heart failure. *Ann Intern Med* 1985;103:1-6.
57. Uretsky BF, Lawless CE, Verbalis JG, et al: Is converting enzyme inhibition associated with decreased sympathetic nervous system activity and arginine vasopressin secretion? *Circulation* 1985;72(suppl 3):283.
58. Goldsmith SR, Francis GS, Cowley AW, et al: Hemodynamic effects of infused arginine vasopressin in congestive heart failure. *J Am Coll Cardiol* 1986;8:779-783.
59. Nicod P, Waeber B, Bussien JP, et al: Acute hemodynamic effects of a vascular antagonist of vasopressin in patients with congestive heart failure. *Am J Cardiol* 1985;55:1043-1047.
60. Manning M, Sawyer WH: Antagonists of vasopressor and antidiuretic responses to arginine vasopressin (editorial). *Ann Intern Med* 1982;96:520-522.
61. Ishikawa S, Goldberg J, Schrier D, et al: Interrelationship between subpressor effects of vasopressin and other vasoactive hormones in the rat. *Miner Electrolyte Metab* 1984;10:184-189.
62. Tabrizchi R, King K, Pang C: Vascular role of vasopressin in the presence and absence of influence from angiotensin-II or α-adrenergic system. *Can J Physiol Pharmacol* 1986;64:1143-1148.
63. Ribiero A, Mulinasi R, Garras I, et al: Sequential elimination of pressor mechanisms in severe hypertension in humans. *Hypertension* 1986;8(suppl 1):169-173.
64. Stone CR, Imai N, Thomas A, et al: Hemodynamic effects of vasopressin inhibition in congestive heart failure. *Clin Res* 1986;34:632A.

65. Arnolda L, McGrath BP, Cocks M, et al: Vasoconstrictor role for vasopressin in experimental heart failure in the rabbit. *J Clin Invest* 1986;78:674-679.
66. Jamieson JD, Palade GE: Specific granules in atrial tissue. *J Cell Biol* 1964;23:151-172.
67. deBold AJ, Borenstein HB, Veress AT, et al: A rapid and potent natriuretic response to intravenous injection of atrial myocardial extract in rats. *Life Sci* 1981;28:89-94.
68. Laragh JH: Atrial natriuretic hormone, the renin-aldosterone axis and blood pressure-electrolyte homeostasis. *N Engl J Med* 1985;313:1300-1340.
69. Needleman P, Greenwald JE: Atriopeptin: A cardiac hormone intimately involved in fluid, electrolyte, and blood pressure homeostasis. *N Engl J Med* 1986;314:828-834.
70. Atlas SA, Kleinert HD, Camargo MJF, et al: Purification, sequencing and synthesis of natriuretic and vasoactive rat atrial peptide. *Nature* 1984;309:717-719.
71. Currie MG, Geller DM, Cole BR et al: Purification and sequence analysis of bioactive atrial peptides (atriopeptins). *Science* 1984;223:67-69.
72. Flynn TG, deBold ML, deBold AJ: The amino acid sequence of atrial peptide with potent diuretic and natriuretic properties. *Biochem Biophys Res Commun* 1983;117:859-865.
73. Kangawa K, Matsuo H: Purification and complete amino acid sequence of α human atrial natriuretic polypeptide (α-h ANP). *Biochem Biophys Res Commun* 1984;118:131-139.
74. Dzau VJ, Baxter JD, Cantin M, et al: Nomenclature for atrial peptides. *N Engl J Med* 1987; 316:1276.
75. Dietz JR: Release of natriuretic factor from rat heart-lung preparation by atrial distension. *Am J Physiol* 1984;247:R1093-R1096.
76. Lang RE, Tholken H, Ganten D, et al: Atrial natriuretic factor—a circulating hormone stimulated by volume loading. *Nature* 1985;314:264-266.
77. Schwab TR, Edwards BS, Heublein DM et al: The role of atrial natriuretic peptide in volume expansion natriuresis. *Am J Physiol* 1986;251:R310-R313.
78. Bates ER, Shenker Y, Grekin RJ: The relationship between plasma levels of immunoreactive atrial natriuretic hormone and hemodynamic function in man. *Circulation* 1986;73:1155-1161.
79. Raine AEG, Erne P, Burgisser E, et al: Atrial natriuretic peptide and atrial pressure in patients with congestive heart failure. *N Engl J Med* 1986;315:533-537.
80. Rodeheffer RJ, Tanaka J, Imada T, et al: Atrial pressure and secretion of atrial natriuretic factor into the human central circulation. *J Am Coll Cardiol* 1986;8:18-26.
81. Epstein M, Loutzenhiser RD, Friedland E, et al: Increases in circulatory atrial natriuretic factor during immersion-induced central hypervolemia in normal humans. *J Hypertens* 1986;4(suppl 2):S93-S99.
82. Hodsman GP, Tsunoda K, Ogawa K, et al: Effect of posture on circulating atrial natriuretic peptide. *Lancet* 1985;2:1427-1428.
83. Espiner EA, Crozier IG, Nicholls MG, et al: Cardiac secretion of atrial natriuretic peptide. *Lancet* 1985;2:398-399.
84. Hollister AS, Tanaka I, Imada T, et al: Sodium loading and posture modulate human atrial natriuretic factor plasma levels. *Hypertension* 1986;8(suppl 2):106-111.
85. Sagnella GA, Markandu ND, Shore AC, et al: Effects of changes in dietary sodium intake and saline infusion on immunoreactive atrial natriuretic peptide in human plasma. *Lancet* 1985;2:1206-1211.
86. Edwards BS, Ackermann DM, Wold LE, et al: Presence of ventricular immunoreactive "atrial" natriuretic factor (ANF) in heart failure (abstract). *Kidney Int* 1987;31:268.

87. Cody RJ, Atlas SA, Laragh JH, et al: Atrial natriuretic factor in normal subjects and heart failure patients: Plasma levels and renal, hormonal and hemodynamic responses to peptide infusion. *J Clin Invest* 1986;78:1362-1374.

88. Camargo MJF, Kleinert HD, Atlas SA, et al: Ca-dependent hemodynamic and natriuretic effects of atrial extract in isolated rat kidney. *Am J Physiol* 1984;246:F447-F456.

89. Burnett JC, Granger JP, Opgenorth TS: Effects of synthetic atrial natriuretic factor on renal function and renin release. *Am J Physiol* 1984;247:F863-F866.

90. Huang CL, Lewicki J, Johnson LK, et al: Renal mechanism of action of rat atrial natriuretic factor. *J Clin Invest* 1985;75:769-773.

91. Maack T, Marion DN, Camargo MJF, et al: Effects of auriculin (atrial natriuretic factor) on blood pressure, renal function and the renin-aldosterone system in dogs. *Am J Med* 1984;77:1069-1075.

92. Ichikawa I, Dunn BR, Troy JL, et al: Influence of atrial natriuretic peptide on glomerular microcirculation *in vivo* (abstract). *Clin Res* 1985;33:487A.

93. Ballerman BJ, Dunn BR, Mendez RE, et al: Renal actions of atrial natriuretic peptides, in Mulrow PW, Schrier R (eds): *Atrial Hormones and Other Natriuretic Factors*. Bethesda, Md, American Physiological Society, 1987, pp 83-96.

94. Maack T, Camargo MJF, Kleinert HD, et al: Atrial natriuretic factor: Structure and functional properties. *Kidney Int* 1985;27:607-615.

95. Sonnenberg H, Cupples WA, deBold AJ, et al: Intrarenal localization of the natriuretic effect of cardiac atrial extract. *Can J Physiol Pharmacol* 1982;60:1149-1152.

96. Burnett JC, Opgenorth TJ, Granger JP: The renal action of atrial natriuretic peptide during control of glomerular filtration. *Kidney Int* 1986;30:16-19.

97. Zimmerman RS, Schirger JA, Edwards BS, et al: Cardiorenal-endocrine dynamics during stepwise infusion of physiologic and pharmacologic concentrations of atrial natriuretic factor in the dog. *Circ Res* 1987;61;63-69.

98. Currie MG, Geller DM, Cole BR, et al: Bioactive cardiac substances: Potent vasorelaxant activity in mammalian atria. *Science* 1983;221:71-73.

99. Kleinert HD, Maack T, Atlas SA, et al: Atrial natriuretic factor inhibits angiotensin-, norepinephrine-, and potassium-induced vascular contractility. *Hypertension* 1984;6(suppl 1):143-147.

100. Winquist RB, Faison EP, Waldman SA, et al: Atrial natriuretic factor elicits an endothelium-independent relaxation and activates particulate guanylate cyclase in vascular smooth muscle. *Proc Natl Acad Sci USA* 1984;81:7661-7664.

101. Bolli P, Muller FB, Linder L, et al: The vasodilatory potency of atrial natriuretic peptide in man. *Circulation* 1987;75:221-228.

102. Cody RJ, Kubo SH, Atlas SA, et al: Direct demonstration of the vasodilator properties of atrial natriuretic factor in normal man and heart failure patients. *Clin Res* 1986;34:476A.

103. Muller FB, Erne P, Raine AE: Atrial antipressor natriuretic peptide: Release mechanisms and vascular action in man. *J Hypertens* 1986;4(suppl 2): S109-S114.

104. Kleinert HD, Volpe M, Odell G, et al: Cardiovascular effects of synthetic atrial natriuretic factor in anesthetized and conscious dogs. *Hypertension* 1986;8:312-316.

105. Sasaki A, Kida O, Kangawa K, et al: Hemodynamic effects of α human atrial natriuretic polypeptide (α-HANP) in rats. *Eur J Pharmacol* 1985;109:405-407.

106. Volpe M, Odell G, Kleinert HD, et al: Antihypertensive and aldosterone-lowering effects of synthetic atrial natriuretic factor in renin-dependent renovascular hypertension. *J Hypertens* 1984;2(suppl 3):313-315.

107. Carson PE, Carlyle PF, Cohn JN: Cardiac and regional vascular effects of atrial natriuretic peptide in awake dogs. *Clin Res* 1986;34:707A.

108. Opgenorth TJ, Burnett JC, Granger JP, et al: Effects of atrial natriuretic peptide on renin secretion in non-filtering kidney. *Am J Physiol* 1986;250:F798-F801.

109. Scriven TA, Burnett JC: Effects of synthetic atrial natriuretic peptide on renal function and renin release in acute experimental heart failure. *Circulation* 1986;72:892-897.
110. Atarashi K, Mulrow PJ, Franco-Saenz R, et al: Inhibition of aldosterone production by an atrial extract. *Science* 1984;224:992-994.
111. Goodfriend TL, Elliot ME, Atlas SA: Actions of synthetic atrial natriuretic factor on bovine adrenal glomerulosa. *Life Sci* 1984;35:1675-1682
112. Dusting GJ, Moncada S, Vane JR: Prostaglandins, their intermediates and precursors: Cardiovascular actions and regulatory roles in normal and abnormal circulatory systems. *Prog Cardiovasc Dis* 1979;21:405-430.
113. Oliver JA, Sciacci RR, Pinto J, et al: Participation of the prostaglandins in the control of renal blood flow during acute reduction of cardiac output in the dog. *J Clin Invest* 1981;67:229-237.
114. Terragno NA, Terragno DA, McGiff JC: Contribution of prostaglandins to the renal circulation in conscious, anesthetized and laparotomized dogs. *Circ Res* 1977;40:590-595.
115. Heinrich WL, Anderson RJ, Berns AS, et al: The role of renal nerves and prostaglandins in control of renal hemodynamics and plasma renin activity during hypotensive hemorrhage. *J Clin Invest* 1978;61:744-750.
116. Blasingham MC, Nasjletti A: Differential renal effects of cyclooxygenase inhibition in sodium replete and sodium deprived dog. *Am J Physiol* 1980;239:F360-F365.
117. Nasjletti A, Malik KU: Interrelationship among prostaglandins and vasoactive substances. *Med Clin North Am* 1981;65:891-914.
118. Horton R, Zipser R, Fichman M: Prostaglandins, renal function and vascular regulation. *Med Clin North Am* 1981;65:891-914.
119. Junstad M, Wennmalm A: On the release of prostaglandin E_2 from the rabbit heart following infusion of noradrenaline. *Acta Physiol Scand* 1973;87:573-574.
120. McGiff JC, Crowshaw K, Terrango NA, et al: Differential effect of noradrenaline and renal nerve stimulation on vascular resistance in the dog kidney and the release of a prostaglandin E-like substance. *Clin Sci* 1972;42:223-233.
121. Needleman P, Bronson SD, Wyche A, et al: Cardiac and renal prostaglandin I_2: Biosynthesis and biological effects in isolated perfused rabbit tissues. *J Clin Invest* 1978;61:839-849.
122. Dzau VJ, Packer M, Lilly LS, et al: Prostaglandins in heart failure: Relation to activation of the renin-angiotensin system and hyponatremia. *N Engl J Med* 1984;310:347-352.
123. Punzengruber C, Stanek B, Sinzinger H, et al: Bicyclo-prostaglandin E_2 metabolite in congestive heart failure and relation to vasoconstrictor neurohormonal principles. *Am J Cardiol* 1986;57:619-623.
124. Corwin HL, Bonventre JV: Renal insufficiency associated with nonsteroidal anti-inflammatory agents. *Am J Kidney Dis* 1984;4:147-152.
125. Olivari MT, Levine TB, Cohn JN: Evidence for a direct renal stimulating effect of prostaglandin E_2 on renin release in patients with congestive heart failure. *Circulation* 1986;74:1203-1207.
126. Dzau VJ, Swartz SL, Creager MA: The role of prostaglandins in the pathophysiology and therapy for congestive heart failure. *Heart Failure* 1986;2:6-13.
127. Yun J, Kelly G, Bartter FC, et al: Role of prostaglandins in the control of renin secretion in the dog. *Circ Res* 1972;40:459-464.
128. Patrono C, Pugliese F, Ciabattoni G, et al: Evidence for a direct stimulating effect of prostacyclin on renin release in man. *J Clin Invest* 1982;69:231-239.
129. Levin RI, Jaffe EA, Weksler BB, et al: Nitroglycerin stimulates synthesis of prostacyclin by cultured human endothelial cells. *J Clin Invest* 1981;67:762-769.
130. Moore TJ, Crantz FR, Hollenberg NK, et al: Contribution of prostaglandins to the antihypertensive action of captopril in essential hypertension. *Hypertension* 1981;3:168-173.

131. Rubin LJ, Lazar JD: Influence of prostaglandin synthesis inhibitors on pulmonary vasodilatory effects of hydralazine in dogs with hypoxic pulmonary vasoconstriction. *J Clin Invest* 1981;67:193-200.

132. Swartz SL, Williams GH: Angiotensin converting enzyme inhibition and prostaglandins. *Am J Cardiol* 1982;49:1405-1409.

133. Dzau VJ, Swartz SL, Williams GH, et al: Dissociation of renin-angiotensin and prostaglandin systems during captopril therapy in congestive heart failure (abstract). *J Am Coll Cardiol* 1983;1:727.

134. Goldberg LI, Rajfer SI: Dopamine receptors: Applications in clinical cardiology. *Circulation* 1985;72:245-248.

135. Stemple DR, Kleiman JH, Harrison DC: Combined nitroprusside-dopamine therapy in severe chronic congestive heart failure: Dose related hemodynamic advantages over single drug infusion. *Am J Cardiol* 1978;42:267-275.

136. Covit AB, Laragh JH, Cody RJ: Endogenous dopamine activity in chronic heart function (abstract). *Clin Res* 1983;31:175A.

137. Viquerat CE, Daly P, Swedberg K, et al: Endogenous catecholamine levels in chronic heart failure: Relation to the severity of hemodynamic abnormalities. *Am J Med* 1985;78:455-460.

138. Pierpont GL, Francis GS, DeMaster EG, et al: Elevated left ventricular myocardial dopamine in pre-terminal idiopathic dilated cardiomyopathy. *Am J Cardiol* 1983;52:1033-1035.

139. Sole MJ, Helke CJ, Jacobowitz DM: Increased dopamine in the failing hamster heart: Transvesicular transport of dopamine limits the role of norepinephrine synthesis: *Am J Cardiol* 1982;49:1682-1690.

140. Beregovich J, Bianchi C, Rubler S, et al: Dose related hemodynamic and renal effects of dopamine in congestive heart failure. *Am Heart J* 1974;87:550-557.

141. Maskin CS, Ocken S, Chadwick B, et al: Comparative systemic and renal effects of dopamine and angiotension-converting enzyme inhibition with enalapril in patients with heart failure. *Circulation* 1985;72:846-852.

142. Francis GS, Parks R, Cohn JN: The effects of bromocriptine in patients with congestive heart failure. *Am Heart J* 1983;106:100-106.

143. Rajfer SI, Rossen JD, Douglass FL, et al: Effects of long-term therapy with oral ibopamine on resting hemodynamics and exercise capacity in patients with heart failure: Relationship to the generation of N-methyldopamine and to plasma norepinephrine levels. *Circulation* 1986;73:740-748.

144. Ren JH, Unverferth DV, Leier CV: The dopamine congener, ibopamine, in congestive heart failure. *J Cardiovasc Pharmacol* 1984;6:748-755.

145. Young JB, Leon CA, Pratt CM, et al: Hemodynamic effects of an oral dopamine receptor agonist (fenoldopam) in patients with congestive heart failure. *J Am Coll Cardiol* 1985;6:792-796.

146. Rajfer SI, Anton AH, Rossen JD, et al: Beneficial hemodynamic effects of oral levodopa in heart failure: Relation to the generation of dopamine. *N Engl J Med* 1984;310:1357-1362.

ROBERT J. CODY, MD, and
JOHN H. LARAGH, MD

4

The Renin-Angiotensin-Aldosterone System in Chronic Heart Failure: Pathophysiology and Implications for Treatment

In 1946 Merrill and co-workers[1] reported an increased concentration of renin in blood samples obtained from renal veins of patients with chronic heart failure. At that time, it was speculated that this finding was the manifestation of decreased renal blood flow and, hence, a compensatory response of renin. Over a decade later, the potential pathogenic role of renin-angiotensin-aldosterone (RAA) system activation in the vasoconstriction and sodium retention of heart failure was suggested.[2,3] Although the contribution of this system to heart failure was easy to understand on a theoretical basis, it was difficult to demonstrate in physiologic studies because of the paucity of animal models of heart failure and the inability to block the RAA pathway specifically.

Early clinical studies of converting-enzyme inhibitors played a major role in identifying the extent of RAA system activity and the clinical benefit arising from blockade of this system.[4-10] Since the first edition of this text, additional studies have demonstrated further important points: evidence of functional improvement of both mild and severe heart failure as a result of RAA system inhibition,[11-13] the influence of inhibiting RAA activity on metabolic and target organ function,[14-17] and, perhaps most important, the favorable effect on survival of inhibiting RAA activity in the congestive heart failure population.[18]

The purpose of the present chapter is to delineate the extent of RAA system activity in chronic congestive heart failure; to demonstrate its pathophysiologic effects in heart failure; and to discuss the hemodynamic, hormonal, and clinical improvement resulting from inhibiting angiotensin-mediated vasoconstriction and aldosterone-mediated sodium retention.

RENIN-ANGIOTENSIN-ALDOSTERONE SYSTEM IN CHRONIC CONGESTIVE HEART FAILURE

Renin-Angiotensin-Aldosterone Pathway

Angiotensinogen, a 14-amino-acid α_2-globulin of hepatic origin, is the substrate for the rate-limiting enzyme renin (Fig. 4-1). Renin cleaves four amino acids from angiotensinogen, resulting in production of the decapeptide angiotensin-I. Two additional amino acids are subsequently cleaved from this decapeptide by angiotensin converting enzyme, a carboxypeptidase that was originally identified in the pulmonary circulation,[19] but subsequently has also been identified in blood vessel walls.[20] A carboxypeptidase of similar activity is responsible for degradation of the vasodilator bradykinin. More recently, the key elements of the renin system have been identified in a variety of tissues, which suggests the importance of local tissue regulation of the pathway.[21] Angiotensin-II, the octapeptide generated by converting enzyme, is the most potent endogenous vasoconstrictor. In a situation in which an inappropriate increase of vascular tone may accompany severe reduction of left ventricular function, the elaboration of angiotensin-II would result in further impedance to forward flow, thereby further reducing cardiac output and regional flow. The manifestations of such reduced flow depend on the vascular bed affected. In addition to producing intense vasoconstriction, angiotensin-II directly stimulates aldosterone release from the adrenal gland,[22] resulting in sodium and water retention. Sodium retention and volume expansion not only produce pulmonary and systemic venous congestion but are also implicated in increased vascular stiffness.[23] Aldosterone release also directly stimulates potassium excretion by the kidney. In the setting of intense diuretic therapy, when hypokalemia may be present, this additional stimulus for kaliuresis may predispose to ventricular arrhythmias, which are now recognized as an independent predictor of mortality in heart failure.[24] These considerations are not simply theoretical; the actual extent of RAA system activity in heart failure has been directly identified.

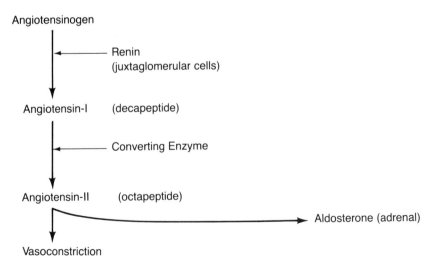

Fig. 4-1. The renin-angiotensin-aldosterone pathway. Renin is the rate-limiting enzyme for this cascade. Factors that stimulate or suppress its release in congestive heart failure are discussed in the text.

Factors Influencing Basal Renin-Angiotensin-Aldosterone System Activity

Stimulation: A variety of factors stimulate renin release (Table 4-1). Reduction of renal blood flow and perfusion pressure consequent to severe left ventricular failure is of primary importance. This is analogous to the reduction of perfusion pressure and flow distal to the fixed lesion of renal artery stenosis.[25] Unlike renal artery stenosis, however, in which the lesion is anatomically fixed, the situation in congestive heart failure is functional; therefore, it is conceivable that the extent of renin release can be altered by any factor that increases or decreases renal blood flow. Such alterations play an important role in the long-term renal outcome of chronic RAA system inhibition (see below).

Table 4-1. Factors that stimulate or suppress renin-angiotensin-aldosterone system activity in chronic heart failure

Factors that stimulate renin release

Decreased renal perfusion
Decreased delivery of sodium to the macula densa
Enhanced sympathetic activity
Aberrant reflex regulation
Reduction of intracellular calcium
Pharmacologic therapy
    Diuretics
    Some vasodilators

Factors that suppress renin release

Sodium repletion
Digoxin therapy
Atrial natriuretic factor

Sympathetic nervous system activity as a stimulus for renin release is well documented. Sympathetic activity is generally increased in heart failure,[26-29] and it is reasonable to assume that this increased sympathetic tone may modulate renin release. However, sympathetic responsiveness is itself inappropriately blunted in heart failure.[27] Thus it is difficult to identify a strong correlation with renin activity.[28,30] The low-pressure mechanoreceptors of the cardiopulmonary vasculature are a reflex regulator of renin release. For instance, it is known that a sudden reduction of right atrial pressure because of upright posture and other factors that decrease venous return will stimulate renin release.[31,32] However, this response is abnormal in heart failure.[33,34] A rapidly growing body of data has provided an appropriate reemphasis on the role of abnormal sympathetic nervous system activity in heart failure,[35,36] indicating a need for additional analysis of this influence on renin release.

An additional powerful stimulus for renin release is a reduction of renal tubular sodium delivery to the macula densa within the nephron.[37] Because of enhanced proximal tubular sodium reabsorption, patients with chronic heart failure have decreased sodium delivery to the macula densa of the distal tubule.[38] This decrease is erroneously perceived by the kidney as a reduction of intravascular volume, and renin release is therefore stimulated.

The release of renin from the juxtaglomerular apparatus may be influenced by intracellular calcium in juxtaglomerular cells.[39] This influence can be demonstrated by the increase of plasma renin activity subsequent to the acute administration of calcium entry inhibitors in patients with heart failure, in whom substantial increases of renin occur within minutes of calcium channel antagonism.[40,41] Likewise, increasing intracellular calcium by digitalis preparations may suppress renin release.[39,42]

Pharmacologic therapy for heart failure may directly stimulate renin release. Diuretic therapy, especially with drugs acting on the loop of Henle, is a potent stimulus for release of renin.[43-45] Diuretics are prescribed for most patients with heart failure at early stages of the disease; therefore it can be anticipated that in more chronic stages of the disease diuretics would be a major stimulus for renin release, potentially attenuating the initial benefits associated with diuretic use. Some vasodilators frequently used for the chronic treatment of congestive heart failure, such as hydralazine, prazosin, and minoxidil, can result in an increase of circulating renin.[46-48]

Suppression: Factors that may suppress renin system activity in patients with congestive heart failure have been overlooked. At least three distinct factors can be identified (Table 4-1). Increasing sodium intake by dietary means suppresses renin system activity in normal subjects.[49] Similar suppression has been shown in patients with heart failure not receiving diuretic treatment whose daily dietary sodium intake is increased from 10 to 100 mEq.[50] While this increase of dietary sodium intake causes an overall suppression of RAA activity, the extent to which it is suppressed depends on delivery of sodium to the macula densa. That is, in patients who continue to avidly retain sodium, there remains a relative increase of renin activity.

Digoxin, the most commonly used drug in congestive heart failure, suppresses renin system activity (Fig. 4-2).[42] In response to a single intravenous bolus of digoxin 0.50 mg in patients previously not receiving digoxin therapy, there was a time-dependent reduction of both plasma aldosterone and plasma renin activity, which resulted in a 50% reduction of RAA activity at approximately two to three hours after bolus administration. Both plasma aldosterone and plasma renin activity returned toward baseline by seven hours, when serum digoxin levels were maximally decreased.

A new and exciting finding regarding congestive heart failure is the identification of an endogenous hormone secreted by the heart known as atrial natriuretic factor (ANF). This hormone causes natriuresis and diuresis in normal subjects[51] and suppresses renin system activity when given as an exogenous infusion.[52] In patients with congestive heart failure, in whom the natriuretic effect of the hormone is blunted, there is nonetheless an influence on RAA activity (Fig. 4-3). Plasma renin activity does not decrease, which probably reflects a failure of ANF administration to enhance natriuresis and the delivery of sodium to the distal nephron. Nonetheless, there is a rapid and significant reduction of plasma aldosterone, which is felt to represent a direct suppression of adrenal synthesis of aldosterone.[51]

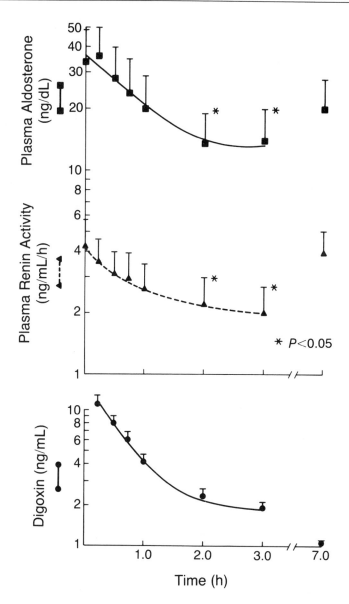

Fig. 4-2. Effect of a single 0.50-mg intravenous bolus of digoxin in patients with congestive heart failure who have not previously been treated. Digoxin administration resulted in a significant suppression of plasma aldosterone and plasma renin activity. Details are discussed in the text. (Adapted from Covit et al, *Am J Med* 1983;75:445-447, with permission.)

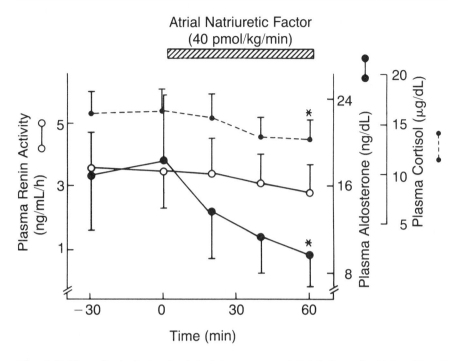

Fig. 4-3. The effect of steady-state intravenous administration of atrial natriuretic factor (ANF) at a rate of 40 pmol/kg/min (equivalent to mg/mL/min). In patients with congestive heart failure in whom natriuresis has not improved on ANF administration, renin is not suppressed, probably because of the inability to deliver sodium to the distal nephron. Since ANF has a direct suppressing effect on aldosterone synthesis, plasma aldosterone levels fall significantly during ANF administration. (Adapted from Cody et al.[52] Reproduced from *The Journal of Clinical Investigation* 1986;78:1362-1374 by copyright permission of the American Society for Clinical Investigation.)

Extent of Activity of the Renin-Angiotensin-Aldosterone System

Considering the wide range of plasma renin activity, a uniform contribution of the RAA system to the pathophysiology of heart failure in all patients would not be anticipated. Because sodium intake is a major factor determining the level of plasma renin activity, it is important to analyze the resting level of plasma renin in relation to sodium intake. However, most patients with severe heart failure are receiving diuretic therapy, or are avidly retaining sodium.[38, 53-55] A "normal" range of renin has not, and cannot, be determined for the heart failure population, unless diuretics are withheld, sodium intake is controlled, and neutral balance (sodium intake = sodium excretion) is established. Unfortunately, such requirements would exclude all but the mildest forms of heart failure from analysis. Therefore, analyses must be based on the range of RAA activity, or arbitrary cut points. In most diuretic-treated patients, RAA activity is increased.[56-58] Figure 4-4 provides an example of the overall range of plasma renin activity and its correlation with urinary aldosterone in 35 patients with heart failure. When the data from all 35 patients were analyzed, there was a good correlation between plasma renin and aldosterone ($r = 0.784, P < 0.001$). Plasma renin activity ranged from 0.12 to 130 ng/mL/h. Although many patients with heart failure have plasma renin activity within

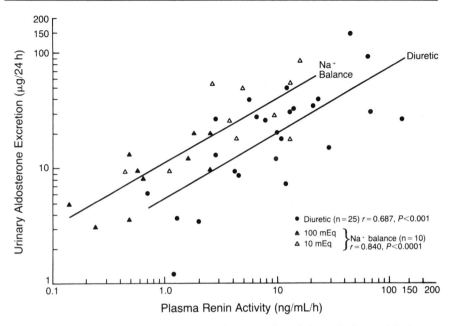

Fig. 4-4. Correlation between the baseline plasma renin activity and urinary aldosterone excretion. In congestive heart failure, there is a strong correlation between baseline plasma renin activity and 24-hour urinary aldosterone excretion (overall correlation $r = 0.784$, $P < 0.001$). The discrete difference between the regression lines for diuretic-treated subjects and for those studied during sodium imbalance probably reflects the aldosterone-suppressing effect of hypokalemia in the diuretic-treated group.

the range of normal stimulated plasma renin, two extremes are readily apparent. A large number of patients show plasma renin activity that is markedly elevated (>10 ng/mL/h), in contrast to those in whom plasma renin activity is markedly suppressed (<1.0 ng/mL/h). Plasma renin activity of the former group is analogous to that observed in patients with hypertension caused by renal artery stenosis; that in the latter group is analogous to the levels of suppressed plasma renin observed in hypertension resulting from primary hypersecretion of aldosterone. Thus it is possible to have "normal" renin levels in moderate to severe heart failure. When the correlation for patients receiving diuretic therapy was compared with that for patients in whom sodium balance studies were performed, two discrete lines of regression paralleling one another were observed. For any given level of plasma renin activity, patients receiving diuretic therapy had urinary aldosterone excretion approximately one half of that observed in patients in sodium balance. Generally, patients receiving diuretic therapy experience a total body potassium deficit. Because hypokalemia may suppress aldosterone release, the lower urinary aldosterone excretion in diuretic-treated patients may reflect reduction of total body potassium. Patients in sodium balance, whose daily potassium intake is closely regulated, would not demonstrate this additional mechanism of aldosterone suppression. Recent data indicate that in symptomatically mild to moderate heart failure, the RAA system is not activated in the absence of diuretics.[59,60]

    To analyze renin system characteristics further as they relate to congestive heart failure patients, we arbitrarily divided 108 consecutive

patients with congestive heart failure according to their baseline plasma
renin activity (Fig. 4-5). We used cut points that are typical of those used to

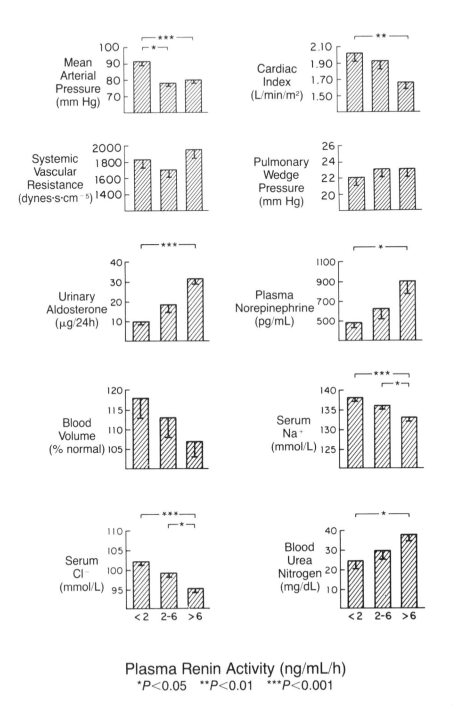

Plasma Renin Activity (ng/mL/h)
*P<0.05   **P<0.01   ***P<0.001

Fig. 4-5. Hemodynamic, hormonal, and metabolic characteristics of 108 patients with
chronic congestive heart failure, according to baseline plasma renin activity.

classify hypertensive patients: plasma renin activity less than 2, 2 to 6, and greater than 6 ng/mL/h. Comparing patients with low-renin versus high-renin heart failure, we found that patients with the greatest activation of the renin system had lower mean arterial pressure and cardiac index, even though systemic vascular resistance and pulmonary wedge pressure were virtually identical for all subgroups. These findings suggest that mechanisms other than angiotensin-II may be responsible for vasoconstriction and increased left ventricular end-diastolic pressure in the low-renin heart failure group. Besides these hemodynamic characteristics, we also studied hormonal and metabolic characteristics of RAA activity by this subgroup analysis. Urinary aldosterone excretion tracked plasma renin activity, being much greater in individuals with high renin values, as were plasma norepinephrine levels. While blood volume, expressed as percent of predicted normal, was relatively low in the high-renin group, it still remained above the normal level. Both serum sodium and serum chloride were much lower in the high-renin group, showing a stepwise decrement compared with the low-renin heart failure patients. Blood urea nitrogen, a plasma marker of prerenal azotemia and renal insufficiency, was greater in the high-renin group. While this subgroup analysis did not establish a cause-and-effect relationship between renin and the variables identified, it nonetheless illustrates the important correlates that are typically seen in heart failure patients when the RAA system is activated: hypotension, increased sympathetic nervous system activity, and marked metabolic derangements. The low-renin state of congestive heart failure is complex but can be influenced by the state of sodium balance[50] or the presence of recent decompensation, as shown in the chronic stages of experimental heart failure[61] or in patients with active cardiac decompensation.[62] In the latter state, in which pulmonary congestion and all the signs and symptoms of severe heart failure are present, marked sodium retention can suppress the renin system in a manner analogous to that observed with sodium loading in metabolically balanced studies.[50]

RENIN-ANGIOTENSIN-ALDOSTERONE SYSTEM AND VASCULAR TONE
The dependence of vascular tone on angiotensin-mediated vasoconstriction can be identified in both animal models and clinical studies. Sodium depletion brings out this dependence, as has been shown in dogs,[63,64] rats,[65] and primates[27] by the use of converting-enzyme inhibitors. In the state of sodium repletion, converting-enzyme inhibitors demonstrate minimal to moderate reduction of blood pressure in animal models. However, in sodium depletion, in which the renin system is activated, a marked reduction of blood pressure occurs after converting-enzyme inhibition. This effect has also been demonstrated in normal human subjects.[66-68] In the sodium repleted state, minimal reduction of blood pressure is observed after converting-enzyme inhibition; in the sodium depleted state (renin system activated), marked hypotension, to the point of fainting and syncope, is evoked by converting-enzyme inhibition. In patients with congestive heart failure, this phenomenon has been studied using the additional stimulus of head-up tilt to evaluate the circulatory adaptation to postural gravitational stress.[69] In diuretic-treated patients who underwent long-term converting-enzyme inhibition, a moderate reduction of blood pressure was seen. However, when these patients were tilted, a greater hypotensive response was noted.[33,35] In patients with marked hypotension, this abnormal

response was attenuated, when tilt was repeated, after the acute, rapid administration of saline into the central circulation. The dependence of vascular tone on angiotensin-mediated vasoconstriction was more clearly demonstrated during a balanced sodium intake study in ten patients, in which diuretics were withheld and tilt studies were performed during sodium depletion (10 mEq) and sodium repletion (100 mEq), each of one week's duration (Fig. 4-6). In the sodium depleted state under baseline conditions, four of ten patients demonstrated a greater than 15% reduction of mean arterial pressure during tilt. After a 25-mg dose of captopril, six patients demonstrated at least a 15% reduction of mean arterial pressure during tilt. Of the six, four patients had a reduction of mean arterial pressure to a level of 38 to 50 mm Hg. In the sodium repleted state, only two of ten patients demonstrated a 15% reduction of mean arterial pressure during tilt under basal conditions. After a 25-mg dose of captopril, three of ten patients demonstrated a 15% reduction of mean arterial pressure, and in only one patient did blood pressure fall to a level less than 60 mm Hg. The renin system had been activated during the 10-mEq diet and was suppressed during the 100-mEq diet. These findings were the first clear evidence of the dependence of vascular tone on angiotensin-mediated vasoconstriction in patients with congestive heart failure. When these observations are coupled with the results in diuretic-treated patients, they *define* the concept of angiotensin-dependent vascular tone in congestive heart failure patients, in whom sodium depletion by means of diuretics typifies the vast majority of the patient population.

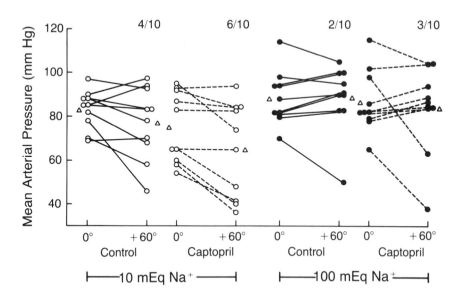

Fig. 4-6. The effect of dietary sodium depletion versus repletion on the blood pressure response to the supine position (0°) and 60° head-up tilt (+60°). The open triangles represent mean values. Tilt studies were performed during sodium depletion, and repeated during sodium repletion, in ten subjects with moderate to severe congestive heart failure. The tilt was repeated after a single 25-mg dose of oral captopril in all subjects in each dietary condition (see text for details). (Adapted from Cody et al.[50] Reproduced from *The Journal of Clinical Investigation* 1986;77:1441-1452 by copyright permission of the American Society for Clinical Investigation.)

RENIN-ANGIOTENSIN-ALDOSTERONE SYSTEM AND SODIUM EXCRETION

The control of sodium excretion in humans depends on two variables of renal function: glomerular filtration rate and sodium reabsorption.[70] Glomerular filtration rate is abnormal in congestive heart failure, as discussed in greater detail in Chapter 5. Sodium reabsorption is controlled by several factors, including sympathetic nervous activity, aldosterone, and, to a lesser degree, intrarenal distribution of blood flow, the balance of hydraulic and oncotic pressure, and atrial natriuretic factor, which may be the elusive "third factor" that has been postulated for many years.

Of all the factors that influence sodium reabsorption, aldosterone is the most important. Because the vast majority of the filtered load of sodium is reabsorbed in the proximal tubule, the modulation of aldosterone activity at the distal tubule accounts for the maintenance of the balance between dietary sodium intake and excretion on any given day. In the pathophysiologic condition of congestive heart failure, in which aldosterone levels are increased (see Fig. 4-4), little if any detectable sodium escapes into the urine. One would therefore expect to find a clear relationship between the extent of RAA activity and urinary sodium excretion. In reality, this relationship is obscured by diuretic therapy. In patients receiving diuretics, it is virtually impossible to find a close relationship between urinary sodium excretion and plasma renin activity (Fig. 4-7). However, this relationship can be seen in patients in whom diuretics are withheld and sodium intake is balanced (Figs. 4-8 and 4-9). Both plasma renin activity and urinary aldosterone excretion are increased during a low sodium intake. As urinary sodium excretion increases with an increase of sodium intake to 100 mEq, both plasma renin and urinary aldosterone excretion are suppressed. However, in those subjects who continue to retain sodium avidly during oral loading, RAA

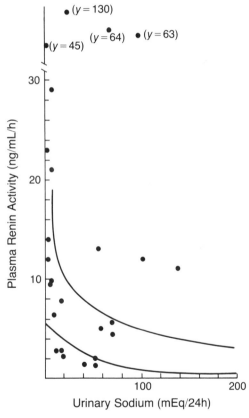

Fig. 4-7. Relationship between urinary sodium excretion and plasma renin activity in normal subjects (indicated by the area enclosed by the solid lines) and congestive heart failure patients receiving diuretics, shown as individual data points. Note the lack of a clear correlation between urinary sodium excretion and plasma renin activity in the diuretic-treated CHF patients.

activity remains increased. These data provide compelling evidence for the preservation of the macula densa signal for renin release in congestive heart failure. When the ingested sodium load is able to reach the macula densa, there is a reduction of the signal for renin release by the juxtaglomerular apparatus, with subsequent reduction of aldosterone secretion, so that the ingested sodium load can be excreted. The difference between the subjects who avidly retained sodium and those who reach neutral balance is not clear. Whether this is a hemodynamic phenomenon, a function of the glomerular filtration rate and its influence on proximal tubule sodium reabsorption, or the influence of other hormonal factors such as prostaglandins or atrial natriuretic factor is not known.

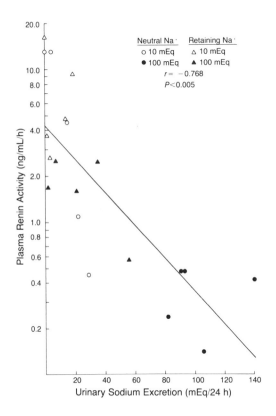

Fig. 4-8. Relationship of urinary sodium excretion to plasma renin activity during balanced sodium intake in patients with congestive heart failure not receiving diuretics. On 100-mEq diet, five patients reached balance (solid circles), while five patients continued to avidly retain sodium (solid triangles). Their respective values during the 10-mEq diet are shown by the open symbols. During the 100-mEq sodium diet, patients who were capable of delivering the ingested sodium to the distal nephron were able to suppress renin system activity and excrete the dietary load. Patients who continued to retain sodium avidly continued to have relative activation of the renin-angiotensin-aldosterone system. (Adapted from Cody et al.[50] Reproduced from *The Journal of Clinical Investigation* 1986;77:1441-1452 by copyright permission of the American Society for Clinical Investigation.)

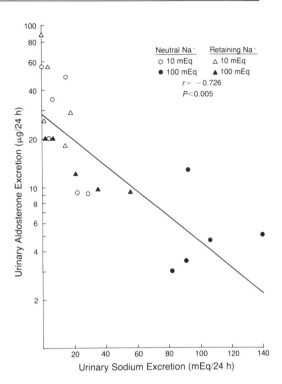

Fig. 4-9. Relationship of urinary sodium excretion to urinary aldosterone excretion during balanced sodium intake. Details are as described in Fig. 4-8. As with plasma renin activity, the extent of urinary aldosterone excretion is a function of the ability to deliver sodium to the distal nephron. (Adapted from Cody et al.[50] Reproduced from *The Journal of Clinical Investigation* 1986;77:1441-1452 by copyright permission of the American Society for Clinical Investigation.)

INHIBITION OF RENIN-ANGIOTENSIN-ALDOSTERONE SYSTEM ACTIVITY IN CHRONIC CONGESTIVE HEART FAILURE

Sites of Potential Pharmacologic Inhibition

If the RAA system is inappropriately activated in chronic congestive heart failure, then blockade of this pathway should result in hemodynamic improvement. The renin cascade can be interrupted at several levels (Fig. 4-10). Release of renin by the juxtaglomerular apparatus can be inhibited by sympatholytic agents. This mechanism may partially explain the beneficial results observed when β-adrenergic blocking agents are administered to patients with severe heart failure.[36,71] The rate-limiting activities of renin may also be inhibited if an analog of angiotensinogen is administered. Such peptides would compete with endogenous angiotensinogen for renin binding sites, thereby preventing the subsequent generation of angiotensin-II. Such competitive inhibitors, which offer a new approach to RAA system inhibition, have been studied *in vivo*,[72-74] and clinical trials have recently been initiated.

The next step for potential inhibition of the renin cascade is at the level of converting enzyme. The beneficial effects of converting-enzyme inhibition in heart failure were initially identified with the nonpeptide teprotide.[5] Teprotide, however, required intravenous administration and is not practical for long-term therapy. Subsequently, the oral converting-enzyme inhibitors captopril and enalapril were developed and extensively studied in heart failure.[16,17,75]

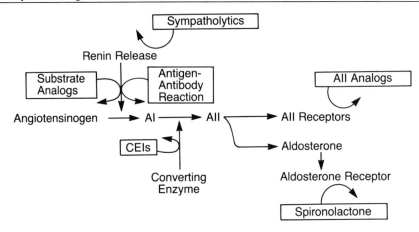

Fig. 4-10. Sites in the RAA cascade where pharmacologic inhibition has been evaluated. See text for details. (AI = angiotensin-I; AII = angiotensin-II; CEIs = converting-enzyme inhibitors.)

Angiotensin-II analogs provide another means of renin system inhibition by directly competing with angiotensin-II for tissue binding sites. Saralasin, the prototypic angiotensin-II analog, has been used for physiologic studies in heart failure.[10,76] There are two major reasons why these agents are difficult to use in patients with heart failure. First, they have a very short half-life[77] and require continuous intravenous infusion. Second, their physiologic activity depends on the basal level of endogenous angiotensin-II at the receptor. That is, when the endogenous angiotensin-II levels are low, these drugs act in an agonist fashion, mimicking the effects of exogenously administered angiotensin-II and producing vasoconstriction. In situations of high endogenous angiotensin-II activity, however, the drugs displace the more potent endogenous angiotensin-II from the receptor, and this antagonist activity results in a reversal of vasoconstriction. The potential agonist effect, which increases vascular resistance, makes this group of drugs impractical for uniform treatment of heart failure.

Finally, spironolactone may be considered a competitive inhibitor of aldosterone at its binding sites in the distal nephron.[78] In theory, such an inhibitor would provide a specific means of blocking the sodium-retaining properties of aldosterone. In general, spironolactone has not been found to be sufficiently potent for long-term reduction of sodium retention. From a practical standpoint, angiotensin converting-enzyme inhibitors remain the most practical approach to renin system inhibition.

Reversal of Angiotensin-Mediated Vasoconstriction If angiotensin-II is contributing to the increased systemic vascular resistance or impedance to ventricular outflow in chronic congestive heart failure, then inhibition of angiotensin-II generation should result in reduction of systemic vascular resistance and increased cardiac output. This, of course, is presumptive, as vascular tone is subject to the influence of both systemic and regional mechanisms that can obscure a direct correlation. Nonetheless, the evidence is compelling. We observed a close correlation among baseline plasma renin activity, reduction of systemic resistance and pulmonary wedge pressure, and increases of both cardiac index and stroke volume index, following captopril administration (Fig. 4-11).[56] Thus, as basal plasma renin activity increased, so did the magnitude of hemodynamic improvement after converting-enzyme inhibition with captopril. Conversely, in patients with plasma renin activity less than 1 ng/mL/h, there was virtually no immediate hemodynamic improvement after converting-enzyme inhibition. This finding suggests that angiotensin-mediated vasoconstriction occurred in most, but not all, patients with heart failure.

That the inhibitory effect is rapid and unequivocal can be observed after the intravenous administration of enalaprilat, the de-esterified active metabolite of enalapril.[79,80] We demonstrated an immediate normalization of circulating levels of angiotensin-II and reversal of vasoconstriction. The

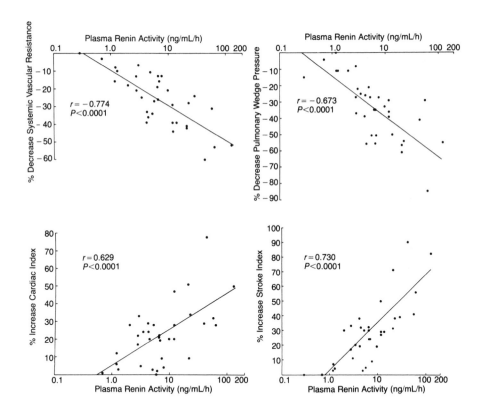

Fig. 4-11. Hemodynamic response to a single dose of oral captopril (25 mg), as related to baseline plasma renin activity in 35 diuretic-treated patients with congestive heart failure. It is clear that the initial response to converting-enzyme inhibitor therapy was related to the basal degree of renin system activation. (Adapted from RJ Cody, JH Laragh, Use of captopril to estimate renin-angiotensin-aldosterone activity in pathophysiology of chronic heart failure, *Am Heart J* 1982;104:1184-1188.)

response in heart failure patients with minimal renin system activity was negligible. While it is difficult always to establish a clear relationship between basal renin system activity and the reversal of vasoconstriction, carefully conducted clinical trials have confirmed these observations.[28,81,82] This relationship is clarified in strictly controlled metabolic studies in which sodium intake is regimented and diuretics are withheld (Fig. 4-12).[50] Under these conditions, captopril produced a modest but significant reversal of vasoconstriction during 10 mEq sodium intake (when renin activity was increased), but virtually no reversal of vasoconstriction during 100 mEq sodium intake (when renin activity was suppressed). This differential hemodynamic response is not due to differences in the plasma levels of converting-enzyme inhibitor achieved with oral administration. Figure 4-13, derived from studies of the pharmacokinetics of captopril,[83] demonstrates this point. Reversal of vasoconstriction occurred only in the presence of increased plasma renin activity, despite comparable plasma captopril levels. Furthermore, the use of the agonist-antagonist saralasin strengthens these observations.[84] In the setting of prior converting-enzyme inhibition, saralasin, acting as an agonist, restored systemic resistance to precaptopril levels, because of the absence of endogenous angiotensin-II, which demonstrates that the vasodilator effect of captopril was due to its reduction of angiotensin-II levels.

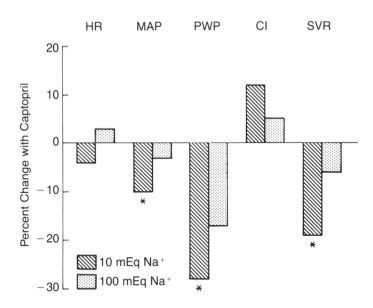

Fig. 4-12. Hemodynamic response to a 25-mg oral dose of captopril in ten patients studied during a 10-mEq and a 100-mEq sodium diet. Changes in heart rate (HR), mean arterial pressure (MAP), pulmonary wedge pressure (PWP), cardiac index (CI), and systemic vascular resistance (SVR) are shown. During the 10-mEq sodium diet, there was a modest, favorable hemodynamic response to converting-enzyme inhibitor therapy. During the 100-mEq sodium diet, when the renin activity was suppressed, there was minimal hemodynamic response to converting-enzyme inhibitor, which confirms that the initial response to captopril depends on RAA system activity. Asterisks indicate a significant response, to a level of at least $P < 0.05$. (Adapted from Cody et al.[50] Reproduced from *The Journal of Clinical Investigation* 1986;77:1441-1452 by copyright permission of the American Society for Clinical Investigation.)

Fig. 4-13. Relationship of pharmacokinetics to RAA system activity (plasma renin activity, PRA) and hemodynamic response to captopril in patients with congestive heart failure. The reduction of systemic vascular resistance during captopril therapy is a function of RAA activity, and not the circulating level or blood concentration of captopril that was achieved. Patient 1 had minimal RAA activation and demonstrated minimal response to captopril. Patient 2 had marked elevation of RAA activity in the baseline state (21.0 ng/mL/h), which increased to 77 ng/mL/h at peak concentrations of captopril. Associated with this response was a reduction of sys-

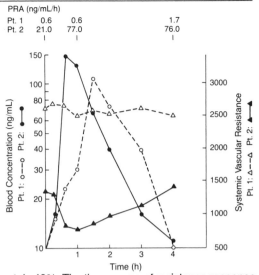

temic vascular resistance of approximately 40%. The time course of resistance response tracked the drug levels. Blood concentration of captopril is expressed in nanograms per milliliter. It should be noted that patient 1, with minimal renin system activation (0.6 ng/mL/h) had minimal hemodynamic response, but nonetheless had a blood concentration of captopril similar to that of patient 2.

Suppression of Aldosterone Secretion

Suppression of aldosterone secretion during RAA system inhibition may be more readily apparent than the reactive increase of plasma renin. It is postulated that angiotensin-II production inhibits renin release by completing a negative feedback loop.[63] Whether the negative feedback loop theory fully explains the large increase of renin is not known. In a group of 38 patients, inhibition of angiotensin-II generation by captopril produced a significant increase of plasma renin activity, from 9.4 to 27.0 ng/mL/h (Fig. 4-14). There was a concomitant reduction of aldosterone secretion from 19 to 11 ng/dL. This pattern of hormonal response was maintained during long-term therapy, in which captopril therapy produced a reactive increase of renin and suppression of urinary and plasma aldosterone (Fig. 4-15). Both acute and chronic suppression of aldosterone have been demonstrated with enalaprilat and enalapril.[79,80,85]

Dose-Response Relationship of Converting-Enzyme Inhibitor Therapy

Unfortunately, the dose-response relationship of converting-enzyme inhibitors to full suppression of RAA system activity has not been fully defined in the congestive heart failure population and may be difficult to determine in pharmacokinetic studies.[86] Defining this relationship is complicated by the multiple interactions that can influence RAA activity at any time, as this is a dynamic, not a static, condition and is greatly influenced by factors such as renal perfusion and diuretic therapy. Based on data in normal subjects, the dosage of captopril and enalapril commonly used for the treatment of heart failure is sufficient to reduce angiotensin to negligible levels. Failure to respond to a converting-enzyme inhibitor probably indicates that the RAA system is not activated in the patient, rather than the result of insufficient drug dosage. Hypotension may ultimately be the key factor that determines chronic dosage in the clinical setting.

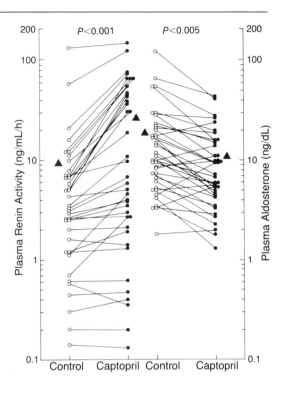

Fig. 4-14. Acute hormonal response to 25-mg oral dose of captopril in patients with congestive heart failure. There was a significant reactive increase of renin and a significant reduction of plasma aldosterone. The solid triangles represent mean values.

Fig. 4-15. Sequential determination of plasma renin activity and urinary aldosterone excretion in patients with congestive heart failure, during long-term captopril therapy. Also shown is urinary sodium excretion, urinary potassium excretion, and serum potassium. The absence of an adverse effect of captopril on renal function is demonstrated by stable values of blood urea nitrogen and serum creatinine. The reactive increase of plasma renin activity was demonstrated at one week of therapy and maintained through eight weeks of therapy. Urinary aldosterone excretion was significantly decreased by one week of therapy, and this effect remained apparent throughout the eight weeks of therapy.

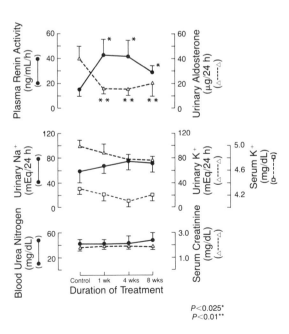

ASSESSMENT OF LONG-TERM OUTCOME DURING RENIN-ANGIOTENSIN-ALDOSTERONE SYSTEM INHIBITION

Once long-term converting-enzyme inhibitor therapy is initiated, one cannot assume that anything short of complete vigilance will result in a successful outcome. Many physicians remain surprised and perplexed that the long-term response to a converting-enzyme inhibitor cannot be correlated with a baseline plasma renin activity determination. To expect such a relationship would be analogous to anticipating that one could predict the long-term response to insulin therapy with a single baseline measurement of blood glucose. As with diabetes, the management of congestive heart failure with converting-enzyme inhibitor therapy is a dynamic process that is influenced by many factors (Table 4-2).

Several factors can continue to perturb the RAA system despite converting-enzyme inhibitor therapy, and these factors may in turn influence the clinical response. It is difficult clinically to judge the optimal diuretic dosage in patients treated with converting-enzyme inhibitors, and excessive diuretics will continue unnecessarily to stimulate renin release by the kidney. General indications for reducing the dose of diuretics include the development of progressive prerenal azotemia, hyponatremia, and hypotension. There are no firm guidelines as to what constitutes hypotension. Many physicians feel that a systolic blood pressure of 90 to 95 mm Hg can be tolerated in this patient population, and that lower levels are occasionally necessary in the most severe cases of heart failure. Below a systolic blood pressure of 90 mm Hg, excessive hypotension by itself or in association with further renal hypoperfusion will result in further stimulation of renin release by the kidney. Because congestive heart failure is a progressive disease with a very

---

Table 4-2. Therapeutic considerations in long-term converting-enzyme inhibition

Response of RAA system during converting-enzyme inhibition

Persistent stimulation
  Excessive diuretics
  Hypotension
  Renal hypoperfusion
  Progressive cardiac impairment

Suppression
  Improved renal perfusion
  Enhanced sodium delivery to the distal nephron
  Decreased sympathetic nervous system activity

Estimating the extent of RAA system blockade

Functional improvement
Correction of hyponatremia
Measurement of renin or aldosterone

Reasons for apparent lack of efficacy

Sodium overload
Adverse events: marked hypotension, renal impairment
RAA-independent pathophysiology
Concurrent clinical events: silent myocardial ischemia, mechanical cardiac defect
Noncompliance
Poor absorption

high mortality, progressive cardiac impairment should be anticipated, and RAA system stimulation may progress over time.

The long-term suppression of the RAA system during converting-enzyme inhibition is, for the most part, the determinant of the favorable outcome produced by this class of pharmacologic agents. Converting-enzyme inhibitors can favorably and directly influence the three major stimuli of renin release. Improving renal perfusion, enhancing the amount of sodium delivered to the distal nephron, and decreasing sympathetic nervous system activity will all act, by the favorable hemodynamic effect of converting-enzyme inhibition, to suppress endogenous release of renin.

Estimating the extent of RAA system blockade is particularly difficult in the clinical setting and cannot be strictly assessed by pharmacokinetic techniques.[86] However, the clinical response provides some degree of reassurance that treatment is effective. Certainly, the improvement of functional capacity—as judged by New York Heart Association classification, exercise performance, and physical findings—is in general a good index of response. As early as 1970 an inverse relationship between serum sodium levels and plasma renin was identified in congestive heart failure,[87] and this observation has been confirmed by several investigators.[88-91] Correction of hyponatremia has emerged as a useful clinical marker for the reversal of the adverse effects of the RAA system in congestive heart failure.[58]

Measurement of the appropriate biochemical markers of the RAA system would be the ideal approach, but this may not be widely applicable outside the research environment. Nonetheless, such assays provide direct information that may be very useful, particularly in refractory cases or cases in which converting-enzyme inhibitor therapy does not appear efficacious. Long-term converting-enzyme inhibitor therapy will cause a reactive increase of plasma renin activity (see Figs. 4-14 and 4-15). Results from at least one study suggest that the magnitude of the reactive increase of renin during long-term captopril therapy provides a guide to hemodynamic outcome.[92] That is, the patients with the largest reactive increase of renin tended to have the most favorable hemodynamic response. It might be even more practical to measure either plasma or urinary aldosterone levels. As aldosterone is the last step in the RAA cascade, one would expect that effective converting-enzyme inhibitor therapy would be associated with measurable and significant reductions of aldosterone. In contrast, marked persistent elevation of aldosterone secretion would suggest that converting enzyme has not been sufficiently inhibited.

An apparent lack of response to converting-enzyme inhibition, or decompensation in a case that was initially responsive, may be explained by several factors. The most common factor would be sodium overload, most typically induced by dietary sodium indiscretion. Even a modest excess of retained sodium on a daily basis can accumulate sufficiently to suppress the renin system, thereby markedly attenuating the previously favorable response to converting-enzyme inhibitor. It is important that patients be counselled to continue a moderate sodium intake (2 to 3 g of sodium) *despite* addition of converting-enzyme inhibitor therapy. Lack of efficacy may also result from the adverse effects of marked hypotension and progressive renal impairment.[14,93,94] It should be apparent that the RAA system is not continuously activated in all heart failure patients. In an RAA-independent state, one would not anticipate an impressive clinical or hemodynamic response to converting-enzyme inhibitors. A lack of long-term efficacy may also develop as a result of changes in concurrent disease, such as silent myocardial ischemia in patients with known coronary disease, or progression of a mechanical cardiac defect such as mitral regurgitation. Finally, noncompliance and poor drug absorption (eg, because of bowel edema) must also be considered.

CONCLUSION   The data summarized in this chapter strongly support the following ideas: (1) The RAA system is activated in most diuretic-treated patients with moderately to severely symptomatic congestive heart failure. (2) This activation has adverse pathophysiologic effects. (3) Converting-enzyme inhibitors can reverse or favorably attenuate the adverse contribution of the RAA system to this pathophysiology. (4) In mildly symptomatic heart failure, particularly in the absence of diuretics, RAA activity may be "normal" and the response to converting-enzyme inhibitors may be attenuated. Despite earlier concepts that RAA activity is markedly increased at the onset of congestive heart failure, preliminary data suggest that despite significant left ventricular impairment, the RAA system may not be activated in the early stages of heart failure in the absence of diuretic therapy. These findings suggest at least two considerations for future studies in heart failure. First, the early neurohormonal events associated with the onset of congestive heart failure should be better defined. Second, a more critical approach should be taken to the use of diuretics in congestive heart failure, to avoid the counterproductive influences that diuretics may provoke. A more judicious approach to the use of diuretics is particularly appropriate now, with the availability of specific inhibition of aldosterone secretion by converting-enzyme inhibitors. Finally, it cannot be overemphasized that the relationship between converting-enzyme inhibitors and diuretic-induced sodium depletion is dynamic. Excessive sodium intake will adversely attenuate the favorable effects of converting-enzyme inhibitors, and, conversely, large fixed doses of converting-enzyme inhibitors will evoke excessive hypotension and renal compromise. In the absence of more objective criteria to determine the optimal relationship between converting-enzyme inhibitors and sodium depletion, physicians must exercise considerable diligence and attention to these factors that will ultimately affect clinical outcome during therapy that inhibits the RAA system.

REFERENCES

1. Merrill AJ, Morrison JR, Brannon ES: Concentration of renin in renal venous blood in patients with congestive heart failure. *Am J Med* 1946;1:468-472.
2. Davis JO: Mechanisms of salt and water retention in congestive heart failure: The role of aldosterone. *Am J Med* 1960;29:486-491.
3. Laragh JH: Hormones in the pathogenesis of congestive heart failure: Vasopressin, aldosterone and angiotensin II. *Circulation* 1962;25:1015-1023.
4. Ader R, Chatterjee K, Ports T, et al: Immediate and sustained hemodynamic and clinical improvement in chronic heart failure by an oral angiotensin converting enzyme inhibitor. *Circulation* 1980;61:931-937.

5. Curtiss C, Cohn JN, Vrobel T, et al: Role of the renin-angiotensin system in the systemic vasoconstriction of chronic congestive heart failure. *Circulation* 1978;58:763-770.

6. Davis R, Ribner HS, Keung E, et al: Treatment of chronic congestive heart failure with captopril, an oral inhibitor of angiotensin-converting enzyme. *N Engl J Med* 1979;301:117-121.

7. Dzau VJ, Colucci WS, Williams GH, et al: Sustained effectiveness of converting enzyme inhibition in patients with severe congestive heart failure. *N Engl J Med* 1980;302:1373-1379.

8. Levine TB, Franciosa JA, Cohn JN: Acute and long-term response to an oral converting enzyme inhibitor, captopril, in congestive heart failure. *Circulation* 1980;62:35-41.

9. Tarazi RC, Fouad FM, Ceimo JK, et al: Renin, aldosterone and cardiac decompensation: Studies with an oral converting enzyme inhibitor in heart failure. *Am J Cardiol* 1979;44:1013-1018.

10. Turini GA, Brunner HR, Ferguson RK, et al: Congestive heart failure in normotensive man: Haemodynamics, renin and angiotensin II blockade. *Br Heart J* 1978;40:1134-1142.

11. Captopril Multicenter Research Group: A placebo-controlled trial of captopril in refractory chronic congestive heart failure. *J Am Coll Cardiol* 1983;2:755-763.

12. Creager MA, Massie BM, Gaxon DP, et al: Acute and long-term effects of enalapril on the cardiovascular response to exercise and exercise tolerance in patients with congestive heart failure. *J Am Coll Cardiol* 1985;6:163-170.

13. The Captopril-Digoxin Multicenter Research Group: Comparative effects of therapy with captopril and digoxin in patients with mild to moderate heart failure. *JAMA* 1988;259:539-544.

14. Powers ER, Bannerman KS, Stone J, et al: The effect of captopril on renal, coronary and systemic hemodynamics in patients with severe congestive heart failure. *Am Heart J* 1982;104:1203-1210.

15. Creager MA, Halperin JL, Bernard DB, et al: Acute regional circulatory and renal hemodynamic effects of converting-enzyme inhibition in patients with congestive heart failure. *Circulation* 1981;64:483-489.

16. Romankiewcz JA, Brogden RN, Heel RC, et al: Captopril: An update review of its pharmacological properties and therapeutic efficacy in congestive heart failure. *Drugs* 1983;25:6-40.

17. Todd PA, Heel RC: Enalapril: A review of its pharmacodynamic and pharmacokinetic properties in therapeutic use in hypertension and congestive heart failure. *Drugs* 1986;31:198-248.

18. CONSENSUS Trial Study Group: Effects of enalapril on mortality in severe congestive heart failure. *N Engl J Med* 1987;316:1429-1435.

19. Ng KKF, Vane JR: Fate of angiotensin I in the circulation. *Nature* 1968;218:1142-1144.

20. Oparil S, Koerner T, O'Donoghue JK: Mechanism of angiotensin I converting enzyme inhibition by SQ 20881 (Glu-Trp-Pro-Arg-Pro-Glin-Ile-Pro-Pro) *in vivo*: Further evidence for extrapulmonary conversion. *Hypertension* 1979;1:13-22.

21. Dzau VJ: Implications of local angiotensin production in cardiovascular physiology and pharmacology. *Am J Cardiol* 1987;59:59A-65A.

22. Laragh JH, Sealey JE: The renin-angiotensin-aldosterone hormonal system and regulation of sodium, potassium and blood pressure homeostasis, in Orloff J, Berliner RW (eds), *Handbook of Physiology*, Section 8: Renal Physiology. Baltimore, Williams & Wilkins, 1973, pp 831-908.

23. Zelis R, Delea CS, Coleman HN, et al: Arterial sodium content in experimental congestive heart failure. *Circulation* 1970;41:213-219.

24. Holmes J, Kubo SH, Cody RJ, et al: Arrhythmias in ischemic and nonischemic dilated cardiomyopathy: Prediction of mortality by ambulatory electrocardiography. *Am J Cardiol* 1985;55:146-151.

25. Goldblatt H: Renal vascular hypertension due to renal ischemia. *Circulation* 1965;32:1-4.
26. Chidsey CA, Harrison DC, Braunwald E: Augmentation of the plasma norepinephrine response to exercise in patients with congestive heart failure. *N Engl J Med* 1962;267:650-654.
27. Cody RJ, Rodger RF, Hartley LH, et al: Acute hypertension in a non-human primate: Humoral and hemodynamic mechanisms. *Hypertension* 1982;4:219-225.
28. Levine TB, Francis GS, Goldsmith SR, et al: Activity of the sympathetic nervous system and renin-angiotensin system assessed by plasma hormone levels and their relation to hemodynamic abnormalities in congestive heart failure. *Am J Cardiol* 1982;49:1659-1666.
29. Thomas JA, Marks BH: Plasma norepinephrine in congestive heart failure. *Am J Cardiol* 1978;41:233-243.
30. Kluger J, Cody RJ, Laragh JH: The contributions of sympathetic tone and the renin-angiotensin system to severe chronic congestive heart failure: Response to specific inhibitors. *Am J Cardiol* 1982;49:1667-1674.
31. Kiowski W, Julius S: Renin response to stimulation of cardiopulmonary mechanoreceptors in man. *J Clin Invest* 1978;62:656-663.
32. Oparil S, Vassoux C, Sanders CA, et al: Role of renin in acute postural homeostasis. *Circulation* 1970;41:89-95.
33. Cody RJ, Franklin KW, Kluger J, et al: Mechanisms governing the postural response, and baroreceptor abnormalities in chronic congestive heart failure: Effects of acute and long-term converting enzyme inhibition. *Circulation* 1982;66:135-141.
34. Lilly LS, Dzau VJ, Williams GH, et al: Hyponatremia in congestive heart failure: Implications for neurohormonal activation and responses to orthostasis. *J Clin Endocrinol Metab* 1984;59:924-930.
35. Cohn JN, Levine TB, Olivari MT, et al: Plasma norepinephrine as a guide to prognosis in patients with chronic congestive heart failure. *N Engl J Med* 1984;311:819-824.
36. Fowler MG, Laser JA, Hopkins GL, et al: Assessment of the β-adrenergic receptor pathway in the intact failing human heart: Progressive receptor down-regulation and subsensitivity to agonist response. *Circulation* 1986;74:1290-1302.
37. Vander AJ, Miller R: Control of renin secretion in the anesthetized dog. *Am J Physiol* 1964;207:537-546.
38. Cannon PJ: The kidney in heart failure. *N Engl J Med* 1977;296:26-32.
39. Churchill PC: Possible mechanism of the inhibitory effect of ouabain on renin secretion from rat renal cortical slices. *J Physiol* 1979;294:123-134.
40. Prida XE, Kubo SH, Laragh JH, et al: Evaluation of calcium-mediated vasoconstriction in chronic congestive heart failure. *Am J Med* 1983;75:795-800.
41. Ryman KS, Kubo SH, Shaknovich A, et al: Influence of baseline hemodynamic status and sympathetic activity on the response to nicardipine, a new dihydropyridine, in patients with hypertension or chronic congestive heart failure. *Clin Pharmacol Ther* 1987;41:483-489.
42. Covit AB, Schaer GL, Sealey JE, et al: Suppression of the renin-angiotensin system by intravenous digoxin in chronic congestive heart failure. *Am J Med* 1983;75:445-447.
43. Ikram H, Chan W, Espiner EA, et al: Haemodynamic and hormone response to acute and chronic furosemide therapy in congestive heart failure. *Clin Sci Mol Med* 1980;59:443-449.
44. Nicholls MG, Espiner EN, Donald RN, et al: Aldosterone and its regulation during diuresis in patients with gross congestive heart failure. *Clin Sci Mol Med* 1974;47:301-315.
45. Francis GS, Siegal RM, Goldsmith SR, et al: Acute vasoconstrictor response to intravenous furosemide in patients with chronic congestive heart failure. *Ann Intern Med* 1985;103:1-6.

46. Colucci WS, Williams GH, Alexander RW, et al: Mechanisms and implications of vasodilator tolerance in the treatment of congestive heart failure. *Am J Med* 1981;71:89-99.
47. Mitchell HC, Pettinger WA: Long-term treatment of refractory hypertensive patients with minoxidil. *JAMA* 1978;239:2131-2136.
48. Ueda H, Kaneko Y, Takeda T, et al: Observations on the mechanism of renin release by hydralazine in hypertensive patients. *Circ Res* 1970;26 & 27 (suppl 2):201-206.
49. Millar JA, McGrath PB, Mathews PG, et al: Acute effects of captopril on blood pressure and circulatory hormone levels and salt-replete and depleted normal subjects and essential hypertensive patients. *Clin Sci* 1981;61:75-83.
50. Cody RJ, Covit AB, Schaer GL, et al: Sodium and water balance in chronic congestive heart failure. *J Clin Invest* 1986;77:1441-1452.
51. Cody RJ, Atlas SA, Laragh JH: Physiological and pharmacological studies of atrial natriuretic factor, a human natriuretic and vasoactive peptide. *J Clin Pharm* 1987;27:927-936.
52. Cody RJ, Atlas SA, Laragh JH, et al: Atrial natriuretic factor in normal subjects and heart failure patients: Plasma levels and renal, hormonal, and hemodynamic responses to peptide infusion. *J Clin Invest* 1986;78:1362-1374.
53. Braunwald E, Plauth WH, Morrow AG: A method for the detection and quantification of impaired sodium excretion: Results of an oral sodium tolerance test in normal subjects and in patients with heart disease. *Circulation* 1965;32:223-229.
54. Chonko AM, Bay WH, Stein JH, et al: The role of renin and aldosterone in salt retention of edema. *Am J Med* 1977;63:881-889.
55. Cody RJ, Franklin KW, Laragh JH: Postural hypotension during tilt with chronic captopril therapy of severe congestive heart failure. *Am Heart J* 1982;103:480-484.
56. Cody RJ, Laragh JH: Use of captopril to estimate renin-angiotensin-aldosterone activity in pathophysiology of chronic heart failure. *Am Heart J* 1982;104:1184-1188.
57. Francis GS, Goldsmith SR, Levine TB, et al: The neurohormonal axis in congestive heart failure. *Ann Intern Med* 1984;101:370-377.
58. Packer M, Lee MH, Kessler PD, et al: Role of neurohormonal mechanisms in determining survival in patients with severe chronic heart failure. *Circulation* 1987;75(suppl 4):80-92.
59. Bayliss J, Norell M, Canepa-Anson R, et al: Untreated heart failure: Clinical and neuroendocrine effects of introducing diuretics. *Br Heart J* 1987;57:17-22.
60. Kubo SH, Clark M, Laragh JH, et al: Identification of normal neurohormonal activity in mild congestive heart failure and stimulating effect of upright posture and diuretics. *Am J Cardiol* 1987;60:1322-1328.
61. Watkins L, Burton JA, Haber E, et al: The renin-angiotensin-aldosterone system in congestive heart failure in conscious dogs. *J Clin Invest* 1976;57:1606-1614.
62. Dzau VJ, Colucci WS, Hollenberg NK, et al: Relation of the renin-angiotensin-aldosterone system to clinical state in congestive heart failure. *Circulation* 1981;63:645-651.
63. Samuels AE, Miller ED Jr, Fray CS, et al: Renin-angiotensin antagonists and the regulation of blood pressure. *Fed Proc* 1976;35:2512-2520.
64. Hall JE, Guyton AC, Smith MJ Jr, et al: Chronic blockade of angiotensin II formation during sodium deprivation. *Am J Physiol* 1979;237:F424-F432.
65. Gavras H, Brunner HR, Vaughan ED Jr, et al: Angiotensin-sodium interaction in blood pressure maintenance of renal hypertensive and normotensive rats. *Science* 1973;180:1369-1371.
66. Sancho J, Re R, Burton J, et al: The role of the renin-angiotensin-aldosterone system in cardiovascular homeostasis in normal human subjects. *Circulation* 1976;53:400-405.

67. Haber E: The role of renin in normal and pathological cardiovascular homeostasis. *Circulation* 1976;54:849-861.
68. Niarchos AP, Pickering TG, Case DB, et al: Role of the renin-angiotensin system in blood pressure regulation. *Circ Res* 1979;45:829-837.
69. Kubo SH, Cody RJ: Circulatory autoregulation in chronic congestive heart failure: Response to tilt in 41 patients. *Am J Cardiol* 1983;52:512-518.
70. Vander AJ: *Renal Physiology.* New York, McGraw-Hill, 1985, pp 131-134.
71. Swedberg K, Waagstein F, Hjalmarson A, et al: Prolongation of survival in congestive cardiomyopathy by beta-receptor blockade. *Lancet* 1979;1:1374-1376.
72. Burton J, Cody RJ, Herd JA, et al: Specific inhibition of renin by an angiotensin analog: Studies in sodium depletion and renin-dependent hypertension. *Proc Natl Acad Sci* 1980;77:5476-5479.
73. Cody RJ, Burton J, Evin G, et al: A substrate analog inhibitor of renin that is effective *in vivo. Biochem Biophys Res Commun* 1980;97:230-235.
74. Zusman RM, Burton J, Christensen D, et al: Hemodynamic effects of a competitive renin inhibitory peptide in humans: Evidence for multiple mechanisms of action. *Trans Assoc Am Physicians* 1983;96:365-374.
75. Cody RJ: Haemodynamic responses to specific renin-angiotensin inhibitors in hypertension and congestive heart failure: A review. *Drugs* 1984;28:144-169.
76. Cody RJ, Franklin KW, Kluger J, et al: Sympathetic responsiveness and plasma norepinephrine during therapy of chronic congestive heart failure with captopril. *Am J Med* 1982;72:791-797.
77. Turker RK, Page IH, Bumpus FM: Antagonists of angiotensin II, in Page IH, Bumpus FM (eds), *Angiotensin,* New York, Springer-Verlag, 1974, pp 162-169.
78. Liddle GW: Specific and non-specific inhibition of mineralocorticoid activity. *Metabolism* 1961;10:1021-1030.
79. Kubo SH, Cody RJ, Laragh JH, et al: Immediate converting enzyme inhibition with intravenous enalapril in chronic congestive heart failure. *Am J Cardiol* 1985;55:122-126.
80. Cody RJ: Conceptual and therapeutic approaches to inhibition of the renin-angiotensin system in chronic congestive heart failure. *J Cardiovasc Pharmacol* 1986;8(suppl 1):S58-S65.
81. Packer M, Medina N, Yushak M, et al: Usefulness of plasma renin activity in predicting hemodynamic and clinical responses and survival during long-term converting enzyme inhibition in severe chronic heart failure. *Br Heart J* 1985;54:298-304.
82. Mettauer B, Rouleau J-L, Bichet D, et al: Differential long-term intrarenal and neurohormonal effects of captopril and prazosin in patients with chronic congestive heart failure: Importance of initial plasma renin activity. *Circulation* 1986;73:492-502.
83. Cody RJ, Schaer GL, Covit AB, et al: Captopril kinetics in chronic congestive heart failure. *Clin Pharmacol Ther* 1982;32:721-726.
84. Cody RJ, Covit AB, Schaer GL, et al: Estimation of angiotensin II receptor activity in chronic congestive heart failure. *Am Heart J* 1984;108:81-89.
85. Cody RJ, Covit AB, Schaer GL, et al: Evaluation of a long-acting converting enzyme inhibitor (enalapril) for the treatment of chronic congestive heart failure. *J Am Coll Cardiol* 1983;1:1154-1159.
86. Kubo SH, Cody RJ: Clinical pharmacokinetics of angiotensin converting enzyme inhibitors: A review. *Clin Pharmacokinet* 1985;10:377-391.
87. Brown JJ, Davies DL, Johnson VW, et al: Renin relationships in congestive cardiac failure, treated and untreated. *Am Heart J* 1970;80:329-342.
88. Levine TB, Franciosa JA, Vrobel T, et al: Hyponatremia as a marker for high renin heart failure. *Br Heart J* 1982;47:161-166.
89. Schaer GL, Covit AB, Laragh JH, et al: Association of hyponatremia with increased renin activity in chronic congestive heart failure: Impact of diuretic therapy. *Am J Cardiol* 1983;51:1635-1638.

90. Dzau VJ, Hollenberg NK: Renal response to captopril in severe heart failure: Role in natriuresis and reversal of hyponatremia. *Ann Intern Med* 1984;100:777-782.
91. Packer M, Medina N, Yushak M: Correction of dilutional hypernatremia in severe chronic heart failure by converting enzyme inhibition. *Ann Intern Med* 1984;100:782-789.
92. Packer M, Medina N, Yushak M: Efficacy of captopril in low-renin congestive heart failure: Importance of sustained reactive hyperreninemia in distinguishing responders from non-responders. *Am J Cardiol* 1984;54:771-777.
93. Mujais SK, Fouad FM, Textor SC, et al: Transient renal dysfunction during initial inhibition of converting enzymes in congestive heart failure. *Br Heart J* 1984;52:63-71.
94. Packer M, Lee WH, Medina N, et al: Functional renal insufficiency during long-term therapy with captopril and enalapril in severe congestive heart failure. *Ann Intern Med* 1987;106:346-354.

NORMAN K. HOLLENBERG, MD, PhD

5

The Role of the Kidney in Heart Failure

The relationship between the heart, the kidney, and the clinical expression of disease has long been recognized. The Yellow Emperor's Classic of Internal Medicine, published over 4,500 years ago, makes a series of astonishingly modern statements based on clinical observation[1]: "The heart rules over the kidney. . . . If too much salt is used in food . . . there are dropsical swellings. . . . The water of the kidneys . . . causes the troubled breathing." The kidney clearly plays a prominent role in the pathogenesis and expression of congestive heart failure. It can be a primary factor through the production of hypertension; more commonly, it represents a contributory factor through sodium retention and edema formation, or through its influence on body chemistry, especially involving potassium, magnesium, and water homeostasis.

Claude Bernard opened the homeostasis-oriented modern era over a century ago. He pointed out that the medium in which our cells live is not the external world; rather, it is the blood and tissue fluid, the internal milieu. An elaborate system has developed to protect the chemical constitution and volume of that isolated internal fluid; the kidneys play the central regulatory role. Indeed, excretory function is incidental to the regulatory process.

Homer Smith,[2] in what still stands as the classic analysis of the contribution of reduced sodium excretion and resultant fluid retention to the pathogenesis of congestive heart failure, reminded us of an often forgotten element in Starling's analysis: failure of renal sodium excretion due to reduced myocardial reserve leads not only to dependent edema and pulmonary congestion, but may also contribute to the increased venous and chamber pressures and volumes. Indeed, the engorgement may lead to further cardiac dilatation and exaggerate the failure of the already incompetent heart. With tongue in cheek, Smith asked " . . . how much, if anything, the heart has to do with chronic congestive heart failure."

The kidney, of course, is not the culprit; the renal response is appropriate in relation to the information it receives. What is inappropriate are the signals being transmitted to the kidney. Sodium retention is initially responsible for edema and, with increasing failure, for pulmonary congestion and the resultant exertional dyspnea, orthopnea, and paroxysmal nocturnal dyspnea. As myocardial reserve becomes further compromised, hyponatremia and azotemia often supervene. New and more potent natriuretic agents are particularly prone to precipitate azotemia and hyponatremia. Until the terminal stages of the process, it is possible, with increasing doses of furosemide and with diuretic combinations, to initiate a diuresis. The price that is paid, especially in the late stages, is a progressive rise in blood urea nitrogen and serum creatinine as volume is compromised and renal perfusion and glomerular filtration rate fall.

The purpose of this chapter is to provide an overview of renal structure and function as they bear on the pathogenesis and expression of congestive heart failure. Other relevant topics that are mentioned in this chapter, but reviewed in depth elsewhere in this book, include hypertension, the renin-angiotensin-aldosterone system, the pharmacology of the available agents used for treatment, vascular function, the state of the autonomic nervous system and its relationship to circulatory function, and the relation of electrolyte disarray to sudden death. Some redundancy is necessary to make the presentation logical and comprehensive.

RENAL STRUCTURE IN RELATION TO FUNCTION

The important relationship between structure and function is a truism that is broadly applicable, but nowhere more compelling. The kidney can be thought of as a series of concentric organs, each with a highly specialized structure, function, and blood supply.[3] Blood flow in the renal cortex where the glomeruli and proximal and distal tubules all lie, is about 4 to 5 mL/g/min. This is considerably greater than the requirements for local metabolism, but appropriate for the delivery to the glomeruli of large volumes of plasma for ultrafiltration. Moreover, the very low vascular resistance that such a flow rate reflects permits the transmission of the force initiating filtration (ie, hydrostatic pressure) to the glomerular capillary level.

The Inner Cortex

Nephrons that originate in the inner cortex are specialized.[4] Their tubules extend into the medulla for variable distances and thus are considerably longer than those of the outer cortex. The efferent arterioles of inner cortical nephrons, the vasa recta, also descend into the medulla.

The Renal Medulla

It is in the medulla that the critical role of renal architecture is best seen. The countercurrent arrangement of the tubules and vessels makes it possible to concentrate the medullary interstitium and thus the urine to an osmolality more than four times that of plasma in humans. Again, the blood supply is modified to a level appropriate to local function. Renal papillary perfusion is in the neighborhood of 0.2 mL/g/min, considerably less than the flow to most metabolically active organs.

Nephron Heterogeneity   The million nephrons that make up the human kidney have traditionally been viewed as though the function of each nephron unit were identical. This convention, although convenient, denies the characteristic differences of inner and outer cortical nephrons. Evidence is accumulating that not only structural, but also functional heterogeneity exists.[5-7] The contribution of regional heterogeneity to water handling is unequivocal. A possible contribution to sodium handling and abnormalities of sodium handling in edematous states, including congestive heart failure, remains a matter of debate.

Glomerular Filtration   The creation of urine begins in the glomerulus, where an ultrafiltrate of plasma is separated from the blood perfusing the glomerular capillaries. The force promoting filtration is hydrostatic pressure in the glomerular capillaries. Early indirect estimates of glomerular capillary pressure suggested a level about two thirds that of arterial pressure.[3] Direct measurements, which require exposure of the kidney, suggest a somewhat lower level for at least the superficial nephrons.[8] Regardless of which estimate is correct, it is the highest capillary pressure in the body, adequate to offset the forces that retard filtration, plasma oncotic, and intratubular pressures. The critical role of capillary hydrostatic pressure as the first step in initiating nephron function underscores the importance to the kidney of overall cardiovascular function and local hemodynamic events.

Renal Perfusion   The kidneys in a normal adult weigh less than 300 g, and yet receive about 20% of the cardiac output. The resultant blood flow, 3 to 5 mL/g/min, is among the highest in the body. As cardiac output falls, this fraction of cardiac output provides a reservoir for the maintenance of perfusion in tissues such as the heart and brain, which tolerate poorly a reduction in blood flow. The corollary is that cardiovascular events that result in a reduction in cardiac output, hypotension, and active renal vasoconstriction must have a profound influence on renal function well beyond the effects of inadequate delivery of oxygen or substrate for metabolism. To illustrate, if renal blood flow is reduced by half, the flow rate per gram in the renal cortex still considerably exceeds that to the heart and brain, which averages about 1.0 mL/g/min. The functional consequences of inadequate perfusion to the kidney, unless extreme, are primarily reflected in inadequate delivery of pressure to the level of the glomerular capillary, rather than cell injury or death. This concept, so different from that relating myocardial perfusion and performance, for example, is central to understanding reduced renal function in congestive heart failure. A reduction in arterial blood pressure or an increase in renal vascular resistance—especially when it involves the afferent arteriole—act in concert to reduce glomerular capillary pressure and thus the rate of glomerular filtration. Such an increase in preglomerular resistance may be induced by sympathetic nervous system activity, circulating catecholamines, or locally generated angiotensin-II. To the extent that an increase in the postglomerular response occurs, the reduced blood flow is not matched by a parallel fall in glomerular filtration rate. The fraction of plasma flowing to the kidney that is filtered, the "filtration fraction," is increased, although the total amount filtered is reduced.

Renal Perfusion and Function: Intrarenal hemodynamic events may influence renal function through avenues in addition to the control of the glomerular filtration rate.[9] If 120 mL/min is normally filtered and 1 mL/min is excreted, it is obvious that 119 mL/min must be reabsorbed. Removal of the reabsorbed filtrate by the blood supply represents one rate-limiting factor for net sodium reabsorption. That, in turn, is determined by peritubular capillary hydrostatic and oncotic pressures. An increase in filtration fraction, common in patients with congestive heart failure,[10,11] results in increased peritubular capillary oncotic pressure, enhanced sodium reabsorption, and a further contribution to the pathogenesis of the edema.

Moreover, it is possible that an unchanged renal plasma flow and filtration rate influences net renal function by redistributing glomerular filtrate to nephrons with a different functional capacity. This possibility was first put forward by Goodyer and Jaeger,[12] to account for enhanced renal sodium reabsorption following rapid hemorrhage in dogs. It was later applied to the kidney in congestive heart failure by Barger and his co-workers[13] and has been examined repeatedly for over 20 years, although the importance of redistribution of glomerular filtration remains controversial.

Sodium and Potassium Handling by the Kidney
Sodium and chloride are actively reabsorbed throughout the entire length of the nephron, but the characteristics of their reabsorption and its functional implications vary in different parts of the nephron.[6] The proximal tubule removes about 80% of the filtered sodium and chloride, and a larger fraction of the filtered bicarbonate. Water follows and the reabsorption is isosmotic. Potassium is also actively absorbed at this point, and over 80% of filtered potassium is removed from the filtrate.

In the ascending limb of the loop of Henle, an additional 10% to 15% of the filtered sodium load is reabsorbed, primarily due to active absorption of the anion chloride. Here, however, a parallel water shift does not occur. Thus, a concentration gradient is achieved between hypertonic medullary interstitium and hypotonic residual tubular fluid. This gradient is critical in the creation of both a dilute and a concentrated urine by the kidney, and thus for water homeostasis. Reduced sodium reabsorption in this portion of the nephron, because of enhanced proximal reabsorption, contributes to the pathogenesis of hyponatremia, which frequently occurs in advanced congestive heart failure. It is at this level that the "loop diuretics," furosemide and ethacrynic acid, work. When they reduce sodium reabsorption in the loop, they also limit the diluting capacity of the kidney, and thus contribute to hyponatremia.

About 5% to 10% of filtered sodium is delivered to the distal tubule. This contribution of the distal tubule to sodium reabsorption becomes apparent when viewed quantitatively: 10% of the filtered sodium represents 2,500 mEq of sodium every day, an amount close to the normal total body sodium content. In the distal tubule a portion of the reabsorbed sodium is accompanied by the remaining, easily absorbed anion, chloride. Because the other anions are bulky, polar, and relatively poorly absorbed, further sodium reabsorption results in charge separation and the generation of an electrical potential. It is this potential, with the tubular lumen becoming electrically negative, that results in the shift of potassium and hydrogen ion into the distal tubular fluid. Aldosterone enhances this process, accounting for the hypokalemia and metabolic alkalosis seen with secondary aldosteronism in the patient with congestive heart failure. For convenience of discussion this interaction is called "exchange," but it does not represent a true exchange process: it is neither tightly linked, nor carrier mediated.

Water Handling   The kidneys' ability to concentrate and dilute the urine occurs in the loop of Henle, where sodium and chloride transport occurs in a segment that is impermeable to water. Isotonic tubular fluid, a small fraction of the total glomerular filtrate, enters the medulla via the descending limb of the loop of Henle. Because this segment is permeable to water, the tubular fluid becomes progressively more concentrated as it traverses the hypertonic inner medulla. In the ascending limb, the concentrated fluid enters the region where chloride and sodium are actively pumped out. The impermeability to water in this portion of the nephron results in progressive dilution of the tubular fluid. It is primarily sodium and chloride that are pumped out, and this accounts for the progressive hypertonicity of the medulla. A dilute fluid thus enters the distal convoluted tubule. Further reabsorption of sodium occurs in the collecting duct, where permeability to water is variable and under the direct influence of antidiuretic hormone (ADH). In the absence of ADH, the collecting duct is impermeable to water, and a copious dilute urine with minimal osmolality of 40 to 50 mOsm/L is formed. In the presence of ADH, the collecting duct becomes permeable to water, and the tubular fluid is partly reabsorbed, running down the gradient into the concentrated medulla. A small volume of concentrated urine is thus formed, with a maximal osmolality of about 1,200 mOsm/L.

The function of the loop has several important clinical implications. For the countercurrent system to work, sufficient sodium chloride must be delivered to the loop in order to create the hypertonic milieu of the inner medulla. An increase in sodium reabsorption proximal to the loop, in the proximal convoluted tubule, reduces the ability of the kidney to both concentrate and dilute the urine. This may well contribute to the pathogenesis of hyponatremia in the patient with congestive heart failure.[14,15] Any factor that interferes with sodium and chloride reabsorption in the loop will interfere with both functions. Because loop diuretics have their primary action here, their use may also contribute to the pathogenesis of hyponatremia.

**THE NORMAL
DEFENSE OF
EXTRA-
CELLULAR
FLUID
AND PLASMA
VOLUME**
As stated earlier, the kidney is not a culprit, but rather a victim. Its response is appropriate to the signal it receives. What initiates the signal? The forces that dominate the kidney involve the defense of extracellular fluid and plasma volume. Because edematous states appear to reflect activation of these systems, it seems most appropriate to discuss that aspect next.

Why should defense of extracellular fluid have primacy for the kidney? The answer probably lies in phylogeny.[2] In the progressive move from salt to fresh water, to air temporarily, and then permanently—a series of moves that were presumably motivated by survival forces—the kidney's primary responsibility has been to handle the increasingly difficult burden of preserving these volumes. Because volume conservation is so critical for cardiovascular function and survival, the response of the kidney and of the afferent elements responsible for volume homeostasis are keyed to preventing and reversing volume deficits. The reduction in cardiac output—and, to the extent that it occurs, fall in blood pressure—which characterizes the marginal myocardium is, presumably, perceived as a volume deficit by the sensing system.

The Renal Response to Hemorrhage

Hemorrhage represents the simplest model of a volume deficit, and few phenomena have been more widely studied. During hemorrhage, unless very abrupt, blood pressure does not fall until a 5- to 10-mL/kg volume is removed. Thereafter blood pressure begins to fall, but at a slower rate than the reduction in blood volume because of activation of compensatory vasoconstrictor forces. Pharmacologic interruption or surgical ablation of the sympathetic nervous system, or the renin-angiotensin system, results in an enhanced fall in blood pressure. Antidiuretic hormone plays a quantitatively minor role.

During very rapid hemorrhaging, over a few seconds or minutes, the anticipated renal vasoconstriction does not occur.[16] Rather, with the rapid fall in blood pressure, renal blood flow is unchanged. The simplest explanation, although as yet unproved, is that the forces responsible for renal vascular autoregulation dominate the response in this setting. No information appears to be available on renal sodium handling during the transient response.

With more gradual hemorrhage, renal blood flow, glomerular filtration rate, and sodium excretion all fall.[12] The fall in glomerular filtration rate, until severe hypotension supervenes, is smaller than the fall in renal plasma flow, so that filtration fraction increases. Hypotension is not necessary for sodium retention, as with the very slow rates of hemorrhage a sharp drop in sodium excretion is well documented to occur prior to a fall in blood pressure, renal plasma flow, or glomerular filtration rate. The reduction in sodium excretion also occurs far too quickly for aldosterone release to make a contribution.

Sodium Retention During Hemorrhage

In the absence of a change in renal plasma flow, glomerular filtration rate, filtration fraction, arterial blood pressure, or a contribution of aldosterone, what factor is responsible for sodium retention? There are two candidates. The first involves changes in intrarenal blood flow distribution or local intrarenal perfusion rates. The second involves hormonal factors other than aldosterone, which are thought to act on the tubule.

Intrarenal Blood Flow Distribution and Perfusion Rates: A host of methods have been applied to assess intrarenal blood flow during hemorrhage and hypotension. The majority reveal an especially sharp reduction in blood flow to the outer cortex. Carriere et al,[17] for example, documented a change in the pattern of krypton transit through the kidney by external monitoring, and interpreted those curves on the basis of carefully timed radioautographs, which showed patchy areas of reduced outer cortical perfusion. Strong support for their interpretation arose from the study of Bell and Harper.[18] They employed a GM tube that monitored a 1-mm depth of the superficial cortex. It showed an especially striking reduction in perfusion in that area, when compared with total renal blood flow measured with a flowmeter. Confirmation also came from the application by Passmore et al[19] of freeze-dissection to the assessment of krypton 85 transit, which showed reasonable concordance with data derived from radioactive microsphere measurements of regional cortical perfusion. Stein et al[20] also showed a sharp reduction in outer cortical blood flow during hemorrhage with radioactive microspheres as the tracer. The only technique that has not documented such a change is that associated with electrode placement in the renal cortex to monitor hydrogen clearance,[21] although this technique revealed patchy outer cortical hypoperfusion in states characterized by more chronic volume deficits.[22]

Whether the regional perfusion rates are associated with regional changes in filtration and function seems likely, but is less well documented. Whether these changes contribute to sodium retention—the central issue in this analysis—is even less well characterized. The critical experiment has not yet been devised.

Additional Hormones: In the 1950s, two factors were known to represent major determinants of sodium handling by the kidney. Renal plasma flow and glomerular filtration rate were the first, and aldosterone was the second factor. In 1961, De Wardener et al[23] devised an experiment documenting that striking changes in sodium handling by the kidney could occur when neither plasma flow, glomerular filtration rate, nor aldosterone could have accounted for it. They pointed out that because the first two groups of factors known to be important in sodium homeostasis were not responsible, a "third factor" must have been operative. This set off two decades of searching for the factor, the accumulation of an enormous amount of literature on the subject, and a debate, which continues to this day.

There is substantial, continuing interest in the implications of this experiment for the pathogenesis of edematous states.[24,25] A host of possible candidates as natriuretic hormones in heart failure include dopamine, kallikrein-kinin, prostaglandin E_2, sodium-potassium ATPase inhibitors, and the atrial natriuretic peptides.[26] It is a common clinical experience, for example, that prostaglandin synthetase inhibitors will lead to sodium retention and decompensation in patients with advanced congestive heart failure.[27]

Recently, for obvious reasons, major attention has been focused on the atrial natriuretic peptides. In the remarkably short time between identification of a potent natriuretic factor in atria[28] to delineation of its structure by several groups in 1983,[29] it was attractive to consider the possibility that the impaired ability of the kidney to handle sodium reflected a true "deficiency state," in which cardiac synthesis or release of natriuretic peptide was limited by heart disease. Yet, a host of studies published in a short period of time have documented that plasma atrial natriuretic peptide concentration is not low in the patient with congestive heart failure. Rather, plasma levels are elevated.[30-33] There are no exceptions among the many reports. Thus, it is clear that the heart does not lose its ability to release atrial natriuretic peptides when heart failure develops. Indeed, the material enters the circulation from the right atrium in heart failure.[33] Rather than a deficiency state, at least in experimental heart failure, the renal vascular response and natriuretic response to synthetic atrial peptide is sharply limited.[34]

Identification and delineation of the actions of atrial natriuretic peptide have not made a major contribution to our understanding of the pathogenesis of congestive heart failure. It is clear that the renal response to the natriuretic peptides is limited, but because the renal response to other natriuretic agents, such as loop diuretics, is also often blunted, this observation lacks specificity.[35] The forces at work limiting sodium excretion by the kidney in advanced heart failure are not easily overridden.[36]

The failure to find a deficiency of atrial natriuretic peptide, or other natriuretic factors, to account for abnormalities in renal sodium handling in heart failure has served to focus attention, once again, on the determinants of renal perfusion.

The Mediators of the Renal Vascular Response   Substantial evidence implicates both the sympathetic nervous system and the renin-angiotensin system in the renal vascular response. Many studies have documented that denervation, α-adrenergic blocking agents, ganglionic blocking agents, or other drugs that interfere with sympathetic nervous system activity result in better sustained renal blood flow during hemorrhage.[37]

An elegant cross-perfusion technique was employed to isolate the action of renal nerves. Following hemorrhage, there was unequivocal retention of sodium by a kidney perfused from a dog in which blood volume was intact; clearly, only neural influences could have been responsible.[38] The fall in sodium excretion was associated with a fall in renal plasma flow, but not glomerular filtration rate, so that filtration fraction rose. The authors discussed the possible contributions of redistribution of filtrate, changes in peritubular capillary hydrostatic and oncotic pressure, and a direct tubular effect of the sympathetic nerves. Evidence has accumulated that the sympathetic nerves may modulate tubular sodium handling by a direct action,[39] but it seems likely that under most circumstances the blood supply is engaged.

Pharmacologic interruption of the renin-angiotensin system also modifies the renal vascular response to hemorrhage.[40,41] The increase in renin secretion and perfusion changes that follow hemorrhage appear, in part, to be due to several factors including the renal baroreceptor and the drop in blood pressure, the action of sympathetic nerves on β-adrenergic receptors, and prostaglandin release.[42,43] Blockade of prostaglandin formation enhances the renal vascular response to angiotensin and to hemorrhage, but the precise contribution of intrarenal prostaglandin formation remains undefined.

THE KIDNEY IN CONGESTIVE HEART FAILURE

The State of the Renal Blood Supply   The application in the 1940s of the then new clearance techniques to assess renal plasma flow and glomerular filtration rate in patients with advanced congestive heart failure demonstrated a profound and consistent reduction in both indices in patients with advanced disease. It was recognized that even a modest fall in glomerular filtration rate represented a very large reduction in sodium load presented to the tubules for reabsorption. Thus, the observed abnormality was apparently sufficient to account for the sodium retention and edema. The studies with a special impact were performed by Merrill[44,45] at Emory University, where Warren, Stead, and their associates were then evolving new concepts on the pathogenesis of congestive heart failure. The observations on the kidney played an unequivocal role in the evolution of their concept of "forward failure" in the pathogenesis. According to this concept, the reduction in cardiac output consequent to an incompetent myocardium resulted in a fall in renal perfusion, which was virtually always present in patients in whom congestive heart failure was overt, and in whom cardiac output was likely to be sharply reduced.

Filtration fraction was increased in most patients, but the influence of the heart failure on glomerular filtration rate was less consistent. In patients in whom cardiac output was about half the anticipated value, the renal blood flow was reduced to about one fifth of normal. Merrill[45] went on to document, in an additional ten patients in whom milder heart failure was not associated with overt edema, that renal plasma flow and glomerular filtration rate were within normal range. Minimal exercise, however, resulted in a sharp reduction in renal plasma flow and a striking reduction in glomerular filtration rate in six of these ten patients. This observation, as discussed below, may have important implications.

Werko et al,[46] in a much larger study involving 72 patients with mitral valve disease, documented that the reduction in renal plasma flow was proportional not only to the severity of the symptoms, but also to the reduction in cardiac output and rise in pulmonary artery and pulmonary wedge pressures. There was, again, a less striking fall in glomerular filtration rate so that filtration fraction rose. This group also confirmed the observation that mild exercise, too mild to induce a renal response in normal subjects, was associated with a striking fall in plasma flow and sodium excretion. Moreover, hydralazine promoted a striking reversal of the fall in renal plasma flow, suggesting that a substantial portion of the fall in renal perfusion was functional.[47] Indeed, the renal vasodilator prevented the renal vascular response to exercise.

By the late 1950s, several dozens of reports appeared, and were summarized by Wesson[11] (Figs. 5-1 and 5-2). Vander et al,[10] in their detailed review of the literature, focused on the consistent fall in renal plasma flow, which was out of proportion to the fall in glomerular filtration rate. They made the then bold suggestion that the impact of the increased filtration fraction could contribute to the enhanced sodium reabsorption. This conclusion received little recognition, as it preceded, by a decade, the popular acceptance of the role of such physical factors.

How early in the course of congestive heart failure does a renal response occur in humans? Symptoms provide a crude index. More sensitive indices, provided by measurement of right ventricular pressure and pulmonary capillary wedge pressure[46] or sodium space,[48] made it clear that renal plasma flow may be reduced before symptoms become overt. Subclinical sodium retention can be present at a stage between the functionally normal individual with heart disease and the patient with overt congestive heart failure.

Much less is known about "high-output heart failure." In otherwise healthy young men with traumatic arteriovenous fistulae, closing the fistula resulted in a prompt increase in sodium excretion, without any systematic change in renal plasma flow or glomerular filtration rate.[49] The investigators concluded that with the expansion of sodium space, hemodynamics had returned to normal. This conclusion preceded by decades the availability of supporting evidence for such an evolution.[50] An acute arteriovenous fistula in animals induces a fall in renal plasma flow, glomerular filtration rate, and sodium excretion despite the increase in cardiac output.[51]

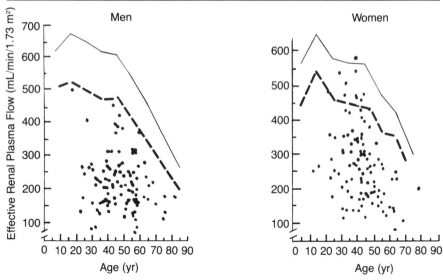

Fig. 5-1. Age-adjusted renal plasma flow in patients with advanced congestive heart failure. Because normal range of plasma flow differs in men and women, data for each sex are presented separately. The solid lines show the mean values for normal men and women as a function of age; the broken lines, SD. (Adapted from Wesson[11] with permission.)

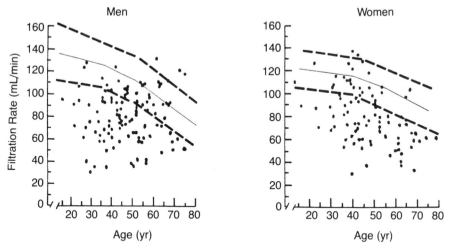

Fig. 5-2. Age-adjusted glomerular filtration rate in patients with advanced congestive heart failure. Because normal range of glomerular filtration rate differs in men and women, data for each sex have been presented separately. (Solid line indicates mean; broken line, range ± SD.) (Adapted from Wesson[11] with permission.)

Distribution of Intrarenal Blood Flow in Patients with Congestive Heart Failure

When renal plasma flow is unchanged in congestive heart failure, is there evidence consistent with a redistribution of intrarenal perfusion? Letteri and Wesson[52] employed glucose titration curves to provide an index of the intrarenal distribution of glomerular filtrate in patients with congestive heart failure, on the premise that an increase in the asymmetry of the titration curve could reflect a shift in the distribution of filtrate

114

among nephrons with a different capacity to handle glucose. The increased "splay" they documented strongly favored a redistribution of blood flow within the kidney in these patients. Diffusible indicator techniques, such as xenon transit, also suggested that cortical perfusion was preferentially reduced in patients with congestive heart failure (Figs. 5-3 and 5-4).[53-55] Indeed, consistent with the observations on total renal blood flow cited above, an excellent correlation was documented between perfusion in the rapid or cortical flow component and end-diastolic pressure in the right ventricle.[54]

The abnormality of renal perfusion is likely to be enhanced in the patient with arrhythmias. Development of the Doppler ultrasonic flowmeter has made it possible to assess phasic flow velocity in humans, where marked beat-to-beat changes have been documented during ventricular arrhythmias.[56]

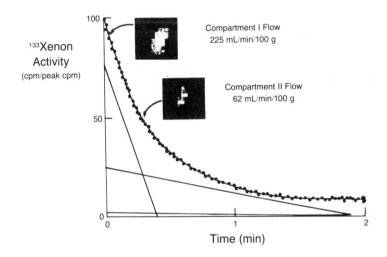

Fig. 5-3. Transit of radioxenon through a kidney in a patient with rheumatic heart disease, but free of congestive heart failure. Insets show scintillation camera images of xenon. The reduction in the size of the kidney image reflects the rapid clearing of xenon from the renal cortex, due to the very high blood flow in that region. (Adapted from MM Kilcoyne, DH Schmidt, PJ Cannon, Intrarenal blood flow in congestive heart failure, *Circulation* 1973;47:786-797, by permission of the American Heart Association, Inc.)

Mediators in Humans   Two studies performed over 20 years ago documented a role for the sympathetic nervous system in the renal response. Spinal anesthesia reversed, in part, the fall in renal plasma flow in some patients with heart failure.[57]

The α-adrenergic blocking agents dibenamine and dihydroergotamine, agents with little influence on the kidney in normal humans, increased renal plasma flow in many patients with congestive heart failure without a consistent influence on glomerular filtration rate.[58] In some, the renal vascular response was associated with a diuresis and natriuresis. The changes in renal vascular state were independent of changes in blood pressure, total peripheral resistance, and cardiac output.

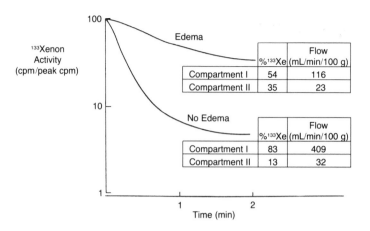

Fig. 5-4. Character of xenon transit in two patients with rheumatic heart disease, one being free of edema and the other having advanced edema. Note the striking reduction in compartment I flow rates, indicative of a reduction in cortical perfusion. (Adapted from MM Kilcoyne, DH Schmidt, PJ Cannon, Intrarenal blood flow in congestive heart failure, *Circulation* 1973;47:786-797, by permission of the American Heart Association, Inc.)

Following hemorrhage, the available evidence suggests that both sympathetic nervous system activity and activation of the renin-angiotensin system contribute to the renal vascular response. By analogy, the available evidence suggests further that both systems contribute to the state of the renal vasculature in congestive heart failure. The development of converting-enzyme inhibitors made it possible to address this issue in humans.

In patients with advanced congestive heart failure, characterized by progressive azotemia due to a sharp reduction in renal plasma flow and glomerular filtration rate, captopril resulted in a systematic increase in renal plasma flow, a smaller but significant increase in glomerular filtration rate, a mild natriuresis, and a striking increase in the renal response to furosemide.[59] These observations suggested that the renal action of angiotensin also contributes heavily to the state of the renal blood supply in congestive heart failure.[59-61]

Are the renal responses to captopril and dibenamine non-specific? Many years ago, Werko et al[47] documented that renal plasma flow increased in patients with mild congestive heart failure after administration of hydralazine. Cogan et al,[62] however, more recently documented the failure of glomerular filtration rate to increase in patients with more advanced congestive heart failure, despite excellent systemic responses to nonspecific vasodilators such as nitroprusside and hydralazine. Therefore, the renal response to captopril and dibenamine are unlikely to have reflected nonspecific vasodilator actions.

Where in the Nephron Does Enhanced Sodium Reabsorption Occur in Congestive Heart Failure?

Two lines of evidence suggest an increase in reabsorption proximal to the ascending limb of the loop of Henle. Osmotic diuretics, which normally reduce the kidney's capacity to generate a dilute urine, paradoxically increase diluting capacity in patients with advanced congestive heart failure.[14] The most straightforward interpretation is that their action at the level of the proximal tubule enhances delivery of sodium to the loop of Henle. Thus, in such patients there must be enhanced proximal tubular reabsorption of sodium.

As a second approach, diuretics that act at various segments within the tubule can be employed to provide an index of regional sodium reabsorption. In this way, Bennett et al[15] provided further evidence for enhanced absorption of sodium in the proximal tubule and loop of Henle in the patient with advanced congestive heart failure. This probably accounts for the observation that the rapid clearing of hyponatremia in patients with heart failure treated with captopril requires concomitant treatment with furosemide.[63] The increase in renal plasma flow and glomerular filtration rate would tend to enhance delivery of sodium beyond the proximal tubule, to the level of the loop of Henle where furosemide exerts its natriuretic action. The increase in distal tubular and collecting duct flow rate, per se, can limit the effective rate of ADH in concentrating the urine.

There is clear evidence of an increase in plasma vasopressin in hyponatremic patients with congestive heart failure.[64] In that study, hyponatremia was associated with mild azotemia, as was the clinical situation in patients in whom captopril reversed hyponatremia.[63] The reversal of hyponatremia with converting-enzyme inhibition is relatively specific, because a comparative assessment with other vasodilators in heart failure, including hydralazine and prazosin, did not reverse hyponatremia.[65]

Studies in Animal Models

In contrast to the relatively uniform reports in animal models of hemorrhage, which are routinely acute studies, and studies in patients with congestive heart failure, considerable heterogeneity is found in reports of animal models of congestive heart failure. From these studies, it is not clear under what conditions the primary process in the heart influences the renal blood supply, what the pattern of the renal vascular response is, where in the nephron enhanced tubular reabsorption occurs, or even whether there is a uniform response to injury until very advanced lesions are produced.

The reason for this may, at least in part, lie in the information reviewed above. It is likely that early in congestive heart failure much of the sodium retention occurs during periods of physical activity. The clinical dictum that the patient with heart failure will rapidly reverse the edema with bed rest may have implications for understanding the pathogenesis. The nature of the technical requirements for detailed studies in animal models has precluded a systematic examination of this factor. Evidence has been presented that shows animals with cardiac injury have an enhanced renal vascular response to exercise[66,67] consistent with this possibility. If this analysis is correct, then the study of the kidney in congestive heart failure provides another example in which clinical investigation has provided more compelling insights than have arisen from the detailed studies conducted in animal models.

IMPLICATIONS FOR THERAPY Withering, in his monograph on foxglove, suggested that the agent might have a primary action on the kidney, since clinical improvement often paralleled the copious diuresis. Certainly, recognition of the role played by sodium retention and the therapeutic implications of reduced sodium intake and effect of diuretics were key advances in treatment. The most recent advance involved the recognition that vasodilator agents, through a reduction in preload and afterload, could result in a striking reversal of clinical symptoms.[68] The utility of this approach in producing symptomatic relief in these patients is now beyond doubt. The foregoing analysis has suggested that selection of the best agent for an individual patient should include a consideration of the action of the agent on the kidney.

The Influence of Diuretics Although there are no placebo-controlled double-blind clinical trials on the influence of furosemide on either symptoms associated with pulmonary congestion and edema, or on natural history, few would deny the ability of diuretic agents to produce symptomatic relief. Although diuretics induce a natriuresis through their action on the kidney, it was recognized early that effective diuresis shifts cardiovascular dynamics toward normal.[69] Acutely, furosemide produces evidence of a reduction in preload,[70,71] whereas with prolonged use the influence of sustained diuresis on ventricular function appears to primarily reflect a reduction in afterload.[72]

Interest in the influence of diuretics on the natural history of heart failure has centered on their negative metabolic effects. Prolonged use of thiazide and loop diuretics in the patient with heart failure results in hyponatremia, hypokalemia, and hypomagnesemia.[73-75] About 40% of patients with a potassium deficit have a concomitant magnesium deficit, which makes the hypokalemia resistant to treatment with a potassium supplement until the magnesium deficit is corrected.[73] The possible contribution of these electrolyte abnormalities to the genesis of arrhythmias and sudden death in the patient with heart failure has been considered recently[76] and is the subject of a detailed evaluation elsewhere in this book.

The Renal Response to Angiotensin Converting-Enzyme Inhibitors In normal humans and other animals, the renal response to pharmacologic interruption of the renin-angiotensin system depends on the conditions under which the assessment has been performed. A consistent increase in renal blood flow generally occurs in response to agents that block angiotensin-II formation and to agents that block the action of angiotensin-II on its receptor[3] when administered after restriction of sodium intake. The striking similarity of response to the two classes of agents in experimental animals and in humans provided a strong line of evidence that reversal of the action of angiotensin was involved. As opposed to earlier available agents, captopril increased renal blood flow in normal human subjects even during ingestion of a substantial amount of sodium, an observation that initially raised questions about captopril's specificity.[77] More recent studies confirmed and extended this observation. Saralasin, the angiotensin antagonist, when infused in a sufficient dose to make a contribution of endogenous angiotensin unlikely, prevents captopril-induced renal vasodilatation.[78,79] Indeed, even in a setting designed to minimize activity of the renin-angiotensin system through a combination of a high-salt diet and treatment with desoxycorticosterone in the rabbit, captopril induced renal vasodilatation through this mechanism.[79] Intrarenal and systemic angiotensin-II formation may not be parallel. Indeed, substantial evidence suggests intrarenal angiotensin-II formation.[3] It is likely that the difference between the renal response to captopril and to those agents that were available earlier reflects the greater effectiveness of captopril in pharmacologic interruption of the system.

A functional response to captopril included a modest natriuresis and little or no change in glomerular filtration rate. When a natriuresis was documented, it was often evident within 20 minutes. This is too soon to reflect the fall in plasma aldosterone, which generally takes a substantially longer time to express its action on the kidney. For this reason, the early natriuresis has generally been attributed to the renal vasodilatation induced by captopril.

In the patient with congestive heart failure, there has been considerable variation in the reported effects of captopril on renal blood flow and function. During acute studies, Dzau et al[59] reported a consistent increase in the renal plasma flow and glomerular filtration rate with a brisk natriuresis. Hyponatremia cleared rapidly in these patients, who had been selected because they were resistant to alternative vasodilators and were extraordinarily ill. During chronic therapy with captopril and enalapril a similar increase in renal plasma flow has been reported.[61,80] On the other hand, in other acute studies, a fall in effective renal plasma flow and glomerular filtration rate has been reported.[81] In these studies the natriuresis did not occur and hyponatremia failed to clear.

Is it possible to discern a difference in these studies? A likely possibility lies in the dose of captopril employed. Dzau et al[59] employed initial doses of 2.5 to 5 mg, with a major goal being to minimize the fall in mean arterial blood pressure in the patients in whom arterial blood pressure was already near the renal "autoregulatory break." Under these conditions, renal function routinely improved (Fig. 5-5). When mean arterial pressure ranges from 85 to 150 mm Hg, arterial pressure per se has little influence on renal perfusion and function because of autoregulation. As mean arterial pressure falls into the range of 80 to 90 mm Hg, renal plasma flow and glomerular filtration rate fall strikingly as blood pressure is reduced.

In the other studies, larger doses of captopril were employed (25 to 100 mg/d). Indeed, the report by Pierpont et al[81] of an inverse correlation between the change in blood pressure and change in creatinine clearance and sodium excretion is consistent with a central role of reduced perfusion pressure in the failure of the kidney to demonstrate a salutary response (Fig. 5-6). The importance of minimizing the fall in blood pressure, both degree and duration, to achieve a salutary response to converting-enzyme inhibition has recently been highlighted in a comparative trial of captopril and enalapril.[82] The greater potency and duration of action of enalapril resulted in a greater frequency of clinical renal failure in patients with advanced congestive heart failure in a study in which large and fixed doses were employed.

Both agents correct hypokalemia and hypomagnesemia in patients with advanced congestive heart failure, presumably because of reversal of secondary aldosteronism.[59,63,80,83] Given the importance of the renal response to converting-enzyme inhibition as a determinant of its overall clinical effectiveness, careful attention to the dose and the blood pressure level is mandatory.

CONCLUSION Available data suggest that renal excretory function plays an important role in the pathogenesis of congestive heart failure and its response to therapy. A substantial portion of the renal functional response reflects active vasoconstriction, in large part due to the local action of angiotensin-II. For that reason, inhibition of angiotensin-II formation by converting-enzyme inhibition contributes to clinical improvement not only through afterload reduction, but also through a salutary action on the kidney. The salutary actions include an improvement in renal perfusion and reversal of the tendency of diuretics to induce azotemia and electrolyte disarray. Captopril also promotes

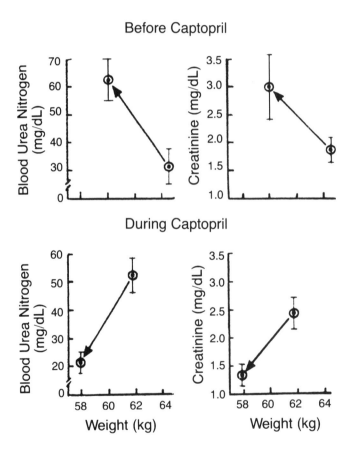

Fig. 5-5. Relation between attempts at diuresis, reflected in the fall in weight, and renal excretory function in patients with advanced heart failure. Note that the patients rapidly developed azotemia when diuretics were administered prior to introduction of captopril. Following introduction of captopril, there was a parallel fall in blood urea nitrogen and creatinine, despite effective diuresis. (Adapted from Dzau et al.[59] Reprinted, by permission of *The New England Journal of Medicine*, 302;1371-1379, 1980.)

a natriuresis, and thus clearing of edema, through its action on the renal blood supply and through reduced aldosterone release. Finally, prevention of secondary aldosteronism reverses the hypokalemia that is commonly found in such patients. The renal actions of captopril promote the rapid reversal of hyponatremia, another important manifestation of advanced congestive heart failure, through facilitation of furosemide-induced diuresis.[63] An important clinical caveat that is emerging from the studies performed in this area is that if the salutary actions on the kidney are to be apparent, close attention must be paid to the dose administered and to limiting the blood pressure fall induced by converting-enzyme inhibitors.

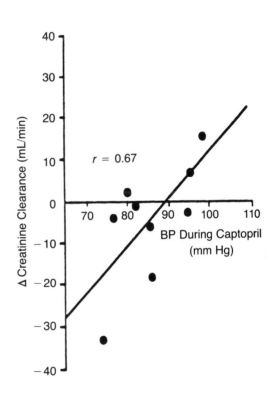

Fig. 5-6. Correlation between the blood pressure (BP) fall induced by captopril and the net change in renal excretory functions. In patients with advanced congestive heart failure, blood pressure is often sufficiently low so that a further drop induced by captopril can interfere with renal excretory function, despite the salutary direct influence of captopril on the kidney. (Adapted from G Pierpont, GS Francis, JN Cohn, Effect of captopril on renal function in patients with congestive heart failure, *Br Heart J* 1981;46:522-527, with permission.)

REFERENCES

1. Ruskin A: *Classics in Arterial Hypertension.* Springfield, Ill, Charles C Thomas, 1956, p 358.
2. Smith HW: Salt and water volume receptors: An exercise in physiologic apologetics. *Am J Med* 1957;23:623.
3. Hollenberg NK: The physiology of the renal circulation, in Black D, Jones NF (eds): *Renal Disease*, ed 4. Oxford, England, Blackwell Scientific Publications, 1979, pp 30-63.

4. Moffat DB: *The Mammalian Kidney*. Cambridge, England, Cambridge University Press, 1957.
5. Bulger RE, Dobyan DC: Recent advances in renal morphology. *Annu Rev Physiol* 1982;44:147-179.
6. Berry CA: Heterogeneity of tubular transport processes in the nephron. *Annu Rev Physiol* 1982;44:181-201.
7. Walker LA, Valtin H: Biological importance of nephron heterogeneity. *Annu Rev Physiol* 1982;44:203-219.
8. Brenner BM, Troy JL, Daugharty TM, et al: Dynamics of glomerular ultrafiltration in the rat: II. Plasma-flow dependence of GFR. *Am J Physiol* 1972;223:1184-1190.
9. Blantz RC, Tucker BJ: Determinants of peritubular capillary fluid uptake in hydropenia and saline plasma expansion. *Am J Physiol* 1975;228:1927-1935.
10. Vander AJ, Malvin RL, Wilde WS, et al: Re-examination of salt and water retention in congestive heart failure (editorial). *Am J Med* 1958;25:497-502.
11. Wesson LG Jr: *Physiology of the Human Kidney*. New York, Grune & Stratton, 1969.
12. Goodyer AVN, Jaeger CA: Renal response to non-shocking hemorrhage: Role of the autonomic nervous system and of the renal circulation. *Am J Physiol* 1955;180:69-74.
13. Barger AC, Herd JA, Sparks HV Jr: The kidney in congestive heart failure, in Blumgart HL (ed): *Symposium on Congestive Heart Failure,* ed 2. New York, American Heart Association, 1966, no. 1, p 49.
14. Bell NH, Schedl HP, Bartter FC, et al: An explanation of abnormal water retention and hypoosmolarity in congestive heart failure. *Am J Med* 1964;36:351-360.
15. Bennett WM, Bagby GC, Antonovic JN: Influence of volume expansion on proximal tubular sodium reabsorption to saline infusion. *Am Heart J* 1973;85:55-64.
16. Hollenberg NK, Schulman C: Renal perfusion and function in the sodium-retaining states, in Seldin DW, Giebisch G (eds): *Physiology and Pathology of Electrolyte Metabolism*. New York, Raven Press, 1985, vol 46, pp 1119-1136.
17. Carriere S, Thoburn GD, O'Morchoe CC, et al: Intrarenal distribution of blood flow in dogs during hemorrhagic hypotension. *Circ Res* 1966:19:167-179.
18. Bell G, Harper AM: Effect of hemorrhage on blood flow through renal cortex of the dog. *J Appl Physiol* 1970;28:583-588.
19. Passmore JC, Leffler CW, Neiberger RE: A critical analysis of renal blood flow distribution during hemorrhage in dogs. *Circ Shock* 1978;5:327-338.
20. Stein JH, Boonjarern S, Wilson CB, et al: Alterations in intrarenal blood flow distribution. *Circ Res* 1973;32:161-172.
21. Aukland K, Kirkebo A, Loyning E, et al: Effect of hemorrhagic hypotension on the distribution of renal cortical blood flow in anesthetized dogs. *Acta Physiol Scand* 1973;84:514-525.
22. Kirkebo A, Tyssebotn I: Effect of dehydration on renal blood flow in dog. *Acta Physiol Scand* 1977;101:257-263.
23. De Wardener HE, Mills IH, Clapham WF, et al: Studies on the efferent mechanism of the sodium diuresis which follows the administration of intravenous saline in the dog. *Clin Sci* 1961;21:249-258.
24. Bricker NS, Donavitch GM: Extracellular fluid volume regulation: On the evidence for a biologic control system, in Epstein M (ed): *The Kidney in Liver Disease*, ed 2. New York, Elsevier Science Publishing Company, Inc, 1983, pp 13-21.
25. Buckalew VM Jr, Gruber KA: Natriuretic hormone, in Epstein M (ed): *The Kidney in Liver Disease*, ed 2. New York, Elsevier Science Publishing Company, Inc, 1983, pp 479-494.
26. Warren S, Dzau V: Natriuretic hormones in heart failure. *Heart Failure* 1982;2:33-39
27. Dzau VJ, Packer M, Lilly LS, et al: Prostaglandins in severe congestive heart failure: Relation to activation of the renin-angiotensin system and hyponatremia. *N Engl J Med* 1984;310:347-352.
28. deBold AJ, Borenstein HB, Veress AT, et al: A rapid and potent natriuretic response to intravenous injection of atrial myocardial extract in rats. *Life Sci* 1981;28:89-94.

29. Atlas SA, Laragh JH: Atrial natriuretic peptide: A new factor in hormonal control of blood pressure and electrolyte homeostasis. *Annu Rev Med* 1986;37:397-414.

30. Tikkanen I, Fyhrquist F, Metsarinne K, et al: Plasma atrial natriuretic peptide in cardiac disease and during infusion in healthy volunteers. *Lancet* 1985;2:66-69.

31. Nakaoka H, Imataka K, Amano M, et al: Plasma levels of atrial natriuretic factors in patient with congestive heart failure (letter). *N Engl J Med* 1985;313:892-893.

32. Shenker Y, Sider RS, Ostafin EA, et al: Plasma levels of immunoreactive atrial natriuretic factor in healthy subjects and patients with edema. *J Clin Invest* 1985;76:1684-1687.

33. Raine AEG, Erne P, Burgisser E, et al: Atrial natriuretic peptide and atrial pressure in patients with congestive heart failure. *N Engl J Med* 1986;315:533-538.

34. Scriven TA, Burnett JC Jr: Effects of synthetic atrial natriuretic peptides on renal function and renin release in acute experimental heart failure. *Circulation* 1985;72:892-897.

35. Brater DC: Resistance to diuretics: Emphasis on a pharmacological perspective. *Drugs* 1981;22:477-494.

36. Goetz KL: Atrial receptors, natriuretic peptides, and the kidney: Current understanding. *Mayo Clin Proc* 1986;61:600-603.

37. Hollenberg NK: *The Role of the Sympathetic Nervous System in the Development of Decompensation During Hemorrhagic Shock*, PhD thesis (pharmacology). University of Manitoba, Winnipeg, Manitoba, 1965.

38. Gill JR Jr, Casper AGT: Role of the sympathetic nervous system in the renal response to hemorrhage. *J Clin Invest* 1969;48:915-922.

39. Dibona GF, Johns EJ: Study of the role of renal nerves in the renal response to 60° head-up tilt in the anesthetized dog. *J Physiol* 1980;299:117-126.

40. Jakschik BA, McKnight RC, Marshall GR, et al: Renal vascular changes during hemorrhagic shock and the pharmacologic modification by angiotensin and catecholamine antagonists. *Circ Shock* 1974;1:231-237.

41. LaChance JG, Arnoux E, Brunette MG, et al: Factors responsible for the outer cortical ischemia observed during hemorrhagic hypotension in dogs. *Circ Shock* 1974;1:131-144.

42. Selkurt EE: Current status of renal circulation and related nephron function in hemorrhagic and experimental hemorrhagic shock: II. Neurohumoral and tubular mechanisms. *Circ Shock* 1974;1:89-97.

43. Henrich WL, Schrier RW, Berl T: Mechanisms of renin secretion during hemorrhage in the dog. *J Clin Invest* 1979;64:1-7.

44. Merrill AJ: Edema and decreased renal blood flow in patients with chronic congestive heart failure: Evidence of "forward failure" as the primary cause of edema. *J Clin Invest* 1946;25:389-400.

45. Merrill AJ, Cargell WH: The effect of exercise on the renal plasma flow and filtration rate of normal and cardiac subjects. *J Clin Invest* 1948;27:272-277.

46. Werko L, Varnauskas E, Eliasch H, et al: Studies on the renal circulation and renal function in mitral valvular disease: I. Effect of exercise. *Circulation* 1954;9:687-699.

47. Werko L, Varnauskas E, Eliasch H, et al: Studies on the renal circulation and renal function in mitral valvular disease: II. Effect of apresoline. *Circulation* 1954;9:700-705.

48. Chobanian AV, Burrows BA, Hollander MD: Body fluid and electrolyte composition in cardiac patients with severe heart disease, but without peripheral edema. *Circulation* 1961;24:743-753.

49. Epstein FH, Post RS, McDowell M: The effect of an arteriovenous fistula on renal hemodynamics and electrolyte excretion. *J Clin Invest* 1953;32:233-241.

50. Watkins L Jr, Burton JA, Haber E, et al: The renin-angiotensin-aldosterone system in congestive failure in conscious dogs. *J Clin Invest* 1976;57:1606-1617.

51. Hilton JG, Kanter DM, Hays DR, et al: The effect of acute arteriovenous fistula on renal functions. *J Clin Invest* 1955;34:732-736.

52. Letteri JM, Wesson LG Jr: Glucose titration curves as an estimate of intrarenal

distribution of glomerular filtrate in patients with congestive heart failure. *J Lab Clin Med* 1965;65:387-405.

53. Dell RB, Sciacca R, Lieberman K, et al: A weighted least-squares technique for the analysis of kinetic data and its application to the study of renal 133 xenon washout in dogs and man. *Circ Res* 1973;32:71-84.
54. Kilcoyne MM, Schmidt DH, Cannon PJ: Intrarenal blood flow in congestive heart failure. *Circulation* 1973;47:786-797.
55. Kinoshita M, Kusukara R, Mashiro I, et al: Intrarenal distribution of blood flow and renin in chronic congestive heart failure. *Jpn Circ J* 1975;38:121-131.
56. Benchimol A, Desser KB: Phasic renal artery blood flow velocity in man during cardiac arrhythmias. *Am J Med Sci* 1977;261:161-166.
57. Mokotoff R, Ross G: The effect of spinal anesthesia on the renal ischemia in congestive heart failure. *J Clin Invest* 1948;27:335-339.
58. Brod J, Fejfar Z, Fejfarova MH: The role of neurohumoral factors in the genesis or renal hemodynamic changes in heart failure. *Acta Med Scand* 1954;148:273-290.
59. Dzau VJ, Colucci WS, Williams GH, et al: Sustained effectiveness of converting-enzyme inhibition in patients with severe congestive heart failure. *N Engl J Med* 1980;302:1373-1379.
60. Creager MA, Halperin JL, Bernard DB, et al: Acute regional circulatory and renal hemodynamic effects of converting-enzyme inhibition in patients with congestive heart failure. *Circulation* 1981;64:483-489.
61. Mujais SK, Fouard FM, Textor SC, et al: Contrasting acute and chronic renal hemodynamic effects of captopril in congestive heart failure. *Clin Res* 1981;29:752A.
62. Cogan JJ, Humphreys MH, Carlson CJ, et al: Renal effects of nitroprusside and hydralazine in patients with congestive heart failure. *Circulation* 1980;61:316-322.
63. Dzau VJ, Hollenberg NK: Renal response to captopril in severe heart failure: Role of furosemide in natriuresis and reversal of hyponatremia. *Ann Intern Med* 1984;100:777-782.
64. Szatalowicz VL, Arnold PE, Chaimovitz C, et al: Radioimmunoassay of plasma arginine vasopressin in hyponatremic patients with congestive heart failure. *N Engl J Med* 1981;305:263-266.
65. Packer M: Sudden unexpected death in patients with congestive heart failure: A second frontier. *Circulation* 1985;72:681-685.
66. Higgins CB, Vatner SF, Franklin D, et al: Effects of experimentally produced heart failure on the peripheral vascular response to severe exercise in conscious dogs. *Circ Res* 1972;31:186-194.
67. Millard RW, Higgins CB, Franklin D, et al: Regulation of the renal circulation during severe exercise in normal dogs and dogs with experimental heart failure. *Circ Res* 1972;31:881-888.
68. Cohn JN, Franciosa JA: Vasodilator therapy of cardiac failure. *N Engl J Med* 1977;297:27.
69. Rader B, Smith WW, Berger AR, et al: Comparison of the hemodynamic effects of mercurial diuretics and digitalis in congestive heart failure. *Circulation* 1964;29:328-345.
70. Franciosa JA, Silverstein SR, Wilen M: Hemodynamic effects of nitroprusside and furosemide in left ventricular failure. *Clin Pharmacol Ther* 1982;32:62-69.
71. Biddle T, Yu PN: Effect of furosemide on hemodynamics and lung water in acute pulmonary edema secondary to myocardial infarction. *Am J Cardiol* 1979;43:86-90.
72. Wilson JR, Reichek N, Dunkman WB, et al: Effect of diuresis on the performance of the failing left ventricle in man. *Am J Med* 1981;70:235-239.
73. Dyckner T, Wester PO: Potassium/magnesium depletion in patients with cardiovascular disease. *Am J Med* 1987;82:S11-S17.
74. Whang R: Magnesium deficiency: Pathogenesis, prevalence, and clinical implications. *Am J Med* 1987;82:S24-S37.
75. Ryan MP: Diuretics and potassium/magnesium depletion: Directions for treatment. *Am J Med* 1987;82:S38-S47.
76. Packer M, Gottlieb SS, Blum MA: Immediate and long-term pathophysiologic

mechanisms underlying the genesis of sudden cardiac death in patients with congestive heart failure. *Am J Med* 1987;82:S4-S10.

77. Hollenberg NK: Renin, angiotensin, and the kidney: Assessment by pharmacologic interruption of the renin-angiotensin system, in Epstein M (ed): *The Kidney in Liver Disease*. New York, Elsevier Science Publishing Company, Inc, 1982.

78. Wong PC, Zimmerman BG, Kraft E, et al: Pharmacological evaluation in conscious dogs of factors involved in the renal vasodilator effect of captopril. *J Pharmacol Exp Ther* 1981;219:646-650.

79. Hollenberg NK, Passan D: Specificity of renal vasodilatation with captopril: Saralasin prevents the response in the DOCA-treated salt-loaded rabbit. *Life Sci* 1982;31:329-334.

80. Cleland JGF, Dargie HJ, Ball SG, et al: Effects of enalapril in heart failure: A double blind study of effects on exercise performance, renal function, hormones, and metabolic state. *Br Heart J* 1985;54:305-312.

81. Pierpont G, Francis GS, Cohn JN: Effect of captopril on renal function in patients with congestive heart failure. *Br Heart J* 1981;46:522-527.

82. Packer M, Lee WH, Yushak M, et al: Comparison of captopril and enalapril in patients with severe chronic heart failure. *N Engl J Med* 1986;315:847-853.

83. Cleland JGF, Dargie HJ, East BW, et al: Total body and serum electrolyte composition in heart failure: The effects of captopril. *Eur Heart J* 1985;6:681-688.

ELLIOT RAPAPORT, MD

6

Congestive Heart Failure: Diagnosis and Principles of Treatment

Cardiac failure may be defined as an inability of the heart to meet the metabolic demands of the peripheral tissues, especially during exercise, despite normal or elevated cardiac filling pressures. Usually, resting cardiac output is chronically low but may be normal or even increased if either peripheral metabolic demands are increased or large systemic vascular shunts or severe normovolemic anemia is present. Recognition of signs and symptoms resulting from an inadequate cardiac output and from systemic and pulmonary congestion is usually accomplished by obtaining a complete history, a physical examination, and routine laboratory analyses. Diagnosis usually does not require use of sophisticated noninvasive or invasive tests (Fig. 6-1).

SYMPTOMS

Dyspnea

The earliest symptom of left ventricular failure usually is dyspnea on exertion. Patients with underlying left ventricular disease who become noticeably short of breath with exertion often have normal central circulatory pressures at rest, but with exercise there is an abnormal increase in left ventricular filling pressure as cardiac output rises.[1] This increase is accompanied by a comparable rise in pulmonary venous and pulmonary capillary pressures. Engorgement of the pulmonary capillary-venous bed appears to be the common denominator for the production of dyspnea in the presence of heart failure. Decreased pulmonary compliance results from the engorgement of the pulmonary vascular bed, which increases the elastic resistance to inspiratory air flow. In turn, the transpulmonary airway gradient required to accomplish a given degree of ventilation increases, producing an increase in the work of breathing. The preexisting length-tension relationships of the intercostal muscles are altered; that is, the patient senses an inappropriate relationship between the volume of breath achieved and the force producing it. This change in length-tension relationship is signaled centrally through afferent impulses from special muscle spindles and is perceived by the patient as an increased effort of breathing, or dyspnea.[2]

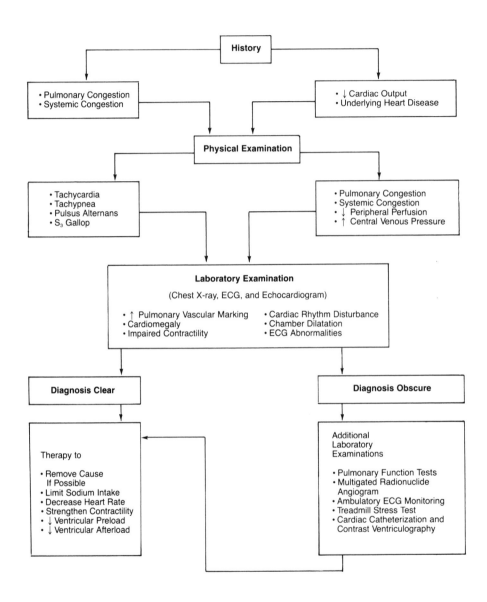

Fig. 6-1. Approach to the diagnosis and therapy of congestive heart failure.

Other mechanisms may also be involved. First, activation of the Hering-Breuer reflex may terminate inspiratory effort before achieving full inspiration, resulting in shallow rapid respirations. Second, pulmonary capillary and venous engorgement may activate the Churchill-Cope reflex, resulting in the sensation of dyspnea. Third, pulmonary vascular engorgement and interstitial fluid accumulation may encroach upon alveoli available for gas exchange, resulting in some degree of restrictive ventilatory insufficiency. In each of these cases, dyspnea appears to be related to the presence of pulmonary capillary hypertension. However, in some patients with cardiac failure, dyspnea may also result from a reduction in cardiac output. Under these circumstances, there may be a direct reduction in blood flow to the muscles of respiration that may lead to an accumulation of acid metabolites and result in the sensation of dyspnea.

Occasionally, dyspnea with exertion may be difficult to identify as a pathologic symptom in contrast to the shortness of breath that may occur in older patients or patients who are obese, sedentary, or have emotional problems. It is therefore helpful to establish that there has been unusual shortness of breath or a change from what previously was present. Furthermore, the dyspnea of cardiac failure is frequently characterized by rapid shallow breathing. This is distinctly different from the deep breathing pattern of psychogenic hyperventilation, which is often associated with a sighing type of respiration as well.

Once dyspnea with exertion resulting from left ventricular failure is obviously present, it rarely disappears. It is likely to progress in severity as left ventricular function deteriorates. The length of time from the onset of dyspnea with excess amounts of exertion to the occurrence of dyspnea with minimal activity and the appearance of other symptoms of pulmonary congestion varies, depending on the underlying pathologic basis for left ventricular failure. Usually, dyspnea progresses insidiously. It may take weeks to months to develop to the point where the patient may be dyspneic with minimal exercise or even at rest.

Orthopnea   Orthopnea is the sensation of dyspnea, or labored breathing, while lying relatively flat in bed. As with dyspnea, orthopnea must be distinguished as a distinct change from the normal experience of the patient. Some patients may have used several pillows for many years in order to sleep comfortably. A history of needing several pillows to avoid shortness of breath during sleep is only of importance if it represents a distinct change from the past. The patient who has usually slept without pillows and only recently requires a pillow to sleep comfortably to avoid shortness of breath may be experiencing true orthopnea. Few patients volunteer this information, and the physician must specifically ask for it in order to determine if this evidence of pulmonary congestion is present.

Orthopnea generally occurs at a later stage in the development of left ventricular failure than dyspnea with exertion, and is usually evident when the patient is having dyspnea with relatively mild exertion. Under these circumstances, assumption of the recumbent position may produce significant changes in hemodynamics. Recumbency results in a rise in the position of the diaphragm, thus decreasing ventilatory reserve. More importantly, with assumption of the recumbent position, there is increased venous return from the dependent portions of the body. There is also increased reabsorption of accumulated dependent extracellular fluid as lessening of the gravitational consequences of venous pooling takes place. This increase in venous return and intravascular volume augments right ventricular output, resulting in further increases in pulmonary capillary and venous blood volume. The engorgement of the lungs under these circumstances produces shortness of breath, presumably by the same mechanisms that result in the symptom of dyspnea.

Some patients may complain of shortness of breath when they lie on their left side, while this symptom is not present when they lie flat or on the right side. The cause of this type of positional dyspnea is uncertain but may be related to hypotension and a resultant fall in coronary perfusion pressure with assumption of the left lateral decubitus position.[3]

Paroxysmal Nocturnal Dyspnea   Paroxysmal nocturnal dyspnea is a frightening symptom to experience. It usually occurs three or four hours after the patient has fallen asleep. Most commonly, patients awaken from sleep suddenly, with a sense of smothering. They immediately sit up, and frequently cough as well as gasp for air. The patient may move to a window to take long breaths of colder air. Assumption of an upright position eventually relieves this symptom, although shortness of breath may persist for many minutes. Subsequently, patients are often so fearful of symptom recurrence that they are unable to go back to sleep. They may try to sleep propped up with pillows or with the head of the bed elevated. The same general mechanism leads to paroxysmal nocturnal dyspnea and orthopnea. The difference is that the former is associated with a deterioration in ventilatory reserve during sleep, which eventually awakens the patient with acute dyspnea. Paroxysmal nocturnal dyspnea may be a precursor to the development of acute pulmonary edema, which is simply a more advanced stage of the same phenomenon and generally causes the patient to seek immediate medical care.

Nocturnal Cough   Nocturnal cough may be another symptom of pulmonary congestion and presumably has the same significance as orthopnea or paroxysmal nocturnal dyspnea. Although the cough generally is inconsequential during the day, when the patient retires at night and assumes a recumbent position, coughing becomes prominent. This type of nonproductive cough may become so frequent and disturbing that it interferes with sleep.

Hemoptysis   Hemoptysis in the patient with congestive heart failure may arise from different causes. If a patient has marked pulmonary congestion or frank pulmonary edema, the expectoration of pink-streaked, frothy sputum or even small amounts of gross blood is common. However, expectoration of large amounts of bright red blood is rare in patients with congestive heart failure, although it is not unusual in tight mitral stenosis. The patient in chronic congestive heart failure has an increased likelihood of having a pulmonary embolism, which could cause him to cough up rusty or dark blood mixed with the sputum. This may occur with or without other symptoms of acute pulmonary infarction. In addition, the patient with chronic congestive heart failure is prone to have associated chronic bronchitis due to the presence of edema of the bronchial wall. This may, in turn, lead to some dark blood streaks in the often purulent sputum.

Symptoms of Systemic Congestion Unexplained weight gain may be the earliest evidence of abnormal salt and water retention. Approximately ten pounds of extracellular fluid will accumulate before it becomes evident as pitting edema. Patients may initially note that by evening their feet are swollen or that the elastic top to their socks causes a pitting or depression of the skin above the ankles because fluid has settled in the most dependent portions of the body. Some patients actually cut off the toes of their bedroom slippers to make them fit. As edema worsens, the skin may become noticeably shiny as it is stretched, and the feet and legs may be noticeably swollen as fluid accumulation becomes grossly evident. Such fluid accumulation tends to subside after a night in bed because with recumbency the fluid shifts to the lumbosacral area.

Dependent edema early in the course of untreated congestive heart failure is inevitably associated with an abnormal elevation of central venous pressure. Men may first notice actual engorgement and/or prominent pulsations of the neck veins as they shave in the morning. A diagnosis of dependent edema in the absence of an increase in central venous pressure is unlikely to be due to congestive heart failure, and other causes of circulatory congestion should be sought.

The gradual development of systemic venous congestion can produce discomfort in the right upper quadrant of the abdomen, particularly after many hours of ambulation, because the hepatic capsule is stretched due to hepatic vascular engorgement. This may also result in noticeable tenderness in that quadrant and some bloating of the abdomen. Anorexia is common in patients with developing congestive heart failure and may occur in response to the abdominal discomfort from hepatic congestion and/or edema of the stomach wall. It is often accompanied by a sense of fullness after meals and at times by nausea. However, the presence of gross ascites in patients with congestive heart failure is usually a late, rather than an early, finding. In patients with severe cardiomyopathy, tricuspid valve disease, or constrictive pericarditis, sufficiently high venous and, therefore, hepatic sinusoidal pressures may occur, resulting in leakage of fluid into the abdominal cavity and, eventually, gross ascites. In the early stages of congestive heart failure, such high central venous pressures are unusual and, consequently, ascites is usually not observed. On the other hand, pleural effusions may occur in the early stages, particularly on the right, and contribute to ventilatory insufficiency and the symptoms of dyspnea and orthopnea.

Other Symptoms Low cardiac output in patients with congestive heart failure is frequently associated with symptoms of easy fatigability and chronic tiredness. This may be the major complaint in some patients as they progress into cardiac decompensation. Fatigability may produce a gradual change in patients' activities with limitation in life-style that may be so gradual as to be initially imperceptible to either the patient or his or her family. However, most patients with congestive heart failure present with a significant restriction in their overall physical activity. Such patients may also begin to experience nocturia at the same time. The nocturia reflects the improvement in renal blood flow at night as renal vascular constriction eases with attenuation of the circulatory demands of normal daily ambulation. Consequently, urine formation accelerates during the night hours. Nocturia may contribute to the presence of insomnia, another frequent complaint in patients with congestive heart failure. It also may play a role in further aggravating the symptoms of chronic tiredness and easy fatigability by interrupting normal sleep. A number of other cerebral symptoms may be seen in patients with heart failure, particularly in the elderly when there is accompanying cerebral atherosclerosis. Mental confusion and impaired memory are particularly common.

PHYSICAL EXAMINATION

General Appearance

In chronic congestive heart failure the patient may be quite comfortable while sitting quietly; however, with relatively mild exertion dyspnea occurs and tachypnea becomes apparent. With severe left ventricular failure the patient will be sitting upright in clear-cut respiratory distress with marked tachypnea. When some respiratory center depression is present, either from the use of drugs or cerebral arteriosclerosis, severe left ventricular failure may result in Cheyne-Stokes respiration. Pronounced prolongation of the circulation time from pulmonary veins to the brain coupled with the depressed responsiveness of the respiratory center results in cyclic periods of apnea and hyperventilation. Patients with cardiac failure generally present with a resting tachycardia, and their pulse is frequently decreased in its force. The pulse may also be irregular, due to chronic atrial fibrillation or to the presence of atrial or ventricular premature beats.

Circulatory Congestion

The signs and symptoms of either peripheral or circulatory congestion are at times mistakenly considered to be synonymous with congestive heart failure. Circulatory congestion in a patient with a normal electrocardiogram and in the absence of cardiomegaly, determined either by physical examination or chest roentgenogram, is usually not congestive heart failure. A classic example of the confusion that can arise is the development of circulatory congestion in the recovery room postoperatively, particularly in the older patient. Not infrequently, such patients have received enormous amounts of blood and fluids producing pronounced and, at times, unrecognized hypervolemia. Increased peripheral and central venous pressures and pulmonary capillary and pulmonary venous hypertension may occur, leading to pulmonary and systemic congestion. Not uncommonly, such patients are thought to suffer from underlying organic heart disease with congestive heart failure. However, the rise in filling pressures under these circumstances simply reflects an increased vascular volume that cannot be accommodated without producing pronounced increases in pressure within the pulmonary and systemic venous systems. The clue that these patients are not suffering from heart failure is the fact that the myocardium responds to such high filling pressures with an augmented stroke work. These patients actually have an extremely hyperkinetic circulation with markedly increased cardiac output reflecting the results of the increased preload.

Similar confusion may arise when a normal blood volume is present but venous tone has been enhanced as a consequence of earlier hypovolemia and a resultant low cardiac output. When cardiac output is reduced chronically, regardless of the cause, the resultant increase in adrenergic stimulation not only results in peripheral arterial vasoconstriction but also in increased venomotor tone. When the cause of the low output state is hypovolemia, the increased venous tone encourages venous return to the heart, compensating in part by helping to restore preload and thus maintain cardiac output. If blood volume is acutely normalized, the restored venous volume is contained in a more restricted venous bed, resulting in high central and pulmonary venous pressures. There should be no confusion regarding the cause of circulatory congestion when normal or low filling pressures are present. When patients have marked peripheral edema and the central venous pressure is low or normal, an extracardiac origin such as cirrhosis or chronic renal disease should be sought.

The patient in heart failure usually has a background of underlying cardiac disease. That is, cardiac decompensation results from the effects of chronic pressure overload, acute or chronic volume overload, or primary myocardial disease (cardiomyopathy) in which cardiac contractility has been impaired due to severe ischemia, inflammatory or metabolic derangements, or the replacement of cardiac muscle with fibrous tissue. The clinician should be wary of attributing unexplained edema to the presence of heart failure.

Cardiac Findings The heart may be relatively normal in size when restrictive cardiomyopathy or constrictive pericarditis results in systemic congestion. However, the overwhelming majority of patients with congestive heart failure have an enlarged heart. The ventricle or atrium or both become enlarged as filling pressures increase and the Starling mechanism attempts to maintain an adequate stroke output. Cardiac enlargement is generally diagnosed by the chest roentgenogram, but it is also usually detectable during the physical examination: the apical impulse is displaced laterally and, at times, downward. The apical impulse may or may not be thrusting in nature, depending on whether or not the cause of cardiac failure is associated with pronounced left ventricular overactivity, such as from a pressure or volume overload. S_1 is usually soft, reflecting the reduced rate of rise of interventricular pressure during isovolumic contraction. A bifid apical impulse may be visible, providing the visual counterpart of an audible S_3, which generally accompanies left ventricular failure. If pulmonary hypertension is present, a sustained systolic parasternal lift is detectable as the hand is pressed along the left sternal border. If it arises from the right ventricle, S_3 frequently becomes augmented with inspiration, and the pulmonic component of the second sound may be accentuated. More commonly, it reflects left ventricular failure and is heard as the bell of the stethoscope is placed lightly against the apical impulse and, particularly, when the patient is turned in the lateral recumbent position. Frequently, an S_4 gallop is also heard, reflecting the presence of decreased ventricular compliance, and is, in itself, not indicative of cardiac decompensation. When the heart rate is sufficiently rapid, these two diastolic gallop sounds may merge into a single loud or summation gallop in mid-diastole.

Left ventricular dilatation may sometimes cause a soft apical murmur of mitral insufficiency. Similarly, tricuspid insufficiency from right ventricular dilatation may cause a soft lower sternal or apical systolic murmur, but these murmurs are usually unimpressive, and their presence is not useful in establishing the diagnosis of congestive heart failure. Pulsus alternans may be detected in patients with left ventricular failure by taking the arterial blood pressure. The presence of alternating 5- to 10-mm-Hg or greater variations in the systolic arterial blood pressure can be detected by lowering pressure in the arm cuff gradually toward the systolic blood pressure level. Initially, one hears Korotkoff's sounds at a rate approximately half that which occurs as the systolic pressure is lowered another 5 to 10 mm Hg and the remaining beats come through. The presence of pulsus alternans indicates severe left ventricular dysfunction, supporting the diagnosis of left ventricular failure. Although a pulmonary arterial pulsus alternans is not detectable by physical examination, a similar alteration in pulmonary arterial and right ventricular systolic pressures can be observed when a cardiac catheter is inserted into the central circulation in patients in whom right ventricular function is compromised and right ventricular failure ensues.

Extracardiac Findings

Pulmonary: Persistently elevated pulmonary capillary pressures result in the transudation of fluid from the capillaries into the interstitial spaces and eventually into the interalveolar spaces. When the rate of flow exceeds the ability of the pulmonary lymphatics to clear the interstitial fluid, the accumulated edema results in fine crepitant pulmonary rales. These will be apparent initially in the most dependent portions of the lungs, namely, the posterior bases. When marked pulmonary capillary hypertension is present, these rales will be present in a more general distribution and may be heard over the entire chest. When rales become diffuse, moist, and loud, the clinical manifestations of early acute pulmonary edema may subsequently ensue. Then the rales become more coarse and may obscure the breath sounds. This degree of fluid transudation may also be associated with bronchospasm and/or edema of the bronchial walls, resulting in generalized wheezing and expiratory rhonchi, as well as coarse and fine inspiratory rales.

Central Venous Pressure: Examination of the neck veins is an important element in the diagnosis of congestive heart failure in the decompensated phase. The presence of an elevated central venous pressure is best determined by adjusting the patient's position in bed to a 45° angle and observing the peak of the maximum venous pulsation within the deep jugular venous system. Normally, the venous pressure should not exceed 2 cm of vertical distance above the sternal angle in this position. If it does, central venous pressure is elevated. The actual height of the central venous pressure in centimeters of blood can be estimated by using the sternal angle as a reference. In general, regardless of the position of the body, the middle of the right atrium lies approximately 5 cm below the sternal angle. Therefore, if one estimates the actual vertical distance of the venous pulse above the sternal angle and adds 5 cm to this value, it is possible to closely approximate the hydrostatic level of the central venous pressure. In addition, examination of the central venous pulse may show filling of the neck veins during inspiration in patients with congestive heart failure. It is not uncommon for Kussmaul's sign to be positive in the presence of congestive heart failure. In addition, the central venous pulse may show a pronounced systolic pulse that reflects the presence of tricuspid insufficiency as right ventricular failure becomes pronounced. Extremely high central venous pressures may prevent observation of the venous pulsations, even with the patient sitting upright in bed. With central venous pressures of 20 cm or more, the venous pulsations may disappear within the cranium and, therefore, the raised central venous pressure may be difficult to detect.

The central venous pressure may be in a borderline area and not unequivocally elevated in patients at the onset of congestive heart failure, prior to initiation of treatment. When this is the case, determination of the presence of a hepatojugular reflux should be attempted. This maneuver is best performed with the patient at a 45° angle. Heavy pressure is exerted with both hands over the abdomen, usually in the right upper quadrant, generally for approximately one minute. The patient should be instructed breathe normally with his mouth open during this period in order to avoid performing Valsalva's maneuver. During the period in which pressure is being exerted, there is displacement of splanchnic blood volume toward the central circulation by the increase in intra-abdominal pressure. If impaired right ventricular function is present, this influx of blood is unable to be accompanied by an appropriate increase in right ventricular stroke output and pressure will rise in the central veins. An elevation in jugular venous pressure of greater than 2 cm of water, which persists throughout the minute or so of abdominal compression, indicates impaired right ventricular function regardless of the presence of an apparently normal resting central venous pressure.[4]

Hepatomegaly: Characteristically, cardiac decompensation results in hepatomegaly. The liver span is increased, and the liver is generally palpable well below the right costal margin as a slightly tender, smooth edge that may pulsate if significant tricuspid insufficiency is present. As cardiac competency is restored, liver size shrinks and the liver edge disappears. Occasionally, cardiac decompensation may produce splenomegaly as well.

Edema: A sudden unexplained weight gain may be the earliest sign that fluid accumulation is taking place in the patient developing congestive heart failure. The progressive loss of body tissue may not be appreciated until the true extent of underlying cachexia becomes apparent following successful diuresis. The suspicion, based on the patient's history, that salt and water retention has occurred and resulted in edema can be confirmed by physical examination. Edema accumulates in the dependent areas. When the patient has been reasonably ambulatory or has been sitting on the side of the bed or in a chair, the presence of edema is confirmed by detectable swelling of the feet or ankles. When a finger is applied against the bony structures of the foot or leg, the displacement of fluid results in a dimple or pit, which disappears in approximately a minute. If the patient has been in bed for several days, however, edema will be confirmed by the presence of pitting over the lumbosacral area, whether or not edema is present in the feet or legs. In the presence of massive edema or anasarca, pitting may not be limited to the sacral area or the ankles and feet, but may be apparent over most of the body, including the chest wall.

Pleural Effusions: Fluid transudation commonly takes place in the pleural space. Bilateral pleural effusions or a right hydrothorax is common, although a unilateral hydrothorax on the left side is unusual and should suggest the possibility of a pulmonary embolism. At times, pleural accumulation of fluid may simply blunt the costophrenic angle. At other times, the effusion may be sufficient to obliterate the lower half or even more of the lung field. This is detected by finding dullness to flatness on percussion over the lower lung fields with absent tactile fremitus and breath sounds. Pleural effusion can be confirmed on chest x-ray. As noted earlier, ascites is generally not seen in the early stages of congestive heart failure. Ascites may be prominent, however, with advanced congestive heart failure, particularly in the presence of cardiomyopathy or if tricuspid valve disease or constrictive pericarditis is present.

Hydropericardium: Hydropericardium also commonly occurs in patients with congestive heart failure. Frequently unrecognized in the nonly identified with the routine use of echocardiography. not of hemodynamic consequence but simply reflect the serous fluid in the pericardial sac, often along with fluid ace. Hydropericardium, as well as hydrothorax, clears as restored.

Cyanosis: Cyanosis is common in patients with heart failure. unt of reduced hemoglobin in the capillary beds results in a of the skin and mucous membranes. This usually reflects the incr.. raction of oxygen as flow is reduced through the capillary beds due to the low cardiac output. At times, a decrease in arterial oxygen resulting from ventilation-perfusion abnormalities associated with pulmonary congestion may contribute to cyanosis. The response by the patient to oxygen administration may be helpful if cyanosis is intense and confusion exists as to whether chronic pulmonary disease or cardiac failure is the cause. Cyanosis in patients with cardiac failure improves little during administration of oxygen because the decrease in peripheral blood flow is likely to remain unaffected. In contrast, if cyanosis is the result of primary pulmonary disease, administration of oxygen generally results in a significant rise in arterial oxygen and a consequent decrease in cyanosis or its disappearance.

Laboratory Findings

Blood Chemistry: Blood urea nitrogen and creatinine are often mildly elevated in patients with heart failure, reflecting decreased renal blood flow and glomerular filtration rate. They are likely to rise significantly with aggressive diuretic therapy, reflecting prerenal azotemia. Serum potassium is usually normal in patients with untreated heart failure. With the use of diuretic therapy, approximately 25% of patients demonstrate a reduced serum potassium level unless a potassium-sparing diuretic has been used.

In advanced congestive heart failure the extreme reduction in glomerular filtration rate results in a very small delivery of total sodium to the distal tubules for exchange with potassium. This combined with the loss of potassium from cellular sites may result in actual hyperkalemia, particularly in those patients who receive potassium supplements with diuretic therapy or receive potassium-sparing diuretics. Serum sodium levels may be normal in untreated heart failure, but hyponatremia is commonly observed due to an impaired ability to excrete free water. Hepatic congestion may result in abnormally elevated liver function values. Aspartate aminotransferase (AST), alanine aminotransferase (ALT), and serum bilirubin are often mildly elevated.

Electrocardiogram: The electrocardiogram is not specifically altered by congestive heart failure but may show abnormalities reflecting the underlying cardiac disease. If sufficient fluid accumulation is present, low-voltage QRS complexes may be seen. There may also be changes on the electrocardiogram that reflect administration of various drugs used to treat cardiac failure, such as digitalis, or the effects of electrolyte abnormalities or both. The presence of a normal electrocardiogram in a patient with clear-cut congestive heart failure should alert the physician to the possibility that the patient has circulatory congestion stemming from another cause.

Chest X-ray: Roentgenographic examination is part of the routine workup for all patients with heart failure. The presence of increased preload and pulmonary capillary hypertension in patients with heart failure is generally evident by the presence of cardiomegaly and increased pulmonary vascular markings (Fig. 6-2). The effects of pulmonary capillary hypertension are most marked in the dependent areas of the lung. Redistribution of pulmonary blood flow towards the apices of the lungs occurs as pulmonary vascular resistance increases in the most dependent areas. This redistribution is apparent on the chest roentgenogram as increased vascularity at the apices. The presence of pulmonary capillary engorgement may also result in lymphatic congestion, indicated by Kerley B lines or horizontal lines extending 1 to 2 cm from the lateral chest wall into the lung fields at the bases. Pleural effusions also occur frequently.

Pulmonary edema without cardiomegaly may occur with acute insult to the myocardium, such as with acute myocardial infarction or when acute valvular insufficiency has been produced, such as from acute infective endocarditis. Unremarkable lung vascular markings with minimal cardiomegaly in the presence of high central venous pressure should suggest the possibility of constrictive pericarditis. When congestive heart failure results in an increase in central venous pressure, the superior vena cava may be dilated, resulting in a widened mediastinal shadow at the base of the heart. If clear-cut pulmonary edema is present, a whiteout of the lung fields may be seen. With lesser degrees of pulmonary edema, prominent vascular markings radiate from the hila out into the lung fields with a butterfly distribution.

Treadmill Exercise Test: Treadmill exercise tests have been increasingly used in assessing not only the severity of congestive heart failure

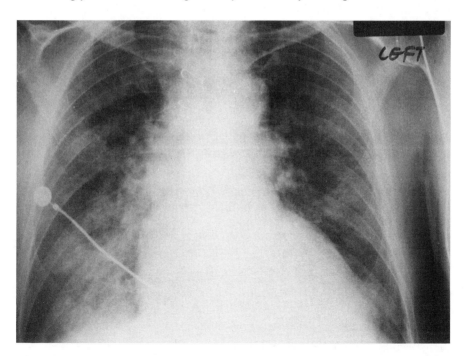

Fig. 6-2. Chest x-ray in a patient in congestive heart failure following bypass surgery. The pulmonic vessels are indistinct because of interstitial fluid around them. Cardiomegaly is evident, and there is haziness of the pulmonary parenchyma radiating from the hilum into the peripheral lung fields due to interstitial edema. Metal sutures are seen in the sternum, and a monitor lead extends across the chest.

but the response to therapy as well. With systems that permit breath-by-breath monitoring of alveolar PO_2 and PCO_2, one can usually identify the anaerobic threshold, that is, the onset of systemic lactate production, as well as measure maximal oxygen uptake. Such efforts require full cooperation of the patient, because it is necessary to gradually increase the treadmill work load (modified Naughton protocol is usually used) to the point of maximally tolerated exercise.

Echocardiogram: The echocardiogram is being increasingly used in the evaluation of the patient with congestive heart failure. It contributes quantitative information regarding ventricular and atrial dimensions, as well as the thickness of the left ventricular posterior wall and the interventricular septum. The echocardiogram also documents the decreased contractile state of the left ventricle. Both the posterior wall and the septum may demonstrate a decrease in systolic displacement, as well as the velocity of contraction. A double diamond configuration to the mitral valve movement is characteristically seen, indicating a low stroke output despite the dilated ventricular chamber. Figure 6-3 is a typical echocardiogram of a patient with congestive heart failure secondary to left ventricular disease.

Although M-mode echocardiography may contribute valuable information, two-dimensional echocardiography affords a more quantitative evaluation. Global function of the left ventricle is more readily estimated, and the ejection fraction can be more accurately quantified. Regional wall motion abnormalities may be identified, as well as left ventricular aneurysms. Two-dimensional echocardiography may also demonstrate the presence of a left ventricular thrombus in some patients with dilated congestive cardiomyopathy.

Radionuclide Angiograms: Multigated radionuclide angiograms are increasingly being utilized to evaluate left and right ventricular function in patients with heart failure. Although information about global function can generally be obtained equally as well through echocardiography, a nuclear ventriculogram is particularly useful when right ventricular volume and function are being evaluated and when chronic lung disease, obesity, or other technical factors may interfere with the likelihood of obtaining an adequate echocardiogram. A multigated radionuclide angiogram also provides the opportunity of looking at regional wall motion, which is more difficult to study with echocardiography, although it can be evaluated with two-dimensional echocardiography.

Ambulatory ECG Monitoring: Ventricular arrhythmias are common in patients with chronic heart failure; furthermore, complex or frequent ventricular premature beats appear to be a risk factor for sudden death in the patient with chronic congestive heart failure. These may be recognized through the use of 24-hour ambulatory electrocardiographic tracings. To the extent that dysrhythmias may contribute to the presence of congestive heart failure, suppression with appropriate antiarrhythmic therapy may prove beneficial; unfortunately, there is no compelling evidence to suggest that the use of antiarrhythmic agents in the management of congestive heart failure alters mortality. The presence of frequent ventricular arrhythmias by physical examination, electrocardiogram, or Holter monitoring should trigger close inspection of the patient's electrolyte status to ensure that electrolyte imbalance is not the initiator or a contributor to the problem.

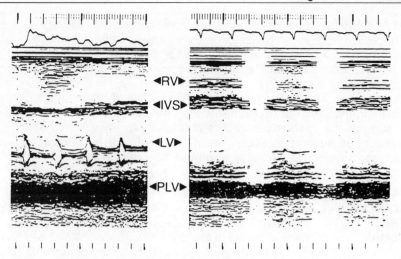

Fig. 6-3. M-mode echocardiogram in a patient with severe congestive heart failure. The dilated left and right ventricular cavities and marked hypokinesis of both the interventricular septum and the posterior left ventricular wall are seen. The characteristic double diamond configuration of the mitral valve is visualized in the left panel. (RV = right ventricle; IVS = interventricular septum; LV = left ventricular cavity; PLV = posterior left ventricular wall.)

Cardiac Catheterization: Cardiac catheterization and contrast ventriculography are rarely indicated to establish the diagnosis of congestive heart failure. If the presence of left ventricular failure is in doubt because a dichotomy exists between the objective findings of impaired cardiovascular function and the symptoms of apparent pulmonary congestion, right heart catheterization may help because it permits estimation of left ventricular filling pressure by measurement of the so-called pulmonary artery wedge pressure. If the wedge pressure is within normal limits at rest, the response to three minutes of steady-state bicycle exercise on the catheterization table will help to establish if left ventricular failure is present. Left ventricular failure can be ruled out if the pulmonary artery wedge pressure remains within normal limits under these circumstances. Similarly, if it is important from a diagnostic standpoint, a catheter may be slipped into the central vein to directly measure venous pressure when marked exogenous obesity prohibits the observer from indirectly judging central venous pressure from the neck veins. Otherwise, catheterization is primarily reserved for those cases in which the patient's response to therapy is being evaluated or when the level of cardiac output is needed to help establish the diagnosis.

In the past, initiation of vasodilator therapy in patients with congestive heart failure was accompanied by monitoring their immediate hemodynamic response. This was done in order to establish that hemodynamic benefit was achieved and to ensure that the dosage was safe and not creating unusual hemodynamic changes. Today, greater experience in the use of vasodilators has alleviated the need for this initial hemodynamic monitoring.

Pulmonary Function Testing: Routine pulmonary function testing is of little value in patients with congestive heart failure. It may be useful periodically, however, to measure the vital capacity in order to estimate the degree of pulmonary congestion. Patients with elevated pulmonary capillary pressures or extracellular accumulation of pulmonary fluid, or both, will exhibit decreased vital capacity, reflecting some degree of restrictive ventilatory insufficiency. As the degree of congestion clears, there will be a corresponding increase in the vital capacity. In addition, analysis of arterial gases is often helpful. Marked arterial hypercapnia may indicate alveolar hypoventilation and suggest that chronic obstructive pulmonary disease is the basic cause of the cardiac decompensation. Similarly, patients with left ventricular failure frequently have some decrease in arterial PO_2 due to ventilation-perfusion abnormalities.

CLASSIFI-CATION OF HEART FAILURE The functional classification of patients with heart disease developed by the New York Heart Association is helpful in evaluating the effects of therapy and in following the natural history of any patient with congestive heart failure. The usefulness of this classification is somewhat limited because treated patients can move from one functional classification to another over a relatively short period of time. Nevertheless, it is a useful classification that is widely applied. The New York Heart Association functional classification is based on the patient's ability to perform physical activity (Table 6-1).

Most physicians have adopted the New York Heart Association functional classification because it is simple and convenient to use. However, a more objective method is desirable in clinical investigation. One that is equally applicable to the clinical management of patients undergoing therapy is the progressive treadmill exercise test,[5] which grades the severity of chronic cardiac failure in terms of the maximal oxygen uptake. One can separate patients into four classes, as shown in Table 6-2. This classification correlates well with reduced maximum cardiac output, and stroke volume during exercise is reproducible.

PRINCIPLES OF TREATMENT

Relief of Underlying Cause One must always be alert to the possibility that the underlying cause of cardiac decompensation may be correctable. This is true particularly in the case of valvular heart disease, in which successful prosthetic valve replacement may restore cardiac competency through the relief of either valvular insufficiency with disappearance of a volume overload or valvular stenosis with elimination of a pressure overload. The development of sudden peripheral vascular collapse, acute pulmonary edema, or congestive heart failure due to acute valvular insufficiency is an indication for emergency surgical valvular replacement. Nearly 90% of patients with congestive heart failure have hypertension or coronary heart disease or both as the antecedent underlying condition.[6]

Ischemic cardiomyopathy producing cardiac failure usually reflects the end stage of severe myocardial destruction from several prior myocardial infarctions and/or the replacement of viable myocardium by fibrous tissue. Normally, such patients are not surgical candidates even if the coronary anatomy is amenable to bypass surgery because the amount of myocardial destruction is excessive. At the time of ventriculography, a patient who has had unloading of the left ventricle accomplished with a large dose of nitroglycerin and still shows a pronounced depression of ejection fraction (under 25%) is generally considered inoperable. However, one must not overlook those patients who have congestive heart failure from coronary artery disease in which there may be a mechanical explanation for the failure, such as the presence of a ventricular aneurysm, a ruptured ventricular septum, or mitral insufficiency secondary to papillary muscle dysfunction or rupture. Heart failure in these cases may improve with surgical management of the mechanical complication. One should also not overlook left ventricular dysfunction produced by reversible myocardial ischemia. One need not have concomitant chest pain when acute pulmonary edema or exacerbation of chronic congestive heart failure results from myocardial ischemia. Revascularization in these patients may prevent future episodes.

Occasionally the underlying etiology of a nonischemic cardiomyopathy becomes apparent and may be amenable to medical therapy. For example, specific medical management may correct cardiac failure among patients with endocrinopathies that impair myocardial performance or in patients with sarcoidosis. Another example is the correction of severe hypertension in the presence of myocardial damage. Adequate control of blood pressure under these circumstances may serve to prevent the subsequent development of clinical heart failure. Again, better management of chronic obstructive pulmonary disease with correction of hypoxia and hypercapnia will help control congestive heart failure. For the most part, however, medical management of heart failure is directed toward palliative treatment of the problem rather than primary relief of the underlying cause.

The primary goals of therapy in congestive heart failure are to reduce the work of the heart, to reduce systemic impedance and ventricular preload, and to improve myocardial contractility.

Restricted Sodium Intake   Dietary sodium should be significantly restricted in patients with cardiac failure. It is difficult to chronically maintain a patient on a severely restricted low-sodium diet. With the availability of potent oral diuretic agents this has become unnecessary. Nevertheless, restriction to approximately 2 g/d is desirable and can be accomplished by ensuring that the patient does not use a salt shaker to add salt to foods and does not add salt during cooking.

Anticoagulants   Patients with dilated congestive cardiomyopathy have a high propensity for thromboembolic complications, leading not only to pulmonary thromboembolism but, at times, to systemic emboli as well. The prevalence of thromboembolic complications is sufficient to warrant the use of chronic anticoagulant therapy whenever severe congestive heart failure is present or in any patient with congestive heart failure in whom a ventricular thrombus is identified by echocardiography. Warfarin is the usual anticoagulant used.

Reduced Work of the Heart   The work of the heart is reduced by lowering myocardial oxygen demand. This is particularly important during the decompensated phase of congestive heart failure. The three major factors that contribute to myocardial oxygen demand are heart size, systolic pressure, and heart rate. Therefore, management of congestive heart failure is directed toward reducing ventricular volume and keeping heart rate low. The purpose of diet and

141

New York Heart Association functional classification

Class I	No limitation. Ordinary physical activity does not cause symptoms.
Class II	Slight limitation of physical activity. Ordinary physical activity will result in symptoms.
Class III	Marked limitation of physical activity. Less than ordinary activity leads to symptoms.
Class IV	Inability to carry on any activity without symptoms. Symptoms are present at rest.

diuretic therapy is to decrease ventricular volume. Digitalis benefits patients with atrial fibrillation by slowing the ventricular rate and thereby reducing the

Table 6-2. Classification of heart failure based on exercise tolerance

Class	Maximal Oxygen Uptake (mL/min/kg)
A	> 20
B	16-20
C	10-15
D	< 10

work of the heart. Significant exercise is to be avoided during cardiac decompensation, because exercise in patients with heart failure increases ventricular volume.[7] Similarly, patients in congestive heart failure tend to have a resting tachycardia and develop an excessive heart rate response to even minimal exercise. For these reasons, during the first several weeks that compensation is being restored, patients are best managed with bed and chair rest. Because of the inherent risk of thromboembolic complications, as well as the psychological benefits that accrue with sitting up by the bed, the patient should not be encouraged to stay in bed excessively. After several weeks and restoration of competency, modest increases in activity become desirable, although resumption of full physical activity is normally inappropriate.

Reduction in Systemic Impedance Vasodilators have been generally accepted as improving both symptoms and exercise tolerance in heart failure. However, recent evidence from randomized clinical trials suggests that vasodilators also prolong survival. The Veterans Administration Cooperative Study on Vasodilator Therapy of Heart Failure (V-HeFT) demonstrated a 28% reduction in mortality among heart failure patients taking digoxin and diuretics when the combination of hydralazine and isosorbide dinitrate was compared with a placebo.[8] Similarly, severe heart failure patients on a "maximal" medical regimen who were randomized to the addition of the angiotensin converting-enzyme inhibitor enalapril had a 40% reduction in mortality after six months compared with those randomized to receive the addition of a placebo in the recently reported Cooperative North Scandinavian Enalapril Survival Study.[9] Whether vasodilators will influence survival and morbid events in patients who have left ventricular dysfunction but are without clinical evidence of congestive heart failure is unknown. This is currently being investigated in a National Heart, Lung and Blood Institute multicenter study comparing enalapril to a placebo.

Vasodilator therapy reverses the excessive systemic impedance resulting primarily from the increased arteriolar resistance associated with congestive heart failure. Although some vasodilators have additional effects, their major action is to reduce the impedance facing the left ventricle during systolic ejection and thereby to decrease the wall force required to empty the ventricle.[10] As a consequence, the contracting ventricle is able to achieve a smaller end-systolic volume from a given end-diastolic volume and thereby increase stroke output. To the extent that some vasodilating agents, such as nitroprusside, also produce pulmonary arteriolar vasodilatation, the impedance facing the right ventricle may decrease as well. Vasodilators are either direct-acting agents on vascular smooth muscle tone or are receptor-dependent agents.[11] Drugs that are pure arterial vasodilators with very little effect on the venous capacitance vessels or on the pulmonary arterioles primarily increase the stroke output with very little change, if any, in left ventricular filling pressures. The arterial pressure, in turn, may or may not remain constant, depending somewhat on patient selection.

Generally, in patients with heart failure, the fall in arteriolar resistance is matched by a comparable rise in stroke output so that arterial pressure generally remains very close to pretreatment levels.

Afterload reduction, with resultant improvement in regional blood flow, may help to reduce the metabolic acidosis that may accompany marked reductions in cardiac output associated with severe congestive heart failure. Acidosis directly decreases myocardial contractility. Thus, afterload reducing agents may secondarily improve contractility by decreasing metabolic acidosis, further improving stroke output.

Increase in Venous Capacitance Venodilator drugs primarily lessen venous return and thereby decrease ventricular filling pressure. In patients with congestive heart failure, this decrease in preload from a pure venodilating drug will have very little effect on the stroke output. This reflects the fact that the patient is on the flat part of the Frank-Starling curve relating stroke output to end-diastolic volume (or transmural distending pressure). Thus, when there are high filling pressures in the failed heart, a decrease in ventricular filling pressure has very little effect on altering stroke output. Use of a venodilating agent in patients who have normal or minimally elevated filling pressure may actually drop stroke output, because these patients are now on the ascending limb of the Starling curve. This effect has been noted in patients with acute myocardial infarction without evidence of pump failure after early administration of nitroglycerin, a potent venodilator. The pulmonary artery wedge pressure can drop to levels as low as 4 to 5 mm Hg. Concomitantly, a decrease in stroke output with a resultant significant tachycardia can occur.

Surprisingly, the use of vasodilators in patients with congestive heart failure has not been generally accompanied by a rise in heart rate. There are probably several explanations for this. First, patients with heart failure tend to already have tachycardia, which reflects the diminished stroke output and the resultant increased adrenergic activity, including sinoatrial node stimulation. Additionally, however, the ability of vasodilators to augment stroke output with little effect on pressure prevents the secondary tachycardia that will be seen when these agents are used in patients with hypertensive disease.

Patients in acute pulmonary edema have frequently ben-
efited dramatically from the administration of morphine. Morphine helps to
allay anxiety, relieve pain, and sedate the patient, but its major benefit relates
to its effect on the peripheral circulation, particularly its venodilating properties.
Thus, morphine helps to reduce venous return to the heart, thereby reducing
pulmonary congestion.

Vasodilators that lower systemic impedance and produce
venodilation result in an increased end-stroke output with a reduction in filling
pressure of the ventricle. These are both highly desirable objectives because
the reduction in filling pressure diminishes the signs and symptoms of pulmonary and systemic congestion, while the increase in stroke output not
only increases tissue perfusion to various organ systems but also decreases
the symptoms of general tiredness and easy fatigability. This helps to reverse
the various compensatory adjustments that have, to some extent, been self-
defeating. In particular, this includes the generalized increase in adrenergic
stimulation.

Diuretics and dietary salt restriction exert their primary
benefit in congestive heart failure by decreasing extracellular water and
intravascular blood volume. Elimination of dependent edema helps reduce
tissue pressure opposing venous pooling and, therefore, improves the capacitance of the venous system. Similarly, decreased intravascular volume,
which ultimately occurs when edema is eliminated, with continued use of
diuretic agents also directly reduces ventricular preload and thereby helps
diminish the filling pressures in both the pulmonary and systemic circulations.
It should be noted that the immediate effects of intravenous furosemide are
direct venodilation that is independent of its effect on decreasing intravascular
volume. Studies of venous capacitance demonstrate that this effect begins
minutes after intravenous injection of the diuretic and long before there is
any significant increase in urinary output that would reflect a reduction in
vascular volume. However, with chronic oral usage, the major beneficial effect
of the drug is achieved through its ability to decrease fluid retention and
intravascular volume.

Improved Myocardial Contractility Positive inotropic agents strengthen myocardial contractility.
Digitalis glycosides, which have been used for over 200
years, are the prototype. They inhibit sodium-potassium
ATPase at the myocardial membrane binding receptor
site and lead to an increase in ionized intracellular calcium,
which serves to increase myocardial contractile tone. More recently, interest
has focused on agents that appear to work by other mechanisms (ie, adre-
noreceptor agonists and drugs that inhibit phosphodiesterase). The resultant
positive inotropic effect with both classes of drugs reflects an increase in
intracellular cyclic AMP. Although a number of these newer agents are still
under active investigation, the initial results of long-term treatment have been
discouraging. Although short-term hemodynamic improvements are universally
demonstrable, long-term benefits are yet to be proven. In some cases there
has been a suggestion that long-term usage may actually have been harmful,
perhaps due to further down regulation of myocardial adrenal receptors,
which are already depleted in chronic congestive heart failure.

Inotropic drugs in the presence of congestive heart failure
also increase stroke output and decrease ventricular filling pressure. The

increase in stroke output is a direct reflection of strengthened myocardial contractility. The extent to which stroke output increases and filling pressure decreases may be moderated by the peripheral effects of the particular inotropic agent being utilized. For example, digitalis is both an arteriolar and venous constricting agent. Its ability to raise stroke output during sinus rhythm in the failed heart, despite these effects on the systemic circulation, reflects its ability to significantly improve the force of the myocardial contraction.[12] A drug like dobutamine, which produces systemic vasodilatation as well as a powerful inotropic effect, will increase cardiac output but at the same time significantly decrease ventricular filling pressure. In contrast, dopamine, which tends to liberate norepinephrine, thereby increasing systemic impedance, will increase stroke output in some heart failure patients in response to its powerful inotropic effect on the myocardium, but it may result in little change in ventricular filling pressure or at times produce an increase in left ventricular filling pressure. Thus, newer oral inotropic agents such as pirbuterol, prenalterol, amrinone, and salbutamol, whether they act on adrenergic receptors or not, must be examined in terms of their effects on the peripheral circulation, as well as their inotropic properties, in order to evaluate their role in the management of congestive heart failure.

Atrial
Natriuretic
Peptides
Atrial natriuretic peptide is a newly discovered hormone secreted by the atrium in response to stretching of atrial myocytes, such as occurs with elevated filling pressures. Plasma levels are elevated in patients with heart failure. This peptide has significant natriuretic, aldosterone-inhibiting, and vasorelaxant properties, which suggest that exogenous administration of additional hormone might be beneficial in the treatment of patients with congestive heart failure. Preliminary studies in patients after administration of a synthetic analog of atrial natriuretic peptide revealed beneficial hemodynamic responses and enhanced diuresis and natriuresis.[13] Future clinical trials can be expected.

Cardiac
Transplantation
Cardiac transplantation has emerged in recent years as a viable option for the management of end-stage congestive heart failure. One-year survival in several centers has been greater than 90% for patients in whom survival of approximately 50% would have been anticipated with traditional medical management. Recent improved results with cardiac transplantation primarily reflect early recognition of rejection with repeated transvenous endomyocardial biopsies and the introduction of cyclosporine for immunosuppression. The major limitations in the widespread applicability of cardiac transplantation are the relative lack of appropriate donors, the strain on available cardiac surgical resources and the large costs involved, end organ damage other than cardiac or other significant systemic disease in the candidate, and unsuitability of transplantation for the older patient. Nevertheless, it is likely that in the future there will be increasing use of this treatment modality for managing severe chronic heart failure.

CONCLUSION
An approach to the diagnosis and treatment of a patient with heart failure is summarized in Figure 6-1. The diagnosis of congestive heart failure is generally made by a careful history and physical examination. Symptoms of pulmonary congestion that point to the diagnosis of heart failure include exertional dyspnea, orthopnea, paroxysmal nocturnal dyspnea, noc-

turnal cough, and hemoptysis. These may be combined with symptoms and signs of systemic congestion and inadequate cardiac output including fatigue, exertional palpitations, unexpected weight gain, dependent edema, hepatomegaly, bibasilar crepitant pulmonary rales, and increased central venous pressure. In addition, cardiac findings of pulsus alternans, S_3 gallop, tachycardia, and ventricular dilatation strongly support the primary role of cardiac failure as the source of pulmonary and systemic congestion. Laboratory criteria include the demonstration of underlying cardiac disease with evidence of impaired left ventricular function, which has resulted in high ventricular filling pressures and a low cardiac output.

Therapy, such as surgical closure of a septal defect or pericardiectomy in the presence of constrictive pericarditis, if correctable, is directed fundamentally toward elimination of the etiology. More often, therapy is palliative. Symptomatic control of heart failure is a prime goal. Recent evidence suggests vasodilators not only improve symptoms but also prolong life in class III and IV patients. Treatment is directed toward restricting sodium intake, strengthening myocardial contractility, reducing ventricular preload, reducing heart rate, and reducing ventricular afterload. Agents that accomplish one or more of these functions help to reduce ventricular filling pressure and to increase stroke output, which are the hemodynamic abnormalities primarily resulting in the symptoms and signs of congestive failure.

REFERENCES

1. Lewis BM, Houssay HEJ, Haynes FW, et al: The dynamics of both right and left ventricles at rest and during exercise in patients with heart failure. *Circ Res* 1953;1:312-320.
2. Rapaport E: Dyspnea: Pathophysiology and differential diagnosis. *Prog Cardiovasc Dis* 1971;13:532-545.
3. Perloff JK: The clinical manifestations of cardiac failure in adults. *Hosp Pract* 1970;5:43-50.
4. Rapaport E: Congestive heart failure: 1. General considerations, in *Practice of Medicine*. Hagerstown, Md, Harper & Row, 1979, vol 6, chap 3.
5. Weber KT: New hope for the failing heart. *Am J Med* 1982;72:665-671.
6. Smith WM: Epidemiology of congestive heart failure. *Am J Cardiol* 1985;55:3A-8A.
7. Rapaport E, Wong M, Ferguson RE, et al: Right ventricular volume in patients with and without heart failure. *Circulation* 1965;31:531-541.
8. Cohn JN, Archibald DG, Ziesche S, et al: Effect of vasodilator therapy on mortality in chronic congestive heart failure: Results of a Veterans Administration Cooperative Study. *N Engl J Med* 1986;314:1547-1552.
9. The CONSENSUS Trial Study Group: Effects of enalapril on mortality in severe congestive heart failure: Results of the Cooperative North Scandinavian Enalapril Survival Study (CONSENSUS). *N Engl J Med* 1987;316:1429-1435.
10. Ribner HS, Bresnahan D, Hsieh AM, et al: Acute hemodynamic responses to vasodilator therapy in congestive heart failure. *Prog Cardiovasc Dis* 1983;25:1-42.
11. Packer M, LeJemtel TH: Physiologic and pharmacologic determinants of vasodilator response: A conceptual framework for rational drug therapy for chronic heart failure. *Prog Cardiovasc Dis* 1982;24:275-292.
12. Arnold SB, Byrd RC, Meister W, et al: Long-term digitalis therapy improves left ventricular function in heart failure. *N Engl J Med* 1980;303:1443-1448.
13. Riegger GAJ, Kromer EP, Kochsiek K: Atrial natriuretic peptide in patients with severe heart failure. *Klin Wochenschr* 1986;64(suppl 6):89-92.

JAMES E. DOHERTY, MD

7

Use of Digitalis and Diuretics in the Treatment of Heart Failure

The importance of digitalis and diuretics in the treatment of heart failure is highlighted by the observation that in 1986 digoxin was the fourth most frequently prescribed drug in the United States, and two of the remaining ten most frequently prescribed drugs were diuretics. In order to define the optimum role of digitalis glycosides and diuretics in the management of cardiac insufficiency, the pharmacodynamics, pharmacokinetics, and adverse drug effects of these classes of drugs are reviewed in this chapter. Subjective (symptomatic) and objective (hemodynamic) benefits in patients with cardiac failure are also evaluated to determine the characteristics of patients most likely to benefit from digoxin and/or diuretic therapy.

DIGITALIS GLY-COSIDES IN CONGESTIVE HEART FAILURE

Although digitalis glycosides have been used for two centuries, the exact mechanism of action is still not completely understood. The beneficial inotropic effect of digitalis is probably related to inhibition of sodium-potassium-adenosine triphosphatase enzyme,[1] as well as its effect upon the cardiac concentration of potassium, sodium, and particularly calcium and magnesium.[2]

Myocardial Actions of Digitalis Glycosides

Digitalis inhibits sodium-potassium-adenosine triphosphatase, the enzyme responsible for generating energy, which enables extrusion of sodium from the myocardial cell following action potentials. This results in gradual accumulation of intracellular sodium and a loss of intracellular potassium. Elevated intracellular sodium concentration increases the availability of calcium to participate in excitation-contraction coupling and to strengthen the force of myocardial contractility.[3-5]

The beneficial effects of digitalis upon the failing myocardium can be demonstrated by the Frank-Starling curve (Fig. 7-1). For any

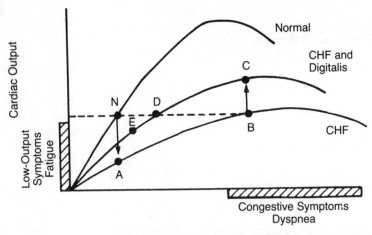

Fig. 7-1. The three curves depict ventricular function in normal subjects and in those with congestive heart failure (CHF) and heart failure after treatment with digitalis. Points N through D represent, in sequence, initial reduction of contractility due to congestive heart failue (N to A); use of Frank-Starling compensation to maintain cardiac output (A to B); increase in contractility when digitalis is administered (B to C); and reduction in the use of Frank-Starling compensation, which digitalis allows (C to D). Any factor that reduces ventricular filling pressure (decreased venous return) will lower cardiac output in spite of an inotropic effect (D to E). Of note is the fact that points N, B, and D all lie on the same line in the vertical axis and, thus, all represent the same cardiac output, but each is on a different end-diastolic pressure on the horizontal axis. The levels at which symptoms of congestion, such as dyspnea, and symptoms of low cardiac output, such as fatigue, occur are represented by the hatched areas. (Reproduced, with permission, from DT Mason, Digitalis pharmacology and therapeutics: Recent advances, *Ann Intern Med* 1974;80:520-530.)

given ventricular state, the force of contraction is increased (up to a limit) when ventricular end-diastolic fiber length is stretched by increased filling pressure. Thus, in the normal heart with an increase in ventricular filling pressure, cardiac output is maintained; however, in the failing heart with depressed contractility, further ventricular dilation is required to maintain cardiac output (points N and B). The inotropic effects of digitalis improve ventricular function toward normal and reduce the need for Frank-Starling preload compensation (point D).[5]

The effects of digitalis upon electrical activity of the myocardium contribute to antiarrhythmic activity and to cardiac toxicity. Digitalis reduces action potential duration, increases the slope of phase 4 depolarization, reduces resting membrane potential, and decreases the maximum rate of rise of phase 0 (V_{max}). Depending on dose, these changes may cause increased automaticity and variable degrees of heart block.[3,5] These effects are similar in atrial and ventricular tissue.

In addition to the direct effects upon electrical activity, digitalis also enhances vagal tone. In the failing heart with compensatorily increased levels of sympathetic tone, vagal activity may be considered therapeutic. Sinus heart rate is slowed and conduction through the atrioventricular node is reduced, which is clearly beneficial in the presence of supraventricular tachyarrhythmias.[3]

Overview of Effectiveness
The use of hemodynamic monitoring techniques has provided objective evidence to confirm over 200 years of clinical experience that digitalis improves cardiac muscle function in patients with heart failure.[6] The "limited" inotropic effect of digitalis is one of its desirable properties, as metabolic cost of this effect is also limited. Chronic digoxin therapy significantly improves left ventricular performance at rest in many patients, as measured by cardiac index, and greater increases during exercise have been noted.[6] Exercise tolerance also improves following digitalis treatment.[7]

The therapeutic value of digitalis in supraventricular tachycardias remains unchallenged,[8] but the need for continued digitalis in patients with normal sinus rhythm has been questioned.[9,10] Several investigators have successfully weaned patients with stable chronic congestive failure and normal sinus rhythm from long-term maintenance regimens of cardiac glycosides. However, suboptimal study design was apparent in some reported series. For example, open protocols were often followed.[11-15] Many patients received subtherapeutic doses of digoxin, and successful drug discontinuation was more likely in patients with serum digoxin concentrations less than 0.8 mg/mL.[15] The initial indication for digitalis was often unclear, and some patients never had evidence of cardiac insufficiency.[11] In addition, discontinuation of digitalis resulted in no change in clinical symptoms despite deterioration in noninvasive hemodynamic parameters.[13,16] This latter discrepancy may be due to the ability of digitalis to augment cardiac output and reduce symptoms only in the presence of congestive heart failure. Because failure was compensated in the stabilized patients, there were no immediate signs of clinical deterioration. Additional well-designed studies are needed to more precisely identify patients who may not require long-term digitalis treatment.[13]

The role of digitalis in cor pulmonale is controversial because of the variable responses associated with different types of pulmonary disease (eg, chronic versus acute, restrictive versus obstructive, presence or absence of left ventricular disease). Further, acute hypoxemia appears to sensitize the myocardium and enhance the risk of digitalis-induced arrhythmias. Digitalis is clearly beneficial in reducing systemic signs of congestion in patients with symptoms of right-sided failure. In patients without failure, the increased cardiac output and elevated pulmonary arterial systolic pressure are likely to enhance the pressure work of the right ventricle.[17] Using noninvasive hemodynamic studies, Mathur et al[18] demonstrated that patients who also have compromised left ventricular function (without overt failure) are more likely to respond to digitalis. The contribution of improved left ventricular function to afterload reduction was proposed as the mechanism for improved right ventricular ejection fraction. The best treatment for congestive heart failure related to pulmonary disease is treatment of the pulmonary pathology itself.

PHARMACO-KINETICS The major limitation of digitalis is the risk of drug toxicity.[19] However, the risk of adverse effects is minimized with application of basic pharmacokinetic principles and an awareness of risk factors for developing toxicity.[20]

"Full digitalizing doses" were recommended in years past for congestive heart failure. This was often taken to mean prescription of increasing amounts of drug until cardiac or extracardiac signs of toxicity appeared, as suggested by Withering[21] in his treatise on the foxglove. The drug was either discontinued until the next bout of congestive failure appeared, as was the custom for a time in Europe,[22] or "backed off" and, when toxic manifestations abated, a "maintenance" dose was restarted. The latter approach was more popular in the United States. The relatively high morbidity and mortality associated with digitalis toxicity in hospitalized cardiac patients has been emphasized by Beller et al,[23] and the wisdom of such an approach to treatment today is doubtful. Prudent application of basic pharmacokinetic principles has minimized the toxicity traditionally associated with digitalis therapy.[20] Digitalis toxicity is much less frequently seen today.[24]

Digoxin Digoxin (12-hydroxydigitoxin) obtained from *Digitalis lanata* is the most popular glycoside in clinical use. Because of its greater polarity in comparison with digitoxin, the bioavailability of digoxin is less than 80%. The new gelatin capsule of digoxin increases bioavailability up to 90% to 95%.[25,26] Therefore, the new formulation necessitates a 20% reduction in digoxin dose, compared with the usual tablet formulation (Table 7-1). This capsule may be useful in patients with malabsorption syndromes and, in

Table 7-1. Usual doses* of digitalis glycosides

Drug	Rapid Digitalization (24 h)	Slow Digitalization	Maintenance
Digoxin			
Tablet	0.5 mg initially, then 0.25 mg q4h × 4 if necessary (do not exceed 2 mg)	0.125-0.50 mg daily × 7	0.125-0.5 mg daily
Gelatin capsule	0.4 mg initially, then 0.2 mg q4h × 4 (do not exceed 1.6 mg)	0.1-0.4 mg daily × 7	0.1-0.2 mg daily
Injection	1.0-1.5 mg IV in divided does over 24 h		
Digitoxin			
Tablet	1.2-1.6 mg in divided doses	0.15 mg daily × 30	0.15 mg daily
Injection	1.0-1.6 mg IV in divided doses over 24 h		

*Specific manufacturer's product information should be consulted before prescribing.

many patients, may eliminate day-to-day variation in bioavailability. Foods and drugs that alter gastrointestinal motility may alter digoxin absorption. These changes are usually not clinically significant.

Pharmacokinetic studies of tritium-labelled digoxin show important pharmacokinetic differences among the various routes of administration. Comparison of serum concentrations following administration of three formulations of digoxin (oral digoxin in an alcoholic solution, 12 patients[27]; intramuscular injection, 10 patients[28]; and intravenous administration, 13 patients[29]) revealed that intramuscular absorption is delayed and associated with slightly lower peak serum concentrations than orally administered digoxin (Fig. 7-2). Serum concentrations of digoxin following intramuscular administration are 83% of intravenously administered digoxin. Because of reduced bioavailability and pain at the injection site, the intramuscular route is not recommended by the author.

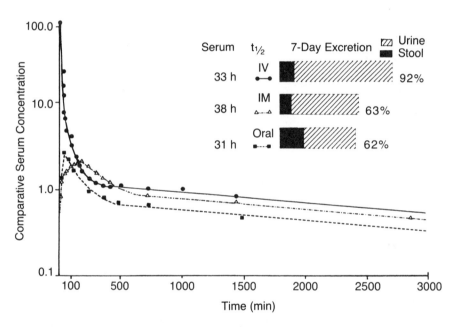

Fig. 7-2. Comparative composite serum levels of digoxin and seven-day excretion rates after oral, intramuscular, and intravenous administration. The serum curves are shown as comparative serum concentration to illustrate the important early differences in serum concentration by the various routes of administration. Excretion rates shown are for patients with normal renal function and clearly show the major route of excretion to be the kidney, regardless of the route of administration. (Adapted from Doherty[139] with permission from the *Journal of the Arkansas Medical Society*.)

It is also important to choose the most appropriate time for determining a serum concentration after administration of digoxin by various routes. One must wait until the equilibration plateau is achieved in order to have a serum concentration that is representative of myocardial concentrations. Thus, two to four hours after an intravenous dose, eight to ten hours after intramuscular dose, and five to six hours after an oral dose are the optimal times to obtain samples for digoxin assay.

Digoxin is widely distributed in tissues, as evidenced by its large volume of distribution (5 to 8 L/kg). It is readily bound to heart and skeletal muscle tissues, whereas adipose tissue contains little digoxin.

The plasma-to-myocardial ratio is remarkably constant, which explains the consistent relationship between serum concentrations and pharmacodynamic effect. Because distribution into adipose tissue is poor, lean or ideal body weight provides a more appropriate basis for calculating volume of distribution. Protein binding is insignificant (25%) and is reduced in renal impairment.[30]

Digoxin is eliminated primarily via renal mechanisms including glomerular filtration and tubular secretion. The latter mechanism can account for up to 50% of the digoxin excreted in the urine. However, tubular secretion is a saturable process at high serum concentrations. Tubular reabsorption can reduce renal clearance of digoxin in patients with cardiovascular disease and prerenal azotemia.[30] Approximately 30% of a dose of digoxin is excreted unchanged into the urine daily. Seven-day excretion of tritiated digoxin by the various routes of administration revealed that 80% to 90% of unchanged digoxin is recovered in the urine (Fig. 7-3). After a single dose, approximately 15% to 20% may be recovered from the stool, depending on the route of administration. The increased polarity of the compound (compared

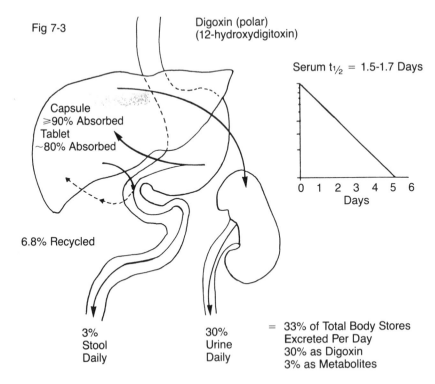

Fig 7-3

Digoxin (polar)
(12-hydroxydigitoxin)

Serum $t_{1/2}$ = 1.5-1.7 Days

Capsule
≥90% Absorbed
Tablet
~80% Absorbed

6.8% Recycled

0 1 2 3 4 5 6
Days

3%
Stool
Daily

30%
Urine
Daily

= 33% of Total Body Stores
Excreted Per Day
30% as Digoxin
3% as Metabolites

Fig. 7-3. Pharmacokinetic diagram for digoxin. Diagrammatically shown are absorption, excretion, and metabolism of this glycoside under circumstances of congestive heart failure and relatively normal renal and thyroid function, without electrolyte disturbances or hypoxia. (Adapted from Doherty et al[140] with permission.)

with digitoxin) probably explains why the large quantitie
recovered unchanged in the urine.[29]

Studies show that a substance with ﹍
noactivity (DLIS) is present in some patients with renal insu.
substance is also found in other disease states and may repre﹍
dogenous human inotropic substance.[32]

Thyroid disease alters digoxin disposition. Elevated serɯ
concentrations corresponding with prolonged elimination half-life have been
observed in hypothyroid patients.[33] In contrast, hyperthyroid patients exhibit
depressed serum levels and enhanced glomerular filtration. It appears that
the relative hypersensitivity or resistance to digoxin in patients with thyroid
disease is due, at least in part, to changes in pharmacokinetics.[34]

Digitoxin   Increased lipid solubility is primarily responsible for the
different pharmacokinetic properties of digitoxin, in comparison with digoxin. Digitoxin is almost completely absorbed from the gastrointestinal tract (Fig. 7-4), resulting
in 90% to 100% bioavailability. Serum concentrations are
usually 15 to 25 ng/mL in the well-digitalized patient. Digitoxin is less preferentially distributed to tissue than digoxin and is avidly bound to serum
albumin (90% to 97%).

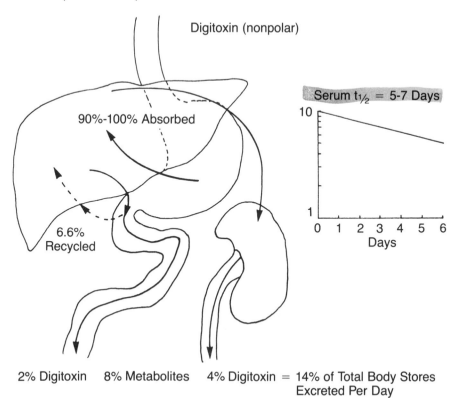

Fig. 7-4. A pharmacokinetic diagram for digitoxin. Note the long half-life of five to
seven days and the extensive metabolism for ultimate excretion in the urine. (Adapted
from Doherty et al[140] with permission.)

Digitoxin is almost totally metabolized in the liver to primarily cardioinactive metabolites. Digoxin has been identified as a metabolite but is quantitatively unimportant.[35] Excretion is via the feces (71%) and urine (29%). The half-life of elimination is five to seven days.[36]

DIGITALIS
INTOXICATION
Digitalis toxicity has largely been reported in hospitalized patients. Its incidence may be exaggerated because this group of patients often has underlying diseases or requires other medications, which may adversely influence the pharmacokinetic behavior of digitalis. A survey taken at the Little Rock Veterans Administration Medical Center revealed that 26% of patients on the medical service were taking digoxin and 6% of these were deemed to be in a toxic state, according to clinical findings and radioimmunoassay serum level determinations. This experience is at the lower end of the 5% to 15% incidence reported in other series,[34] yet it is probably representative of the current lower trend for digitalis toxicity.[24] Reasons for this appear to be multifactorial: greater use of a single glycoside (digoxin), more conservative dosing regimens, frequent monitoring of serum concentrations, better appreciation of limitations of therapeutic response to digitalis, increasing use of alternative agents to improve cardiac performance, and appreciation of special situations that may predispose to toxicity.[37] *Suspicion* is the watchword for prevention (Table 7-2).

Table 7-2. Circumstances in which digitalis toxicity should be suspected

Any change in rhythm

Presence of renal insufficiency

Electrolyte disturbances

Hypothyroidism

Visual symptoms

Elderly patients

Headache

Psychotic symptoms

Pulmonary disease

Recent myocardial infarction

Patient not "doing well"

Adapted from Doherty[132] with permission.

Digitalis toxicity is manifested by cardiac and extracardiac disturbances. Arrhythmias are associated with a higher risk of mortality; therefore, it would be useful if extracardiac symptoms preceded cardiac changes. Unfortunately, surveys of intoxicated patients show that cardiac effects occur before other disturbances in 33% to 50% of cases.[38,39]

Extracardiac
Manifestations
Extracardiac symptoms of digitalis intoxication include gastrointestinal and neurologic disturbances. The mechanism for these manifestations is unclear. However, digoxin has been detected in the cerebrospinal fluid, as well as in brain tissue of patients receiving the drug. It is likely,

therefore, that anorexia, nausea, and vomiting are probably mediated by stimulation of medullary chemoreceptors rather than by direct gastrointestinal irritation.[34] Surveys of inadvertent digitalis overdose have been useful in characterizing the extracardiac manifestations of intoxication. For example, in one series, a tablet containing three times the usual digitalis dose (a tablet containing digitoxin 0.2 mg and digoxin 0.05 mg, instead of digoxin 0.25 mg) that was inadvertently given to hospitalized patients in Holland resulted in a high incidence of extracardiac manifestations (Table 7-3). All of the patients were stabilized on digitalis prior to overdose. Exact doses and serum digitalis concentrations were not reported, and the duration of exposure was not definitely stated but may have been up to ten weeks. Toxicity was successfully managed by drug withdrawal except in seven patients (4%), whose deaths were attributed to digitalis-induced arrhythmia.[40]

Table 7-3. Prevalence of extracardiac toxicity in 179 patients who received inadvertent overdoses of digitoxin

Manifestation of Toxicity	Incidence (%)
Fatigue	95
Visual disturbances	95
Decreased muscle strength	82
Anorexia and nausea	80
Psychic disturbances	65
Death (associated with arrhythmia)	4

Data from Lely and van Enter.[40]

The manifestations of digitalis toxicity included neurologic disturbances (95%) characterized by overwhelming fatigue, muscular weakness, and difficulty walking and raising the arms. Visual disturbances (95%) were manifested as hazy vision, difficulty in reading, and alteration of the color of objects; photophobia, glitterings, moving spots, and flames of yellow, red, green, or dark colors were also reported. Most patients had difficulty in red-green perception. Gastrointestinal disturbances (80%) included anorexia, nausea, and/or abdominal pain. Hallucinations, restlessness, insomnia, apathy, and drowsiness also occurred. Transient psychosis was reported in 7% of subjects. Recent studies indicate significant concentrations of digoxin present in canine peripheral nervous tissue, particularly sympathetic ganglia.[41] The time course of accumulation of digoxin in the sympathetic nervous system suggests very early increases in these areas, which achieve maximum values after ten days. These findings support the hypothesis that some toxic (and perhaps inotropic) activity of digitalis may be neurally mediated.

Cardiac Manifestations   The mechanisms by which digitalis causes arrhythmias are an extension of its pharmacodynamic actions and appear to be the results of alteration of impulse formation or conduction, or both. Digitalis may cause almost every known arrhythmia, and it is common for one patient to demonstrate multiple arrhythmias.[39]

Beller et al[23] documented the prevalence of various rhythms in a prospective survey of nearly 1,000 consecutively hospitalized patients, in which 23% receiving digitalis at the time of admission had definite signs of cardiac toxicity. Arrhythmias associated with increased automaticity were more frequent than either conduction defects alone or in combination. Atrioventricular junctional arrhythmias were observed in 50% of the patients (Table 7-4). Although 14 of 34 definitely intoxicated patients died, electrocardiographic abnormalities were present in only 6 patients at the time of death. Factors associated with toxicity included advanced heart disease, underlying atrial fibrillation, anorexia, pulmonary disease, and renal failure.[23]

Table 7-4. Prevalence of rhythm disturbances observed in 34 hospitalized patients with definite digitalis toxicity

Rhythm	Incidence (%)
Atrioventricular junctional escape rhythm	35
Ventricular bigeminy or trigeminy	35
Nonparoxysmal atrioventricular junctional tachycardia (> 80/min)	29
Ectopic ventricular beats alone (> 5/min)	18
Multifocal ventricular ectopic beats and/or ventricular tachycardia	18
Atrioventricular junctional exit block (Wenckebach type)	15
Paroxysmal atrial tachycardia with atrioventricular block	6
Sinus arrest or sinoatrial exit block	3
Mobitz type I second-degree atrioventricular block	3
Mortality	41

Adapted from Beller et al.[32] Reprinted, by permission of *The New England Journal of Medicine*, 284;990-997, 1971.

Importance and Limitations of Digitalis Serum Concentrations The major indications for monitoring serum digitalis concentrations are to ensure adequate digitalization in a patient who demonstrates a suboptimal response and to rule out intoxication.[42] Digitalis assays are useful in detecting noncompliance, malabsorption, drug interactions, or poor tablet bioavailability as causes of suboptimal clinical response. Assays also confirm the suspicion of toxicity in patients with clinical symptoms of overdose and may be useful in dosing patients with renal failure or another underlying condition that results in drug accumulation. Serum digoxin or digitoxin concentrations correlate with toxicity, and levels have been two to three times those of unintoxicated patients.[34]

Although therapeutic serum concentrations for digitalis glycosides are established, patients with "therapeutic levels" can be intoxicated and patients with "toxic levels" may not demonstrate any manifestations of digitalis intoxication.[43] Subtherapeutic levels of digoxin (< 0.5 ng/mL) indicate a high probability of either noncompliance or malabsorption. Digoxin at therapeutic levels (0.5 to 2 ng/mL) adds little to guide therapy. Digoxin levels above 2 ng/mL do not prove digitalis toxicity; they merely indic. is possible. Serum digitalis concentrations are therefore not a clinical judgment. In combination with clinical judgment, serum (are useful in reinforcing the clinician's suspicion of inappropri. for suggesting the need to search for other causes of undesirabl.

MANAGEMENT OF DIGITALIS INTOXICATION The most common arrhythmias (eg, occasi(beats and atrial fibrillation with a very slow ....ular response or regularization with a junctional mechanism) associated with digitalis intoxication can be managed effectively by stopping the drug and monitoring the electrocardiogram.[5,45] Depending on the initial serum concentration, discontinuing digoxin for 24 hours is usually accompanied by an adequate decline in serum concentrations for reversal of toxicity in a patient with normal renal function. In contrast, digitoxin withdrawal must be maintained for several days because of its longer half-life of elimination.

Arrhythmias that compromise cardiac output (eg, ventricular tachycardia, junctional tachycardia or atrial tachycardia, very frequent premature ventricular contractions, and very slow rhythms) generally require treatment. One must also evaluate factors that affect digitalis elimination, such as renal and hepatic function, as well as other reversible conditions that might lower digitalis tolerance, such as hypoxia, electrolyte or pH disturbances, and myocardial infarction.

Antiarrhythmic Agents Lidocaine is useful for controlling ectopic rhythms associated with digitalis toxicity. It does not slow conduction through the atrioventricular node or cause significant depression of myocardial function. However, lidocaine is not very effective in abolishing the junctional tachycardias associated with digitalis. Lidocaine should be administered in an intravenous bolus dose of 50 to 100 mg and maintained at a continuous infusion of 2 to 4 mg/min. An advantage of lidocaine is its relatively short duration of action. In the event that toxicity appears, the pharmacologic effect usually dissipates within 20 minutes. In the presence of heart failure the half-life of lidocaine is usually increased, and caution should be observed.

Phenytoin is similar to lidocaine in its effect on cardiac electrophysiology. Although occasional myocardial depression has appeared with large doses, this effect is less pronounced than that of quinidine or procainamide. Phenytoin is particularly useful for ventricular arrhythmias caused by digitalis. Phenytoin should be administered by slow intravenous infusion of 50 to 100 mg over five minutes, up to 15 mg/kg body weight or until toxicity appears. This is followed by an oral dose of 5 mg/kg body weight if the arrhythmia is controlled.

Quinidine and procainamide should be avoided in the treatment of arrhythmias associated with digitalis toxicity because of the risk of depressing atrioventricular and His-Purkinje conduction and myocardial contractility. Although propranolol shows similar undesirable depressant properties, its antiadrenergic activity may be useful to oppose digitalis-induced automaticity, and it has been useful in combating atrial tachycardia with block and some ventricular arrhythmias.[46]

Potassium   Potassium therapy for managing digitalis-induced arrhythmias requires cautious administration, because the actions of potassium and digitalis are often additive in conduction tissue. Lesser amounts of potassium are required to decrease conduction in the setting of digitalis toxicity.[47] Thus, potassium should be administered to patients with arrhythmias caused by alteration of conduction only if low serum potassium concentrations exist. Potassium effectively abolishes premature ventricular contractions and other ventricular arrhythmias caused by digitalis. Potassium is also effective treatment for atrial tachycardia with block, but must be administered under continuous electrocardiographic monitoring.[48]

Electrical   *Cardioversion*: Direct current countershock is usually not
Therapy   recommended to manage arrhythmias due to digitalis because of serious arrhythmias that may follow. However, if medical management fails and/or vital signs are unstable because of tachyarrhythmia, cardioversion is indicated and is never withheld for fear of further toxicity. Initiating therapy at lower energy levels can reduce the risk of arrhythmia development.[49] Patients with therapeutic digoxin concentrations may safely undergo cardioversion without the concomitant use of class I antiarrhythmics.[50]

Pacing: Temporary transvenous pacing is indicated in the management of digitalis intoxication if slow heart rate is producing hemodynamic compromise. In addition, pacing is useful for control of ventricular arrhythmias when it is felt that an increase in the basic heart rate will suppress the ventricular arrhythmia. Refractoriness of the atrioventricular node is produced by digitalis; therefore, ventricular pacing is preferred.

Cholestyramine   Steroid-binding resins have been used in an attempt to
and Colestipol   shorten the duration of toxicity due to digitalis glycosides. Both digoxin and digitoxin undergo enterohepatic recirculation; therefore, use of an agent such as cholestyramine or colestipol is rational. These agents significantly shorten the half-life of digitoxin[51] and reduce the duration of symptoms of toxicity.[52] However, results with digoxin, which undergoes much less enterohepatic circulation, are less impressive.[53] Unfortunately, most cases of life-threatening digitalis toxicity require promptly acting agents. Thus, steroid-binding resins are of limited usefulness because of their delayed onset of effect.

Activated   Activated charcoal limits the absorption of many drugs
Charcoal   and toxins. It inhibits the absorption of digitalis and significantly increases digitoxin clearance by reducing its enterohepatic recirculation.[54,55] Activated charcoal is recommended in acute digitalis intoxication, especially in patients with renal impairment.[55,56]

Digoxin   Available for life-threatening toxicity, digoxin antibodies in
Antibodies   the form of Fab fragment (Digibind®) of the original antibody molecule effectively reverse digitalis intoxication due to both digoxin and digitoxin. Smith et al[57] described the successful treatment of 26 patients with either digoxin (23 patients) or digitoxin (3 patients) intoxication with digoxin-specific Fab fragments. All patients had life-threatening arrhythmias (eg, ventricular tachycardia

77%, ventricular fibrillation 35%, atrioventricular block with bradycardia 73%, and/or hyperkalemia 42%) resistant to other modalities. Digoxin and digitoxin serum concentrations averaged 19.1 ng/mL (range: 2 to 100 ng/mL) and greater than 100 ng/mL, respectively. Twenty-one (81%) patients achieved a complete response without additional sequelae, and the remaining patients responded initially but eventually died, either because of damage suffered prior to Fab fragment treatment or because of an inadequate antibody supply. Digoxin-specific Fab fragments were especially useful in reversing the severe hyperkalemia caused by inhibition of the sodium-potassium-adenosine triphosphatase enzyme with subsequent release of intracellular potassium. All 11 patients with average serum potassium concentrations of 6.7 mmol/L responded to digoxin-specific Fab fragments, and some required supplemental potassium. Neither hypersensitivity nor renal toxicity occurred during or after treatment with digoxin-specific Fab fragments.

Wenger et al[58] reported an additional experience with 63 patients (7 excluded) in a multicenter study with 53 of the remaining 56 patients responding favorably to the Fab fragment antibodies. On the basis of this additional experience, digoxin Fab fragment antibodies have been released for use in severe toxicity (eg, hyperkalemia, severe atrioventricular block, asystole, ventricular tachycardia, and ventricular fibrillation).

Because the Fab fragment is one third the size of the original IgG antibody molecule (50,000 versus 150,000 daltons) the Fab fragment-digoxin combination may be excreted in the urine with a half-life of only 9.1 hours. The therapeutic effect of the Fab fragment is usually seen within minutes and is often complete in two hours.

Dosage of digoxin Fab fragments may be calculated from the steady-state serum concentrations of digoxin or digitoxin (SDC) through use of these formulas:

For digoxin:

Total body loading dose (mg) = (SDC) (5.6) (weight in kg)/1,000.

For digitoxin:

Total body loading dose (mg) = (SDC) (0.56) (weight in kg)/1,000.

The volume of distribution for digoxin and digitoxin is 5.6 and 0.56 L/kg, respectively. Each 5-mL vial contains 40 mg of purified digoxin antibody fragments that will bind approximately 0.6 mg of digoxin (or digitoxin). Thus, one can calculate the total number of vials required by dividing the total body load of digoxin or digitoxin in milligrams by 0.6 mg/vial:

$$\text{Dose (in no. of vials)} = \frac{\text{body load (mg)}}{0.6}.$$

The dose administered need not be exactly equimolar; digoxin loading dose calculations are approximate. Table 7-5 shows the dose estimate for Fab fragments from serum concentrations. This drug is given intravenously over a period of 30 minutes through a 0.22-μm membrane filter. If cardiac arrest

Table 7-5. Dose estimates* of Fab fragments based on serum digoxin concentration

Patient Weight (kg)	Serum Digoxin Concentration (ng/mL)						
	1	2	4	8	12	16	20
1	0.5 mg	1 mg	1.5 mg	3 mg	5 mg	6 mg	8 mg
3	1 mg	2 mg	5 mg	9 mg	13 mg	18 mg	22 mg
5	2 mg	4 mg	8 mg	15 mg	22 mg	30 mg	40 mg
10	4 mg	8 mg	15 mg	30 mg	40 mg	60 mg	80 mg
20	8 mg	15 mg	30 mg	60 mg	80 mg	120 mg	160 mg
40	0.5 v	1 v	2 v	3 v	5 v	6 v	8 v
60	0.5 v	1 v	2 v	5 v	7 v	9 v	11 v
70	1 v	2 v	3 v	5 v	8 v	11 v	13 v
80	1 v	2 v	3 v	6 v	9 v	12 v	15 v
100	1 v	2 v	4 v	8 v	11 v	15 v	19 v

*Dose is given in milligrams up to 20 kg of patient weight. Above 20 kg, dose is given in number of vials (v), each of which contains 40 mg Fab.

appears to be imminent, digoxin antibodies may be given by a bolus injection. Hypokalemia often develops during the course of treatment as potassium returns to the cellular compartment; therefore, serum levels should be carefully monitored, and replacement therapy instituted if necessary.

This treatment should be cost-effective, because the duration of intensive care may be markedly reduced through use of Fab fragments. It has been designated an orphan drug because of the limited patient population for application.

DRUG INTER-ACTIONS WITH DIGITALIS GLYCOSIDES Drug interactions with both digoxin and digitoxin have been reported as either case reports or small studies.[38] Any drug that lowers serum potassium concentrations may predispose patients to digitalis toxicity. Drug interactions of clinical significance include the digoxin-quinidine, digitoxin-quinidine, and digoxin-verapamil interactions.

Administration of quinidine to patients receiving digoxin approximately doubles digoxin serum concentrations.[59] The change is proportional to the quinidine dose; however, the mechanism of this interaction is unresolved.[60-63] The reaction occurs in 90% of patients receiving therapeutic doses of digoxin and quinidine.[59] Both extracardiac toxicity and atrioventricular conduction delay, as measured by electrocardiogram, have been described as consequences of this interaction.[62] It begins with the first dose of quinidine, and a new digoxin steady state is achieved by the fifth day of combined treatment. It has been suggested that the dose of digoxin should be halved prior to the addition of quinidine. However, this empiric recommendation does not take into account the large, unpredictable interpatient variation. It may be more prudent to monitor the patient clinically and with electrocardiography until the new steady state is achieved.[59]

Elevation of digitoxin serum concentrations has also been observed when quinidine is administered. The digitoxin-quinidine interaction appears to occur by a different mechanism, possibly because of differences in tissue binding and in routes of elimination. As with digoxin, renal clearance is diminished, resulting in elevated serum digitoxin concentrations, and there is also a trend towards reduced nonrenal clearance. There is no change in the apparent volume of distribution, and the digitoxin half-life is lengthened, whereas that of digoxin is not. At this time, digitoxin cannot be recommended as an alternative for patients with problems due to the digoxin-quinidine interaction.[64,65]

Verapamil also increases digoxin serum levels.[66] The digoxin-verapamil interaction is clinically significant, as the two drugs may have additive pharmacodynamic effects such as inhibition of atrioventricular conduction.[67] Verapamil decreases the active tubular secretion of digoxin by the kidneys; reduced renal digoxin clearance leads to a 70% increase in serum digoxin concentration.[68-72] Klein and Kaplinsky[72] showed that the digoxin-verapamil interaction occurs at all levels of digitalization, is proportional to the dose of verapamil, reaches a peak in 7 to 14 days, and can produce significant digitalis toxicity. Nifedipine and diltiazem may reduce digoxin clearance and increase serum digoxin concentration.[73,74] Unlike the digoxin-verapamil interaction, these interactions are of little clinical significance.

Kuhlmann[75] studied the effects of calcium channel blockers on digitoxin's pharmacokinetics in patients with cardiac insufficiency. Verapamil did not affect renal digitoxin clearance; verapamil reduced total body clearance and extrarenal clearance of digitoxin by 27% and 29%, respectively. Plasma digitoxin concentration increased by 35% during concurrent verapamil administration. Diltiazem increased plasma digitoxin concentration by 20%, whereas nifedipine did not alter plasma digitoxin concentration. Kuhlmann concluded that the risk of digitalis intoxication during concurrent verapamil and digitoxin administration is much less pronounced than during concurrent verapamil-digoxin administration.

Amiodarone, a class III antiarrhythmic drug used in patients with refractory ventricular arrhythmias, may affect the pharmacokinetics of commonly used cardiovascular drugs, including digoxin.[76] Amiodarone-induced increases in serum digoxin concentrations have led to digitalis toxicity. The magnitude of this interaction correlates with plasma amiodarone concentrations. The mechanism is multifactorial, including reduced renal and nonrenal clearance of digoxin and a decrease in digoxin's volume of distribution.[77]

Cimetidine, a drug known to decrease hepatic mixed-function oxidase activity and renal tubular secretion of cationic drugs, does not affect digoxin's pharmacokinetics.[78]

GUIDELINES FOR DIGITALIS USE

Indications

Digitalis is indicated for the management of congestive heart failure. Heart failure associated with depressed ventricular contractility is more responsive to digitalis than is failure caused by mechanical disturbances. The third heart sound remains a reliable predictor of digitalis response.[79]

In patients without clinical evidence of failure but with hypertrophied or dilated hearts on radiologic examination, the indication for digitalis is unclear. Theoretically, increased contractility would enable achievement of the same stroke work and cardiac output with a lower filling pressure, leading to greater inotropic reserve. This concept should be particularly beneficial in borderline patients whose normal resting cardiac output is impaired during exercise. This latter group is difficult to identify; there is no evidence of improved prognosis or delay in the onset of hypertrophy in patients prophylactically treated with digitalis.

Digitalis has also been suggested as prophylactic therapy for patients with diminished cardiac reserve prior to major stress (eg, surgery). This use is controversial. In the case of aortocoronary bypass surgery, in which digitalis allegedly suppresses supraventricular arrhythmias, there was no difference in postoperative outcome between digitalized and untreated patients.[80] In comparison, pre- and postoperative administration of propranolol plus digoxin significantly ($P < 0.005$) reduced the incidence of post-aorto-coronary-bypass supraventricular arrhythmias to 3.1% compared with a 21.4% incidence in untreated patients.[81] Postoperative administration of digoxin does not prevent supraventricular tachycardia after aortocoronary bypass surgery.[82]

Paroxysmal supraventricular tachycardia and atrial fibrillation with rapid ventricular response are major indications for digitalis. Uncontrolled studies in patients with atrial fibrillation and untreated or partially treated congestive failure support the use of digoxin to terminate atrial fibrillation.[83,84] However, Falk and colleagues,[85] in a randomized, placebo-controlled, double-blind trial, showed that spontaneous reversion to sinus rhythm is common in patients with atrial fibrillation of recent onset, and that digitalization did not affect the likelihood of reversion to sinus rhythm. In the absence of coexisting heart failure in patients with atrial fibrillation, digoxin is indicated for rate control only. When the ventricular rate is difficult to control (eg, in thyrotoxicosis), the addition of a β-adrenergic blocking drug may be useful.

Hypomagnesemia is present in approximately 20% of patients with atrial fibrillation, and this reduces digoxin's negative dromotropic effects in this population.[86] Hypomagnesemic patients with atrial fibrillation may require twice as much digoxin to successfully control their ventricular response rate. Thus, replacement of magnesium deficiency may be beneficial in this setting.

Recent studies show that verapamil is superior to digoxin in controlling ventricular response rate and improving exercise capacity in patients with chronic atrial fibrillation.[87] Unlike digoxin, verapamil controls ventricular response rate during exercise. This effect significantly improves exercise capacity. Caution is advised in acute atrial fibrillation, though, as verapamil bolus may result in alarming and resistant hypotension.

Atrial flutter with 2:1 atrioventricular block often necessitates high-dose digitalis treatment. Initial attempts at cardioversion may be preferable prior to sensitizing the myocardium with high-dose digitalis. Wolff-Parkinson-White (WPW) tachyarrhythmias with accessory conduction pathways may be responsive to digitalis, but caution is advised: if atrial fibrillation develops in the presence of WPW, ventricular fibrillation may be precipitated. Many propose that digitalis is contraindicated with WPW.

Digitalis is certainly contraindicated in the presence of digitalis toxicity, advanced heart block (ie, second- or third-degree), and ventricular arrhythmia. Digitalis may exacerbate angina not associated with cardiomegaly and cardiac failure. Likewise, inotropic activity is usually detrimental in idiopathic hypertrophic subaortic stenosis unless overt congestive failure is present.

Dosage of Digitalis Glycosides Dosing of digitalis glycosides depends on the intended purpose and the urgency for their effects. In general, the inotropic effects of digitalis are seen at lower levels, in contrast to the chronotropic effect. Patients with atrial fibrillation, in whom digitalis is being used to control the ventricular rate, tolerate doses above the normal. Thus, the initial doses for achieving these two different effects will vary.

Rapid development of congestive heart failure necessitates acute digitalization, which can be accomplished within 24 hours (see Table 7-1). In contrast, the patient in whom heart failure insidiously develops is usually not a candidate for rapid digitalization and can be given maintenance therapy. The time to reach steady state in this situation is dependent on the half-life of the digitalis glycoside selected. Digitalization can be achieved within seven days of maintenance therapy with digoxin or within a month with digitoxin.

The usual digitalizing doses for digoxin and digitoxin are provided in Table 7-1, along with the recommended maintenance doses. It should be noted that the optimum doses for an individual patient may vary from those listed. For example, elderly patients tolerate less digoxin because of reduced renal function and a smaller lean body mass.[88] Patients with myocardial infarction, cardiomyopathy, myxedema, and other diseases that directly affect heart muscle should receive lower doses of digitalis glycosides, because their sensitivity to it may be increased. Hypoxia and cor pulmonale with attendant changes in blood pH also require caution for similar reasons. Smaller doses are suggested together with primary attention to treating the pulmonary problem.

Because excretion is primarily via the kidneys, digoxin doses must be adjusted in renal insufficiency.[89] Digitoxin is less dependent upon kidney function, and some have considered it the drug of choice in renal insufficiency.[36] However, the increased conversion of digitoxin to cardioactive metabolites in renal failure adds an unpredictable variable.[90] The case for digoxin selection for patients with decreased creatinine clearance can be made on the basis of the predictable effects of renal function on drug elimination and dosing.[45]

ROLE OF DIGITALIS IN THE MAN-AGEMENT OF CONGESTIVE HEART FAILURE Digitalis is effective in heart failure of many etiologies, including acquired valvular regurgitation, congenital heart disease with volume overload, coronary artery disease, cor pulmonale, nonobstructive cardiomyopathy, and systemic hypertension. The benefit of digitalis therapy results from increased cardiac contractility. Increased cardiac output, improved New York Heart Association functional class, and better exercise tolerance have been documented following digitalization. The major limitation of digitalis is its potential for drug toxicity, but this is effectively minimized by application of basic pharmacokinetic principles and judicious monitoring of serum concentrations.

A second limitation of digitalis therapy is the lack of evidence supporting prolonged survival. Reports of successful digitalis weaning in clinically stable patients with normal sinus rhythm have led investigators to question the value of digitalis in maintenance treatment. Objective evidence of deterioration has been noted upon digitalis withdrawal even though symptomatic evidence of inotropic deterioration was not obvious. Reevaluation of patients is certainly advisable, but discontinuation of digitalis should be approached with caution and with careful follow-up. The report by Arnold et al[6] certainly demonstrates continued benefit to patients with normal sinus rhythm and chronic heart failure over time.

In the future, innovative "physiologic" approaches to the management of heart failure with vasodilators, converting-enzyme inhibitors, and more potent inotropic agents may replace traditional digitalis therapy. However, at present, digitalis is first-line therapy for the majority of patients with a failing myocardium. When a case becomes refractory to the beneficial effects of digitalis or more severe pump failure develops, these newer drugs offer adjunctive therapy of great benefit.

DIURETICS IN CONGESTIVE HEART FAILURE

Rationale for Use and Expected Benefits

In congestive heart failure, the failing myocardium is unable to maintain adequate cardiac output. The kidney responds to this relative hypoperfusion by retaining salt and water by one or more of several mechanisms (eg, increased proximal tubular sodium reabsorption due to the increased filtration fraction, redistribution of renal blood flow from the cortex to the salt-conserving medulla, and/or activation of the renin-angiotensin system with elevation of aldosterone; see Chap. 4). Renal conservation of salt and water results in expansion of the extracellular volume and increased left ventricular end-diastolic pressure (preload). If the dilated heart has not achieved its plateau within the Starling curve, then the increased fiber length permits maintenance of cardiac output. Otherwise, the increased preload worsens the symptoms of congestive heart failure.[91-94]

Diuretics are used in congestive heart failure to reverse these physiologic imbalances. By inhibiting solute reabsorption in the renal tubule, diuretics restore salt and water elimination. Some diuretics (eg, furosemide, ethacrynic acid, bumetanide) may enhance renal blood flow and shift the balance toward the renal cortex, which lessens salt conservation.[93] Diuretics, however, have no direct effect upon the intrinsic myocardial activity of the failing myocardium.[34]

The beneficial effects of diuretics are illustrated on the Starling curve (see Fig. 7-1). In patients who have exceeded the plateau phase of the pressure-output curve, diuretic-induced relief of systemic or pulmonary congestion reduces intracardiac filling pressure (preload) and permits reascent along the descending right side of the curve. Cardiac output is thus increased by a reduction in preload in this subset of patients. In contrast, cardiac output is decreased by diuresis in patients on the left side of the plateau.[95]

Recently, this traditional concept of the relationship between diuretics and the Starling curve has been challenged, because the descending limb (right side) of the Starling curve is not detected in canine studies. If the left ventricular filling pressure is mechanically depressed in patients (by decreasing venous return), then cardiac output is decreased instead of increased. Neither acute intravenous nor maintenance oral furosemide consistently improved cardiac output in open studies of patients with chronic heart failure (Table 7-6). As an alternative, Wilson et al[96] proposed that any improvement in cardiac output associated with diuretic therapy is caused by afterload rather than preload reduction.

Overview of Clinical Effectiveness
Acute administration of diuretics is associated with symptomatic improvement of untreated congestive cardiac failure of variable severity. This is documented in both open and controlled trials.[92,93,97-104] Diuretic therapy decreases dyspnea on exertion, orthopnea, paroxysmal nocturnal dyspnea, cough, and peripheral edema. Objective signs of improvement include increased urine volume and decreased weight, abdominal girth, neck vein distension, pulmonary rales, and S_3 gallop. Reductions in hepatomegaly and hepatojugular reflux are not as consistently reported as alleviation of other signs of failure. Improved exercise tolerance is achieved in some patients.[92]

Diuretics are also effective in certain cases of refractory heart failure. Intravenous furosemide is beneficial for the emergency treatment of pulmonary edema. The addition of a diuretic active at a more distal site in the nephron (eg, thiazide, metolazone) often promotes further diuresis by preventing distal sodium reabsorption. The use of spironolactone enhances diuresis in refractory edema associated with hyperaldosteronism.[38] Intermittent acetazolamide may promote additional weight loss in the normokalemic, hypochloremic, alkalotic resistance associated with maintenance furosemide and spironolactone.[105]

Hemodynamic Effect of Diuretics
Hemodynamic studies have clarified the effect of diuresis on congestive heart failure (Table 7-6). Both acute (single-dose intravenous) and chronic (oral for eight days) administration of furosemide reduced preload as measured by pulmonary capillary wedge pressure (range: 12% to 32%) and mean pulmonary artery pressure (range: 0% to 35%). Minimal improvement in overall cardiac output occurred as predicted by the Starling curve.[95] In an investigation of a subset of patients with improved cardiac output, Wilson et al[96] reported that increased stroke volume correlated with decreased systemic vascular resistance. Franciosa and Silverstein[106] also noted that improved cardiac output was associated with reduced blood pressure. It appears that diuretics are capable of enhancing cardiac output only when afterload reduction is feasible; the reproducible decrease in preload does not necessarily improve cardiac performance.

The mechanism of diuretic-induced hemodynamic changes has been evaluated by assessing hemodynamic parameters at five-minute intervals after intravenous furosemide. Left ventricular filling pressure was decreased (27%) and calf venous capacitance was increased (52%) within five minutes after furosemide 0.5 to 1 mg/kg intravenously. These hemodynamic changes preceded peak urine flow (30 minutes) and natriuresis (60 minutes), so diuresis could not account for these hemodynamic changes. The initial response appears to be due to either direct vasodilation and/or peripheral venous pooling, with diuresis further enhancing the response at 30 to 60 minutes.[107] These early extrarenal effects probably contribute to the

Doherty

Table 7-6. Summary of studies assessing hemodynamic effects of furosemide in patients with congestive heart failure

Reference	Number of Patients	Study Design	Daily Dose and Route	Duration of Therapy	Other Drugs	Results*
Biddle and Yu[138]	14	Open, controlled, (5 untreated patients)	0.5 mg/kg IV	Single dose	Oxygen, lidocaine	HR, CI, SWI, no △ PAP ↓ 19% RAP ↓ 34% PCWP ↓ 25%
Dikshit et al[107]	20	Open	0.5-1 mg/kg IV	Single dose	Oxygen, lidocaine	HR, CI, no △ TVR ↓ 20% PCWP ↓ 27% RAP ↓ 14%
Franciosa and Silverstein[106]	13	Open	200 mg IV	Single dose	Digoxin	HR, CI, SV, MPAP, MAP, TRV, no △ PCWP ↓ 12% RAP ↓ 12%
Ikram et al[111]	10	Open	1 mg/kg IV	Single dose	Digoxin	CO ↓ 8% MPAP ↓ 35%
	4	Open	80-240 mg PO	8-10 days	Digoxin	CO, MPAP, no△; then ↓CO, ↓MPAP
Wilson et al[96]	13	Open	†	8 days	Digoxin, thiazides, metolazone	CO, no △ HR ↓ 12% SR ↓ 16% TVR ↓ 13% PCWP ↓ 32% RAP ↓ 40%

*HR = heart rate; CI = cardiac index; SV = stroke volume; SWI = stroke work index; MAP = mean arterial pressure; TVR = total vascular resistance; PCWP = pulmonary capillary wedge pressure; MPAP = mean pulmonary arterial pressure; no △ = no change.
†Patients received diuretics until peripheral edema was absent; catheterization was performed after withholding diuretics for 18 hours.

immediate relief of the symptoms of pulmonary edema by increasing venous capacitance and decreasing mean pulmonary arterial pressure.[108]

Failure to predictably improve cardiac output is a major limitation of diuretics in the management of heart failure. Although effective in relieving the symptoms of congestion, diuretics have no direct effect upon the failing myocardium.[38] Furthermore, diuretic-induced hemodynamic changes are likely to worsen cardiac output[109] unless, as discussed previously, afterload reduction is feasible.

As diuretic agents stimulate diuresis, they provoke regulatory processes that tend to counterbalance their effect, so the response in the intact body is less than predicted. For example, the contraction in plasma volume and resultant decreased cardiac output cause a decline in renal blood flow and glomerular filtration rate, which reduces the effect of diuresis.[109] Renal blood flow is suppressed more than glomerular filtration so that the filtration fraction is increased. This is associated with elevated oncotic pressure within the peritubular space and enhanced sodium reabsorption proximal to the site of action of diuretics.[110] After four to six days of diuresis, the renin-angiotensin-aldosterone system may be activated with gradual elevation of plasma aldosterone. Not only is diuretic-induced sodium elimination inhibited, but peripheral resistance is increased by angiotensin-II, which results in further deterioration of cardiac output.[111]

PHYSIOLOGY OF DIURESIS The sodium that is presented to the kidney for disposition per unit time is called the filtered load. This is the product of glomerular filtration rate and the plasma level of sodium. Alterations in the filtered load are partially compensated by variation in amount of sodium reabsorbed.[112] In most clinical circumstances, the plasma sodium is only slightly changed, and the variation in excretion is related to changes in glomerular filtration rate and renal blood flow.

Sodium transport is also regulated by aldosterone, which promotes reabsorption of sodium from the distal tubule in exchange for potassium and hydrogen ions.[113] When the kidney is underperfused, as it is with depressed cardiac output, the specialized cells of juxtaglomerular apparatus release renin into the circulation. This cleaves angiotensinogen to angiotensin-I, which is converted to angiotensin-II, which in turn stimulates the adrenal release of aldosterone.[114] Other humoral and nonhumoral factors are also important in overall renal sodium reabsorption, so a knowledge of tubular transport sites is pertinent to this discussion.

About 70% of sodium reabsorption occurs in the proximal convoluted tubule (Fig. 7-5, site 1). In this segment, transport depends on active, energy-requiring reabsorption of sodium, which is accompanied either by chloride or by the secretion of hydrogen into the tubular contents, allowing reconstitution of bicarbonate (Fig. 7-5, site 1b).[115] Because this is the major site for sodium, chloride, and bicarbonate transport in the entire tubule system, small changes in reabsorption result in significant changes in ion and fluid transport.[115]

The next site of importance is the thick ascending portion of the loop of Henle (Fig. 7-5, site 2). Chloride is actively transported and sodium passively follows, resulting in sodium chloride reabsorption. This

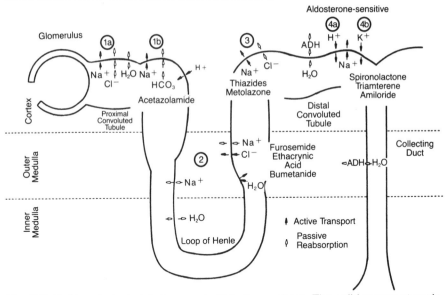

Fig. 7-5. Fluid and electrolyte transport within the nephron. The solid arrows at each locus indicate the actively transported moiety; the open arrows, passive reabsorption. Major sites of action of diuretics are shown. (Adapted from Puschett[137] with permission.)

segment is impermeable to water and thus produces dilute tubular fluid. This portion of the nephron unit receives 30% of filtered sodium load and is capable of reabsorbing up to 50% to 65% of delivered sodium. When urine reaches the early part of the distal convoluted tubule, reabsorption of another 5% to 10% of sodium occurs (Fig. 7-5, site 3).[116]

Activity within the distal convoluted tubule and collecting duct is partially dependent on antidiuretic hormone. When antidiuretic hormone is present, tubular fluid is extracted; when absent or suppressed, both distal convoluted tubule and collecting duct are impermeable to water. The favorable osmotic gradient for the reabsorption of fluid is related to salt and urea transport from the loop and to the normal countercurrent system that provides a hypertonic medullary interstitium.[117]

In the late distal convolution area, and perhaps in the collecting duct, sodium is reabsorbed in exchange for hydrogen and potassium (Fig. 7-5, site 4). This area is regulated by aldosterone (site 4a), although some ionic transfer is independent of its hormone action (site 4b). Only a small amount of sodium (3%) is reabsorbed from this site.

Thiazides   Thiazide diuretics, including chlorthalidone, exert their primary action at the early part of the distal convoluted tubule and possess insignificant carbonic anhydrase activity (Fig. 7-5). Thiazides inhibit sodium reabsorption and evoke potassium secretion. They cause moderate diuresis that is independent of acid-base status (Table 7-7).[118] All thiazides produce similar qualitative and quantitative diuresis but differ in pharmacokinetic properties and dosing regimens. Thiazide diuretics have achieved a prominent place in the management of heart failure, due to convenience of administration and an excellent safety profile. It should be noted that thiazides are not

Table 7-7. Dosage and pharmacokinetic characteristics of diuretics

Drug*	Site of Action†	% Maximum Fractional Na⁺ Excretion‡	Usual Dosage (mg/d)	Onset (h)	Peak (h)	Duration (h)	Most Frequent Complications
Acetazolamide	1	4	250-375	1	2-4	8	Hypokalemia, acidosis, urinary tract calculi, hepatic coma
Amiloride	4	2	5-10	2	4-8	12-24	Hyperkalemia, azotemia
Bumetanide	2,3	23	1-2	1	1-2	4	Hyperuricemia, hypokalemia, alkalosis, deafness, hepatic coma
Chlorothiazide	3	8	500-1,000			6-12	Hyperuricemia, hypokalemia, alkalosis, glucose intolerance, vasculitis, pancreatitis, hepatic coma
Chlorthalidone	3	8	25-100	2	6	24-48	See chlorothiazide
Ethacrynic acid	2,3	23	50-100	0.5 PO 0.25 IV	1-2 0.75	6-8 3	Hyperuricemia, hypokalemia, alkalosis, hyper- and hypoglycemia, gastrointestinal bleeding, deafness, hepatic coma
Furosemide	2,3	23	40-120	1 PO 5 min IV	1-2 0.5	6 2	Hyperuricemia, hypokalemia, alkalosis, glucose intolerance, deafness, hepatic coma
Hydrochlorothiazide	3	8	50-100	2	4	12-18	See chlorothiazide
Metolazone	3	8	5-10	1	2-4	24-48	See chlorothiazide
Spironolactone	4	2	25-200	Gradual	24-48	48-72 after cessation	Hyperkalemia, gynecomastia, acidosis
Triamterene	4	2	100-300	2	6-8	12-16	Hyperkalemia, azotemia, muscle cramps

*Specific manufacturer's package inserts should be consulted before prescribing.
†See Figure 7-5.
‡A measure of effectiveness.

effective in producing a diuresis in patients with moderate renal disease (creatinine clearance < 30 mL/min).[119]

Metolazone is a quinethazone derivative that prevents the reabsorption of sodium at the same site as the thiazides and produces a similar moderate diuresis. In contrast to thiazides, the diuretic effect of metolazone is not affected by declining renal function.[120]

Loop Diuretics   Loop diuretics inhibit chloride transport in the thick ascending loop of Henle and are, therefore, predictably potent diuretics (see Fig. 7-5). At equivalent doses, these agents (furosemide, 40 mg; ethacrynic acid, 50 mg; bumetanide 1 mg) are capable of increasing the fractional sodium excretion by more than 20% (Table 7-7).[98] An indirect result of inhibition of chloride transport within the thick ascending limb is disruption of the gradient, which usually permits passive removal of water from the descending limb at the loop of Henle and medullary collecting duct. This results in increased clearance of free water, whereas other diuretics decrease free water clearance.[116] Loop diuretics also increase the concentration of prostaglandin metabolites in the urine, and their effects are blunted by administration of prostaglandin inhibitors, which suggests a partial action mediated by the prostaglandin system.[121,122] These agents are not affected by the acid-base status or by renal impairment.

Patients with congestive heart failure often become refractory to loop diuretics. Studies show that the response to loop diuretics depends upon the concentration of drug reaching the urine, the time course of its entry into urine, and its pharmacodynamic effect at the loop of Henle.[123] Oral absorption is delayed in patients with bowel edema or intestinal hypoperfusion. Reduced tubular responsiveness to diuretics is observed in some patients. This usually responds to afterload reduction. Frequent dosing or continuous intravenous infusions of furosemide have been advocated as ways to overcome diuretic resistance.[123] Furosemide infusions at rates of 0.25 to 0.75 mg/kg/h produce adequate diuresis in patients who fail to respond to bolus administration.[124]

Potassium-Sparing Diuretics   Spironolactone is a competitive inhibitor of aldosterone and is dependent upon the presence of aldosterone to exert an effect (see Fig. 7-5). Mild diuresis follows administration to patients with heart failure; the effect is enhanced when spironolactone is administered in combination with thiazides or loop diuretics (Table 7-7). Its major benefit is a reduction in the potassium loss associated with these latter agents. The onset of action may take up to 72 hours.

Triamterene and amiloride exert a mild diuretic and anti-kaliuretic effect by blocking a site in the distal convoluted tubule responsible for sodium, potassium, and hydrogen exchange that is independent of the influence of aldosterone (see Fig. 7-5). These agents are more rapid acting, producing an effect within eight hours. As with spironolactone, they are useful in combination with other diuretics for the purpose of diminishing potassium loss.

COMPLICA- TIONS OF DIURETIC THERAPY
When distal tubular delivery of sodium and water occurs during diuretic treatment, potassium and hydrogen ions are also secreted. This results in the generation of bicarbonate and, together with contraction of extracellular fluid volume and increased bicarbonate absorption, leads to hypokalemic metabolic alkalosis. This "contraction" or hypokalemic alkalosis responds to reduction in diuretic dose, reexpansion of extracellular fluid volume, and/or administration of potassium chloride.[125,126] Supplementary use of potassium chloride is often necessary to avoid this complication, which is the most commonly encountered problem in the diuretic treatment of congestive heart failure. Excessive potassium (and magnesium) loss associated with diuresis may lead to serious cardiac rhythm disturbances.

Metabolic acidosis may occur with the use of acetazolamide. Spironolactone, through its antagonizing action on aldosterone, may result in hyperchloremic metabolic acidosis.[127]

Hyponatremia, also a significant complication of diuretic therapy, results from an imbalance between water intake and renal diluting capacity. Furosemide and ethacrynic acid inhibit free water generation and cause excretion of concentrated urine.[128] Bumetanide shares this characteristic. Potassium depletion may also predispose to hyponatremia by enhancing antidiuretic hormone secretion and by causing sodium to move into cells to replace potassium. Total body sodium remains normal or may even be increased in patients with heart failure who are receiving diuretics; therefore, restriction of water intake below external and sensible loss (1,000 mL/d) will suffice to increase the serum sodium concentration. Temporarily stopping diuretics and improving cardiac function through inotropic agents or removal of precipitating causes are also very useful measures. Except for patients with hyponatremia, water restriction has little place in the management of congestive heart failure.

Hyperuricemia is common during chronic administration of thiazide, furosemide, ethacrynic acid, or bumetanide therapy. It is seldom a problem and usually requires no treatment.[129] Should gout develop, allopurinol may be employed with good effect.

Carbohydrate intolerance may occur in patients taking thiazides, less commonly with ethacrynic acid or furosemide. This is often not a problem but deserves attention because it may unmask latent diabetes or even lead to nonketotic hyperosmolar coma.[129]

Hearing loss, usually reversible, may be noted with intravenous and, occasionally, oral ethacrynic acid and furosemide.[130] Slow intravenous administration (over five minutes) is advised to prevent this occurrence. Bumetanide, which has a safety profile that is similar to furosemide's, does not exhibit ototoxicity. Gynecomastia, impotence, and diminished libido may be noted with spironolactone.[131] Thiazides also diminish calcium secretion and may rarely lead to hypercalcemia.

CLINICAL USE OF DIURETICS
Table 7-7 outlines the usual dose of commonly employed diuretics in congestive heart failure. Clinical monitoring of a patient with heart failure routinely requires determination of body weight. Gentle diuresis with loss of 2 to 3 lb daily is best if control of edema is desired. As a general rule,

5 to 7 lb (2 to 3 kg) of weight gain occurs before peripheral edema is noted or symptoms appear if "dry" weight is present. Less change is apparent when a patient's status is compromised. Weight gain or increased symptoms suggest the need for increased diuretic dosage or better control of sodium intake or other precipitating factors. Advising patients to weigh themselves daily and keep a diary provides a method for patients to participate in monitoring their own status. This often reinforces patient education and stresses the importance of sodium restriction. Salt intake should be about 3 g/d for successful treatment with diuretics. Severe salt restriction (500 mg daily) should not be recommended, as it is usually not achievable during outpatient management. More salt may be permitted, but it may provoke increased potassium loss, in addition to making heart failure more difficult to control.

Measurement of electrolyte concentrations should be performed when problems are encountered with heart failure or routinely every 6 to 12 weeks. Routine evaluation is important, particularly if patients are taking digitalis as well as diuretics, because potassium and magnesium deficiency may precipitate digitalis intoxication.[132,133] Urine volume reflects diuresis, and this may be a helpful monitoring parameter in hospitalized patients treated in critical care units. Usually it is unnecessary in the management of ambulatory patients.

ROLE OF DIURETIC THERAPY IN THE MANAGEMENT OF CONGESTIVE HEART FAILURE Diuretics have never occupied a more prominent place in the treatment of heart failure than they do at the present time. The question of whether one should use digitalis first or diuretics first is moot, because both are almost always used together. Diuretics are effective in cardiogenic pulmonary edema, as well as right heart failure and combined ventricular failure.[134] The effectiveness of diuretics in reducing hypervolemia has been demonstrated to establish a downward trend in the increased intravascular pressures responsible for many of the symptoms of heart failure.

Diuretics have no direct effect on cardiovascular performance and in most instances should be used together with cardiac glycosides for optimum effect.[135] In refractory states, diuretics appear to complement the effectiveness of the "unloading" vasodilators.[136] The loop diuretics are often effective in renal insufficiency and may be used in combination with metalozone or acetazolamide when a refractory state exists.[137] Intelligent use of diuretics will improve the quality of life for the patient with heart failure.

CONCLUSION The safe and effective use of diuretic agents in heart failure requires evaluation of the degree of cardiac dysfunction and knowledge of the mechanism and site of action of the diuretic agent. Recognition of potential side effects and hazardous action is essential. Mild congestive failure can usually be managed with a cardiac glycoside alone, moderate failure requires the addition of a thiazide-type agent, while severe or resistant failure often requires a loop diuretic such as furosemide and one of the unloading agents. Complications of diuretic agents often represent an exaggerated pharmacologic response, and care is necessary to prevent or counteract these problems. One should use the smallest effective dose of the appropriate diuretic and avoid the use of a powerful drug when a mild one suffices in achieving the desired therapeutic goal.

REFERENCES

1. Schwartz A, Lindenmayer GE, Allen JC: The sodium-potassium-adenosine triphosphatase: Pharmacological, physiological and biochemical aspects. *Pharmacol Rev* 1975;27:1-134.
2. Farah AE: The effects of the ionic milieu on the response of cardiac muscle to cardiac glycosides, in Fisch C, Surawicz B (eds): *Digitalis*. New York, Grune & Stratton, 1969, p 55.
3. Hoffman BF, Bigger JT: Digitalis and allied cardiac glycosides, in Gilman AG, Goodman LS, Gilman A (eds): *The Pharmacological Basis of Therapeutics*. New York, Macmillan Publishing Co, Inc, 1980, pp 729-760.
4. Katz AM: Congestive heart failure: Role of altered myocardial cellular control. *N Engl J Med* 1975;293:1184-1191.
5. Mason DT: Digitalis pharmacology and therapeutics: Recent advances. *Ann Intern Med* 1974;80:520-530.
6. Arnold SB, Byrd RC, Meister W: Long-term digitalis therapy improves left ventricular function in heart failure. *N Engl J Med* 1980;303:1443-1448.
7. Murray RG, Tweddel AC, Martin W, et al: Evaluation of digitalis in cardiac failure. *Lancet* 1982;1:1526-1528.
8. Shapiro W: Digitalis update. *Arch Intern Med* 1981;141:17-18.
9. McHaffie D, Purcell H, Mitchell-Heggs P, et al: The clinical value of digoxin in patients with heart failure and sinus rhythm. *Q J Med* 1978;47:401-449.
10. Selzer A: Digitalis in cardiac failure: Do benefits justify risks? *Arch Intern Med* 1981;141:18.
11. Dall JLC: Maintenance digoxin in elderly patients. *Br Med J* 1970;2:705-706.
12. Fonrose HA, Ahlbaum N, Bugatch E, et al: The efficacy of digitalis withdrawal in an institutional aged population. *J Am Geriatr Soc* 1974;22:208-211.
13. Griffiths BE, Penny WI, Lewis MI, et al: Maintenance of the inotropic effect of digoxin on long-term treatment. *Br Med J* 1982;284:1819-1822.
14. Hull SM, Mackintosh A: Discontinuation of maintenance digoxin therapy in general practice. *Lancet* 1977;2:1054-1055.
15. Johnson GD, McDevitt DG: Is maintenance digoxin necessary in patients with normal sinus rhythm? *Lancet* 1979;1:567-570.
16. Fleg JL, Gottlieb SH, Lakatta EG: Is digoxin really important in the treatment of compensated heart failure? A placebo-controlled crossover study in patients with normal sinus rhythm. *Am J Med* 1982;73:224-250.
17. Green LH, Smith TW: The use of digitalis in patients with pulmonary disease. *Ann Intern Med* 1977;87:459-465.
18. Mathur PN, Powles P, Pugsley SO, et al: Effect of digoxin on right ventricular function in severe chronic airflow obstruction: A controlled clinical trial. *Ann Intern Med* 1981;95:283-288.
19. Beeson PB: Withering revisited (editorial). *N Engl J Med* 1980;303:1475.
20. Ogilvie RI, Ruedy J: An educational program in digitalis therapy. *JAMA* 1972;222:50-55.
21. Withering W: An account of the foxglove; GGJ and J Robinson, London, 1785; Special Edition (Gryphon, Birmingham, Alabama 1979).
22. Luisada AA: Personal communication, 1974.
23. Beller GA, Smith TW, Abelmann WH, et al: Digitalis intoxication: A prospective clinical study with serum level correlations. *N Engl J Med* 1971;284:990-997.
24. Doherty JE: Unpublished observation, 1987.

25. Lindenbaum J: Greater bioavailability of digoxin solution in capsules. *Clin Pharmacol Ther* 1977;21:278.

26. Doherty JE, Marcus FI, Binnion PF: Multicenter evaluation of the absolute bioavailability of digoxin dosage forms. *Curr Ther Res* 1984;35:301-306.

27. Doherty JE, Perkins WH, Mitchell GK: Tritiated digoxin studies in human subjects. *Arch Intern Med* 1961;108:531-539.

28. Doherty JE, Perkins WH: Studies following intramuscular tritiated digoxin in human subjects. *Am J Cardiol* 1965;15:170-174.

29. Doherty JE, Perkins WH: Studies with tritiated digoxin in human subjects after intravenous administration. *Am Heart J* 1962;63:528-536.

30. Keys W: Digoxin, in Evans WE, Schentag JJ, Jusko WJ (eds): *Applied Pharmacokinetics: Principles of Therapeutic Drug Monitoring.* San Francisco, Applied Therapeutics Inc, 1980, pp 319-349.

31. Graves SE, Brown B, Valdes R: An endogenous digoxin-like substance in patients with renal impairment. *Ann Intern Med* 1983;99:604-608.

32. Deray G, Rieu M, Devynck MG, et al: Evidence of an endogenous digitalis-like factor in the plasma of patients with acromegaly. *N Engl J Med* 1987;316:575-580.

33. Doherty JE, Perkins WH: Digoxin metabolism in hypo- and hyperthyroidism: Studies with tritiated digoxin in thyroid disease. *Ann Intern Med* 1966;64:489.

34. Smith TW, Braunwald E: The management of heart failure, in Braunwald E (ed): *Heart Disease: A Textbook of Cardiovascular Medicine.* Philadelphia, WB Saunders, 1980, pp 509-570.

35. Perrier D, Mayersohn M, Marcus FI: Clinical pharmacokinetics of digitoxin. *Clin Pharmacokinet* 1977;2:292-311.

36. Lukas DS: Some aspects of distribution and disposition of digitoxin in man. *Ann NY Acad Sci* 1971;1979:338-361.

37. Smith TW: Digitalis toxicity: Epidemiology and clinical use of serum concentration measurements. *Am J Med* 1975;58:470-476.

38. Sloman JG, Manolas E: Cardiovascular diseases, in Avery GS (ed): *Drug Treatment.* Sydney, ADIS Press, 1980, pp 554-637.

39. Smith TW: Digitalis glycosides. *N Engl J Med* 1973;288:719-722, 942-946.

40. Lely AH, van Enter CHJ: Non-cardiac symptoms of digitalis intoxication. *Am Heart J* 1972;83:149-152.

41. Cook LS, Doherty JE, Straub KD, et al: Digoxin uptake into peripheral cardiac nerves: A possible mechanism for antiarrhythmic and toxic cardiac actions. *Am Heart J* 1981;101:58.

42. Doherty JE: Digitalis serum levels: Clinical usefulness. *Primary Cardiol* 1982;8:1-9.

43. Smith TW, Haber E: Digoxin intoxication: The relationship of clinical presentation to serum digoxin concentration. *J Clin Invest* 1970;49:2377-2386.

44. Selzer A: Role of serum digoxin assay in patient management. *J Am Coll Cardiol* 1985;5:106A-110A.

45. Doherty JE: Digitalis glycosides: Pharmacokinetics and their clinical implications. *Ann Intern Med* 1973;79:229-238.

46. Gibson D, Souton E: The use of beta-adrenergic receptor blocking drugs in dysrhythmias. *Prog Cardiovasc Dis* 1969;12:16-39.

47. Fisch C, Martz BL, Priebe FH: Enhancement of potassium-induced atrioventricular block by token doses of digitalis drugs. *J Clin Invest* 1960;39:1885-1893.

48. Bigger JT Jr, Strauss HC: Digitalis toxicity: Drug interactions promoting toxicity and the management of toxicity. *Semin Drug Treat* 1972;2:147-177.

49. Lown B, Kleiger R, Williams J: Cardioversion and digitalis drugs: Changed threshold to electric shock in digitalized animals. *Circ Res* 1966;17:519-531.

50. Mann DL, Maisel AS, Atwood JE, et al: Absence of cardioversion-induced ventricular arrhythmias in patients with therapeutic digoxin levels. *J Am Coll Cardiol* 1985;5:882-884.

51. Caldwell JH, Bush CA, Greenberger NJ: Interruption of the enterohepatic circulation of digitoxin by cholestyramine: II. Effect on metabolic disposition of tritium-labeled digitoxin and cardiac systolic intervals in man. *J Clin Invest* 1971;50:2638-2644.

52. Bazzano G, Bazzano GS: Digitalis intoxication: Treatment with a new steroid-binding resin. *JAMA* 1972;220:824-830.

53. Hall WH, Shappell SD, Doherty JE: Effect of cholestyramine on digoxin absorption and excretion in man. *Am J Cardiol* 1977;29:213-216.

54. Mofenson HC, Carccio TR, Greensher J, et al: Gastrointestinal dialysis with activated charcoal and cathartic in the treatment of adolescent intoxications. *Clin Pediatr* 1985;24:678-684.

55. Park GD, Goldberg MJ, Spector R, et al: The effects of activated charcoal on digoxin and digitoxin clearance. *Drug Intell Clin Pharm* 1985;19:937-941.

56. Ekins BR, Watanabe AS: Acute digoxin poisonings: Review of therapy. *Am J Hosp Pharm* 1978;35:268-277.

57. Smith TW, Butler VP, Haber E, et al: Treatment of life-threatening digitalis intoxication with digoxin-specific Fab antibody fragments: Experience in 26 cases. *N Engl J Med* 1982;307:1357-1362.

58. Wenger TL, Butler VP Jr, Haber E, et al: Treatment of 63 severely digitalis-toxic patients with digoxin-specific antibody fragments. *J Am Coll Cardiol* 1985;5(suppl A):118A-123A.

59. Bigger JT: The quinidine-digoxin interaction: What do we know about it? *N Engl J Med* 1981;301:779-781.

60. Doering W: Quinidine-digoxin interaction: Pharmacokinetics, underlying mechanism and clinical implications. *N Engl J Med* 1979;301:400-404.

61. Hager WD, Fenster P, Mayersohn M: Digoxin-quinidine interaction: Pharmacokinetic evaluation. *N Engl J Med* 1979;300:1238-1241.

62. Leahey EG, Reiffel JA, Giardina EGV, et al: The effect of quinidine and other oral antiarrhythmic drugs on serum digoxin: A prospective study. *Ann Intern Med* 1980;92:605-608.

63. Schenck-Gustafsson K, Jogestrand T, Nordlander R, et al: Effect of quinidine on digoxin concentration in skeletal muscle and serum in patients with atrial fibrillation: Evidence for reduced binding of digoxin in muscle. *N Engl J Med* 1981;305:209-211.

64. Fenster PE, Powell JR, Graves PE, et al: Digitoxin-quinidine interaction: Pharmacokinetic evaluation. *Ann Intern Med* 1980;93:698-701.

65. Garty M, Sood P, Rollins DE: Digitoxin elimination reduced during quinidine therapy. *Ann Intern Med* 1981;94:35-37.

66. Somberg JC, Wellins H, Maquite W, et al: Verapamil-digitalis interaction: Effect on cardiac Purkinje fibers and myocardium. *Am J Cardiol* 1982;49:1025.

67. Kounis N: Asystole after verapamil and digoxin. *Br J Clin Pract* 1980;34:57.

68. Belz GG, Aust PE, Munkes R: Digoxin plasma concentration and nifedipine (letter). *Lancet* 1981;1:844-854.

69. Belz GG, Doering W, Munkes R, et al: Interaction between digoxin and calcium antagonists and antiarrhythmic drugs. *Clin Pharmacol Ther* 1983;33:410.

70. Pedersen KE, Pedersen AD, Hvidt S, et al: Digoxin-verapamil interaction. *Clin Pharmacol Ther* 1981;30:311.

71. Klein HO, Lang R, Weiss E, et al: The influence of verapamil on serum digoxin concentration. *Circulation* 1982;65:998.

72. Klein HO, Kaplinsky E: Verapamil and digoxin: Their respective effects on atrial fibrillation and their interaction. *Am J Cardiol* 1982;50:894.

73. Bussey HI: Update on the influence of quinidine and other agents on digitalis glycosides. *Am Heart J* 1984;107:143-146.

74. Rameis H, Magometschnigg D, Ganzinger U: The diltiazem-digoxin interaction. *Clin Pharmacol Ther* 1984;36:183-189.

75. Kuhlmann J: Effects of verapamil, diltiazem, and nifedipine on plasma levels and renal excretion of digitoxin. *Clin Pharmacol Ther* 1985;38:667-673.

76. Marcus FI: Drug interactions with amiodarone. *Am Heart J* 1984;106:924-930.
77. Nademanee K, Kannan R, Hendrickson J, et al: Amiodarone-digoxin interaction: Clinical significance, time course of development, potential pharmacokinetic mechanisms and therapeutic implications. *J Am Coll Cardiol* 1984;4:111-116.
78. Ochs HR, Gugler R, Guthoff T, et al: Effect of cimetidine on digoxin kinetics and creatinine clearance. *Am Heart J* 1984;107:170-172.
79. Lee G, Peng CL, Mason DT, et al: Demonstration of linear dose-response and quantitative attenuation by potassium of inotropic action to digitalis. *Chest* 1982;62:367.
80. Johnson LW, Bickstein R, Fruehan VT, et al: Prophylactic digitalization for coronary artery bypass surgery. *Circulation* 1976;53:819-822.
81. Parker FB, Greiner-Hayes C, Bove EL, et al: Supraventricular arrhythmias following coronary bypass: The effect of preoperative digitalis. *J Thorac Cardiovasc Surg* 1983;86:594-600.
82. Weiner B, Rheinlander HF, Decker EL, et al: Digoxin prophylaxis following coronary artery bypass surgery. *Clin Pharm* 1986;5:55-58.
83. Jennings PB, Makous N, Vander Veer JB: Reversion of atrial fibrillation to sinus rhythm with digitalis therapy. *Am J Med Sci* 1985;235:702-705.
84. Weiner P, Bassan MM, Jarchovsky J, et al: Clinical course of acute atrial fibrillation treated with rapid digitalization. *Am Heart J* 1983;105:223-227.
85. Falk RH, Knowlton AA, Bernard SA, et al: Digoxin for converting recent-onset atrial fibrillation to sinus rhythm: A randomized, double-blinded trial. *Ann Intern Med* 1987;106:503-506.
86. DeCarli C, Sprouse G, LaRosa JL: Serum magnesium levels in symptomatic atrial fibrillation and their relation to rhythm control by intravenous digoxin. *Am J Cardiol* 1986;57:956-959.
87. Lang R, Klein HD, Weiss E, et al: Superiority of oral verapamil therapy to digoxin in treatment of chronic atrial fibrillation. *Chest* 1983;83:491-499.
88. Ewy GA, Kapadia GG, Yao L, et al: Digoxin metabolism in the elderly. *Circulation* 1969;39:449-453.
89. Doherty JE, Perkins WH, Wilson MC: Studies with tritiated digoxin in renal failure. *Am J Med* 1964;37:536-544.
90. Storstein L: The influence of renal function on the pharmacokinetics of digitoxin, in Storstein L (ed): *Proceedings of the International Symposium on Digitalis*. Oslo, Gyldendal Forlag, 1973, p 158.
91. Amann FW, Buhler FR: Vasodilators and diuretics: First line drugs for treatment of hypertensive heart failure. *Cardiology* 1980;65(suppl 1):78-83.
92. Hutcheon D, Nemeth E, Quinlan D: The role of furosemide alone and in combination with digoxin in relief of symptoms of congestive heart failure. *J Clin Pharmacol* 1980;20:59-68.
93. Hutcheon D, Vincent ME, Sandho RS: Clinical use of diuretics in congestive heart failure. *J Clin Pharmacol* 1981;21:668-672.
94. Porter GA: The role of diuretics in the treatment of heart failure. *JAMA* 1980;244:1614-1616.
95. Rader B, Smith WW, Berger AR, et al: Comparison of the hemodynamic effects of mercurial diuretics and digitalis in congestive heart failure. *Circulation* 1974;29:328-345.
96. Wilson JR, Reichek N, Dunkman WB, et al: Effect of diuresis on the performance of the failing left ventricle in man. *Am J Med* 1981;70:235-239.
97. Dixon DW, Barwolf-Gohlke C, Gunnar RM: Comparative efficacy and safety of bumetanide and furosemide in long-term treatment of edema due to congestive heart failure. *J Clin Pharmacol* 1981;21:680-687.
98. Handler B, Dhingra RC, Rosen KM: Bumetanide: A new diuretic. Results of clinical efficacy and safety in patients with congestive heart failure. *J Clin Pharmacol* 1981;21:691-696.
99. Konecke LL: Clinical trial of bumetanide versus furosemide in patients with congestive heart failure. *J Clin Pharmacol* 1981;21:688-690.

100. Levy B: The efficacy and safety of furosemide and a combination of spironolactone and hydrochlorothiazide in congestive heart failure. *J Clin Pharmacol* 1977;17:420-430.

101. Nomura A, Yasuda H, Minami M, et al: Effect of furosemide in congestive heart failure. *Clin Pharmacol Ther* 1981;30:177-182.

102. Smith AGE: Spironolactone in the long-term management of patients with congestive heart failure. *Curr Med Res* 1980;7:131-136.

103. Viherkoski M, Huikko M, Vajoranta K: The effect of amiloride-hydrochlorothiazide combination versus furosemide plus supplementation in the treatment of edema of cardiac origin. *Ann Clin Res* 1981;13:11-15.

104. Walker JF, Cheitlin MD, Arnold J, et al: Multiclinic evaluation of Moduretic in patients with congestive cardiac failure: Comparison with dyazide and hydrochlorothiazide plus potassium chloride. *Curr Ther Res* 1982;32:387-395.

105. Khan MI: Treatment of refractory congestive heart failure and normokalemic hypochloremic alkalosis with acetazolamide and spironolactone. *Can Med Assoc J* 1980;123:883-887.

106. Franciosa JA, Silverstein SR: Hemodynamic effects of nitroprusside and furosemide in left ventricular failure. *Clin Pharmacol Ther* 1982;32:62-69.

107. Dikshit K, Vyden JK, Forrester JS, et al: Renal and extrarenal hemodynamic effects of furosemide in congestive heart failure after myocardial infarction. *N Engl J Med* 1973;228:1087-1090.

108. Heinemann HO: Right-sided heart failure and the use of diuretics. *Am J Med* 1978;64:367-370.

109. Smith TW: Medical treatment of advanced congestive heart failure: Digitalis and diuretics, in Brawnwald E, Mock MB (eds): *Congestive Heart Failure: Current Research and Clinical Applications*. New York, Grune & Stratton, 1982, pp 261-278.

110. Brater DC: Resistance to diuretics: Emphasis on a pharmacological perspective. *Drugs* 1981;22:477-494.

111. Ikram H, Chan W, Espinar EA, et al: Haemodynamic and hormone responses to acute and chronic furosemide therapy in congestive heart failure. *Clin Sci* 1980;59:443-449.

112. Smith TW: *The Kidney: Structure and Function in Health and Disease*. Oxford, England, Oxford University Press, 1951.

113. Sharp GW, Leaf A: Effects of aldosterone and its mechanism of action on sodium transport, in Orloff J, Berliner RW (eds): *Handbook of Physiology*, Section 8: Renal Physiology. Baltimore, Williams & Wilkins, 1973, p 815.

114. Laragh JH, Sealey JE: The renin-angiotensin-aldosterone hormonal system and regulation of sodium, potassium and blood pressure homeostasis, in Orloff J, Berliner RW (eds): *Handbook of Physiology*, Section 8: Renal Physiology. Baltimore, Williams & Wilkins, 1973, p 831.

115. Pitts RF: *Physiology of the Kidney and Body Fluids*, ed 3. Chicago, Year Book Medical, 1974, p 198.

116. Burg MB: Tubular chloride transport and the mode of action of some diuretics. *Kidney Int* 1976;9:189-197.

117. Gottschalk CW, Mylie M: Micropuncture study of mammalian urinary concentrating mechanism: Evidence for countercurrent hypothesis. *Am J Physiol* 1959;196:927-936.

118. Giebisch G: Effects of diuretics on renal transport of potassium, in Martinez-Maldonato M (ed): *Methods in Pharmacology*. New York, Plenum Press, 1976, pp 121-164.

119. Reubi FC: The action and use of diuretics in renal disease, in Freidberg CK (ed): *Heart, Kidney and Electrolytes*. New York, Grune & Stratton, 1962, p 169.

120. Craswell PW, Ezzat E, Kopstein J, et al: Use of metolazone, a new diuretic, in patients with renal disease. *Nephron* 1973;12:63-73.

121. Patak RV, Mookerjee BK, Bentzel CJ, et al: Antagonism of the effects of furosemide by indomethacin in normal and hypertensive man. *Prostaglandins* 1975;10:649-659.
122. Williamson HE, Bourland WA, Marchand GR: Inhibition of ethacrynic acid-induced increase in renal blood flow by indomethacin. *Prostaglandins* 1974;8:297-301.
123. Brater DC: Resistance to loop diuretics: Why it happens and what to do about it. *Drugs* 1985;30:427-443.
124. Krasna MJ, Scott GE, Scholz PM, et al: Postoperative enhancement of urinary output in patients with acute renal failure using continuous furosemide therapy. *Chest* 1986;89:294-295.
125. Kassirer JP, Schwartz WB: Correction of metabolic alkalosis in man without repair of potassium deficiency. *Am J Med* 1966;40:19.
126. Garella S, Chazan JA, Cohen JJ: Saline-resistant metabolic alkalosis or "chloride-wasting nephropathy." *Ann Intern Med* 1970;73:31-38.
127. Manuel MA, Berne GJ, Wagnaild JT, et al: An effect of spironolactone on urinary acidification in normal man. *Arch Intern Med* 1974;134:472-474.
128. Kennedy RM, Earley LR: Profound hyponatremia resulting from thiazide-induced decrease in urinary diluting capacity in a patient with primary polydipsia. *N Engl J Med* 1970;282:1185-1186.
129. Davies DL, Wilson GM: Diuretics: Mechanism of action and clinical application. *Drugs* 1975;9:178-226.
130. Reinock HG, Stein JH: Mechanisms of action and clinical use of diuretics, in Brenner BM, Rector FC (eds): *The Kidney*, ed 2. Philadelphia, WB Saunders Co, 1982.
131. Loreaux L, Menard R, Taylor A, et al: Spironolactone and endocrine dysfunction. *Ann Intern Med* 1976;85:630-636.
132. Doherty JE: Suspicion of digitalis intoxication. *J Am Med Wom Assoc* 1978;33:191-197.
133. Sheehan J, White A: Diuretic-associated hypomagnesemia. *Engl Med J* 1982;285:1157-1159.
134. Robin ED, Cross CE, Zelis R: Pulmonary edema. *N Engl J Med* 1973;288:239-246.
135. Sodums MT, Walsh RT, O'Rourke RA: Digitalis in heart failure: Farewell to foxglove? *JAMA* 1981;242:158-160.
136. Cohn JN, Mathew KJ, Franciosa JA: Chronic vasodilator therapy in the management of cardiogenic shock and intractable left ventricular failure. *Ann Intern Med* 1974;81:777-780.
137. Puschett JB: Physiologic basis for the use of new and older diuretics in congestive heart failure. *Cardiovasc Med* 1977;2:119-134.
138. Biddle TI, Yu PN: Effect of furosemide on hemodynamic and lung water in acute pulmonary edema secondary to myocardial infarction. *Am J Cardiol* 1979;43:86-90.
139. Doherty JE: Determinants of digitalis dosage. *J Arkansas Med Soc* 1969;66:120-125.
140. Doherty JE, Hall WH, Murphy ML: New information regarding digitalis metabolism. *Chest* 1971;59:433-443.

GARY S. FRANCIS, MD

Inotropic Agents in the Management of Heart Failure

The role of nonglycoside inotropic agents in the management of congestive heart failure has become more focused since publication of the previous edition of this book. These drugs are primarily being employed in hospitalized patients who have very advanced or decompensated heart failure and need temporary inotropic support (Table 8-1). Often such patients have decompensated from a previously stable condition, or have New York Heart Association class IV congestive heart failure and are awaiting heart transplantation. They may have suffered acute myocardial infarction and need transient circulatory support, or they may be postoperative with acute heart failure related to perioperative factors.

With the exception of digitalis, inotropic agents are not widely employed to treat patients with chronic, stable heart failure. However, clinical trials with positive inotropic agents are being conducted in patients with less severe forms of heart failure. Until these results are published, inotropic agents will probably continue to be primarily used as temporary support for patients with very advanced or decompensated heart failure.

There are several reasons why newer inotropic agents are being reserved for use in more severe forms of congestive heart failure. For example, the converting-enzyme inhibitor captopril is established as clinically effective therapy for patients with class II to class III heart failure,[1] although the impact on survival in mild to moderate heart failure is still undefined. Some physicians are simply unwilling to employ experimental positive inotropic drugs in class II and class III patients when converting-enzyme inhibitors appear to be clinically efficacious. In addition, the combination vasodilator regimen of hydralazine and isosorbide dinitrate has been reported to strikingly improve survival in patients with chronic heart failure,[2] while no such trend has been observed to date with the use of oral inotropic agents.[3]

it	Mechanism	Response
	Na$^+$-K$^+$ ATPase inhibition	Increased intracellular Na$^+$, enhanced Na$^+$-Ca^{2+} exchange, increased intracellular Ca^{2+} and/or decreased Ca^{2+} efflux leading to increased Ca^{2+} availability to contractile proteins
Norepinephrine	β_1-Stimulation	Increased cyclic adenosine monophosphate (AMP), increased positive intropy
	α_1-Stimulation	Peripheral vasoconstriction
Epinephrine	β_1-Stimulation	Increased positive inotropy
	β_2-Stimulation	Peripheral vasodilation
	α_1-Stimulation	Peripheral vasoconstriction
Isoproterenol	β_1-Stimulation	Increased positive inotropy
	β_2-Stimulation	Peripheral vasodilation
Dopamine		
Low dose ($<$ 2 µg/kg/min)	DA$_1$-stimulation	Increased renal blood flow, natriuresis, vasodilation
	DA$_2$-stimulation	Reduced norepinephrine release
High dose ($\geq$ 2 µg/kg/min)	β_1-Stimulation	Increased positive inotropy
	α_1-Stimulation	Peripheral vasoconstriction
	α_2-Stimulation	Venoconstriction
Dobutamine	β_1-Stimulation	Increased positive inotropy
	β_2-Stimulation	Peripheral vasodilation
	α_1-Stimulation	Peripheral vasoconstriction (probably not clinically important)
Levodopa	Same as dopamine	Same as dopamine
Bipyridine derivatives Amrinone Milrinone	Phosphodiesterase-III inhibition	Increased cellular cyclic AMP, increased positive inotropy, peripheral vasodilation
Imidazoline derivatives Enoximone Piroximone	Phosphodiesterase-III inhibition	Increased cellular cyclic AMP, increased positive inotropy, peripheral vasodilation
Benzimidazole derivatives ARL 115 BS (sulmazole) Pimobendan	Uncertain; probably increased sensitivity of contractile proteins to Ca^{2+}; phosphodiesterase inhibition	Increased positive inotropy
OPC-8212	Unknown	Mildly increased cyclic AMP
DPI 201-106	Prolongs Na$^+$ channel activity; probably increases sensitivity of contractile proteins to Ca^{2+}	Increased positive inotropy
Glucagon Forskolin Histamine	Increase cellular cyclic AMP independent of β_1-stimulation	Increased positive inotropy, peripheral vasodilation

There are persistent concerns that chronic positive inotropy may be deleterious in the therapy of chronic heart failure.[4,5] Many of the positive inotropic agents promote down regulation of the myocardial β-adrenergic receptors during chronic use.[6] This is particularly true of partial β-agonists, and may lead to pharmacologic tolerance.

The side effect profile of some of the inotropic agents can be quite substantial, and initial enthusiasm for these drugs was tempered by negative results from two multicenter trials with oral amrinone, the first of these agents to undergo extensive clinical evaluation.[7,8] Despite these concerns, interest in the new positive inotropic agents persists[9] as there is a clear role for their use in selected patients with severe congestive heart failure. Investigators have learned a great deal about cellular mechanisms of positive inotropy from the study of these drugs. And many small, exploratory studies with inotropic agents of varying mechanisms are currently in progress.

These drugs can be conveniently grouped into one of two categories. First, inotropic drugs limited to intravenous use include the β-adrenergic agonists and amrinone, an inhibitor of cyclic nucleotide phosphodiesterase. Second, orally active inotropic drugs include four classes: digitalis, inhibitors of cyclic nucleotide phosphodiesterase, dopamine analogs, and miscellaneous agents.

INTRAVENOUS INOTROPIC AGENTS

β-Adrenergic Agonists

Norepinephrine, epinephrine, isoproterenol, dopamine, and dobutamine have been extensively studied in patients with congestive heart failure. The positive inotropic effect of these catecholamines is mainly due to stimulation of myocardial β_1-receptors.[10-14] The increased force of contraction usually occurs rapidly. In addition, an increased rate of contraction is typical of almost all positive inotropic agents, as is more rapid myocardial relaxation.

The β-adrenergic agonists are thought to increase myocardial cyclic adenosine monophosphate (AMP), which in turn leads to activation of protein kinases and to phosphorylation of several proteins (Fig. 8-1). Changes in the functional properties of the phosphorylated proteins may alter their ability to bind Ca^{2+} ions, thus altering calcium movement in the sarcoplasmic reticulum and possibly also in the sarcolemma. The net result is to increase the slow Ca^{2+} inward current during the action potential. This may be due to an increase in the number of functional Ca^{2+} channels[15] and to an increase in the probability that Ca^{2+} channels will open during depolarization.[16] The increase in Ca^{2+} via the slow inward current leads to increased Ca^{2+} release from the sarcoplasmic reticulum. β-Adrenergic agonists also increase Ca^{2+} uptake into the sarcoplasmic reticulum, so that more Ca^{2+} is available for release to contractile proteins. This increase in Ca^{2+} uptake by the sarcoplasmic reticulum may also account for the myocardial relaxant effects of the β-adrenergic agonists.

Norepinephrine: Norepinephrine has additional important α_1-adrenergic receptor agonist activity that can cause intense peripheral vasoconstriction. This is not particularly desirable in severe heart failure. The use of norepinephrine is generally restricted to frank cardiogenic shock, when restoration of blood pressure is the immediate objective.

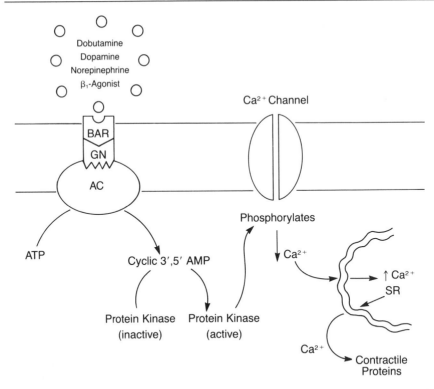

Fig. 8-1. Possible mechanisms whereby β-adrenergic agonists (ie, dobutamine, dopamine, and norepinephrine) enhance the inotropic state of the myocardium. Current evidence suggests that the β-adrenergic receptor (BAR) is a protein in the cell's surface membrane, with a molecular weight of 60,000 to 64,000. Activation of the BAR by an agonist causes the stimulatory guanine nucleotide subunit (GN) to dissociate if a guanine nucleotide is present. The activated stimulatory subunit (GN) then interacts with adenylate cyclase (AC), substantially increasing the activity of the enzyme. Adenosine triphosphate (ATP) is converted by the adenylcyclase to cyclic adenosine monophosphate (AMP), which in turn activates a number of protein kinases. The enzymes then catalyze the transfer of phosphate groups to specific sites on other intracellular proteins, including those responsible for control of the slow inward Ca^{2+} channel. This allows for more Ca^{2+} to enter the cell and enter the sarcoplasmic reticulum (SR), where it is ultimately available for contractile proteins.

Epinephrine: Epinephrine has β_1-, β_2-, and α_1-adrenergic agonist effects. Its marked chronotropic and arrhythmogenic action has greatly diminished its use for congestive heart failure. Epinephrine has, however, become the inotropic agent of choice for the management of cardiac arrest.

Isoproterenol: Isoproterenol has β_1- and β_2-adrenergic properties. Its use is limited by the occurrence of tachycardia, vasodilation (β_2), and ventricular arrhythmias.

Dopamine: Dopamine and dobutamine are the most widely used intravenous β-adrenergic agonists for treatment of severe, decompensated congestive heart failure. Dopamine is a natural, endogenous precursor of norepinephrine. Introduced into clinical practice in the early 1970s, it is frequently used as a cardiac stimulant to treat severe heart failure and cardiogenic shock.[17] Dopamine's positive inotropic effects are principally due to stimulation of cardiac β-adrenergic receptors.

In low doses (< 2 μg/kg/min), dopamine activates vascular dopaminergic (DA_1) receptors, which subserve vasodilatation in the renal, mesenteric, coronary, and cerebral circulations.[18,19] Dopamine can thereby improve renal blood flow when employed in low doses in patients with heart failure. It is natriuretic in doses of less than 0.5 μg/kg/min.[20,21] The mechanism of the natriuresis may be related to redistribution of renal blood flow or result from a direct effect on the tubules.[18] DA_2-receptors are also activated at low dose, which subserves inhibition of norepinephrine release from sympathetic neurons.

Higher doses of dopamine activate β-adrenergic receptors to increase contractility and heart rate. High-dose dopamine stimulates α_1- (peripheral arteriolar constriction) and α_2- (venoconstriction) adrenergic receptors and releases endogenous norepinephrine.

Dopamine was compared with norepinephrine and isoproterenol in early studies of patients with severe left ventricular failure or shock.[22,23] More recently, dopamine has been compared with dobutamine.[24-26] Dopamine and dobutamine have distinctly different hemodynamic profiles (Fig. 8-2). Although both drugs augment stroke volume, dopamine has important peripheral vasoconstrictor properties mediated by α_1-adrenergic receptors, particularly at doses greater than 4 μg/kg/min. This is useful when restoration of blood pressure is of immediate concern. Larger doses of dopamine (5 to 20 μg/kg/min) tend to cause a greater increase in pulmonary

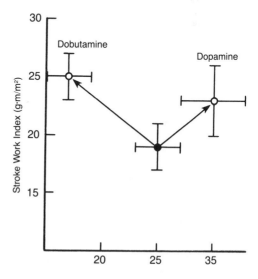

Fig. 8-2. The effect of dobutamine and high-dose dopamine on stroke work index and left ventricular filling pressure in patients with advanced heart failure. (Adapted from HS Loeb, J Bredakis, RM Gunnar, Superiority of dobutamine over dopamine for augmentation of cardiac output in patients with chronic low output cardiac failure, *Circulation* 1977;55:375-381, by permission of the American Heart Association, Inc.)

Left Ventricular Filling Pressure (mm Hg)

capillary wedge pressure than is seen with dobutamine. This may be due to α_2-adrenergically mediated venoconstriction. Once blood pressure is restored, nitroprusside can be added to dopamine therapy to lower pulmonary capillary wedge pressure and further augment cardiac output. Nitroprusside combined with dopamine can effect a greater increase in cardiac output than either agent alone (Fig. 8-3).[27,28]

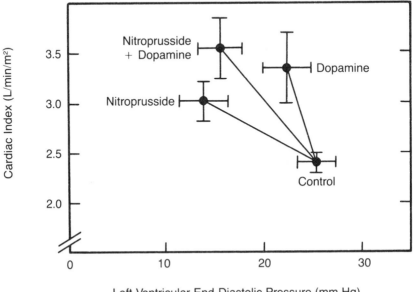

Left Ventricular End-Diastolic Pressure (mm Hg)

Fig. 8-3. The effect of nitroprusside and dopamine, alone and in combination, on left ventricular end-diastolic pressure and cardiac index in patients with advanced heart failure. (Adapted from RR Miller, NA Awan, JE Joye, Combined dopamine and nitroprusside therapy in congestive heart failure: Greater augmentation of cardiac performance by addition of inotropic stimulation to afterload reduction, *Circulation* 1977;55:881-884, by permission of the American Heart Association, Inc.)

Because dopamine can produce an increase in pulmonary capillary wedge pressure in high doses (> 2 μg/kg/min), it is usually employed in low doses to achieve a positive inotropic response in patients with chronic low-output heart failure. Small doses (< 2 μg/kg/min) may be used to increase urine output. At these doses, dopamine appears to be a more potent renal artery vasodilator than converting-enzyme inhibitor therapy.[29] High doses are used in cardiogenic shock. Shock remains the primary indication for high-dose dopamine, where it is the agent of choice for immediate restoration of circulatory integrity. However, high doses of dopamine (10 to 20 μg/kg/min) can cause tachycardia, arrhythmias, and myocardial ischemia. Coronary artery spasm has also been reported with dopamine.[30]

Dobutamine: Dobutamine was introduced into practice in 1978. It exerts potent positive inotropic β_1-adrenergic activity and has less effect on vascular tone than dopamine. It generally produces less heart rate response than dopamine at equivalent doses.[26] Unlike dopamine, dobutamine does not stimulate DA_1-vascular receptors and does not release endogenous norepinephrine. Dobutamine is a racemic mixture of l- and d-isomers, which have different pharmacologic actions.[31] The l-isomer is a potent α_1-adrenergic agonist, but this is offset by the β_1- and β_2-agonist properties of the d-isomer.

The cumulative effect of dobutamine is to increase stroke volume and heart rate. It should not be employed in cardiogenic shock because it has no pressor activity and can only increase blood pressure via an increase in stroke volume.[26] Increasing blood pressure by increasing stroke volume fails to increase diastolic pressure, which is, of course, critical to the perfusion of the ischemic myocardium. Occasionally, dobutamine and dopamine are combined to produce an augmented positive state.[32]

Dobutamine, like nitroprusside, markedly increases stroke volume.[33] Compared with nitroprusside, however, dobutamine has less effect on the lowering of pulmonary capillary wedge pressure (Fig. 8-4), and tends to increase myocardial oxygen consumption by 30% at clinically relevant doses.[34] Dobutamine and nitroprusside in combination result in a higher cardiac output and lower pulmonary wedge pressure than either drug alone.[35]

Dobutamine is widely used to treat severe, chronic congestive heart failure.[36] Long-term (72-hour) infusions can lead to tolerance,[37] but intermittent infusions have been used to maintain clinical improvement.[38-42] This persistent clinical improvement may be related to an increase in the size of myocardial mitochondria observed on myocardial biopsy.[43] Preliminary data, however, indicate that chronic, intermittent, ambulatory dobutamine infusions are only partially successful in improving symptoms and probably do not prolong survival.[44] This form of intermittent infusion therapy is still

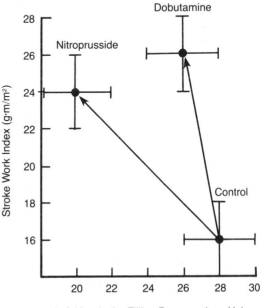

Fig. 8-4. The effect of nitroprusside and dobutamine on stroke work index and left ventricular filling pressure in patients with advanced heart failure. (Adapted from C Berkowitz, L McKeever, RP Croke, et al, Comparative responses to dobutamine and nitroprusside in patients with chronic low output cardiac failure, *Circulation* 1977;56:918-924, by permission of the American Heart Association, Inc.)

being employed in selected patients in some medical centers; but, currently, dobutamine is primarily employed in intensive care units to treat patients with severe heart failure that is refractory to more conventional oral therapy. Short-term infusions may occasionally result in modestly prolonged clinical improvement. The usual dosage is 3 to 20 μg/kg/min.

Amrinone   The selective phosphodiesterase inhibitors are new non-glycoside, noncatecholamine cardiotonic agents, which were developed during the late 1970s and early 1980s (Table 8-2). They demonstrate both vasodilator and positive inotropic properties. Although these drugs are structurally quite dissimilar, they all appear to act by increasing cellular cyclic AMP concentration, presumably by relatively selective inhibition of cyclic nucleotide phosphodiesterase-III (PDE-III).

Table 8-2. Phosphodiesterase-III inhibitors

Amrinone

Milrinone

MDL 17,043 (enoximone)

MDL 19,205 (piroximone)

RO 13-6438

D 13625

Berberine

CI-914

Of the new phosphodiesterase inhibitors, to date only amrinone is approved by the Food and Drug Administration for short-term intravenous use in patients with heart failure. The role of amrinone in patients with severe heart failure is still evolving, but it appears to be most useful in selected patients who do not respond to β-adrenergic agents (eg, dobutamine) because of tolerance (presumably due to reduced β-adrenergic receptor density), or in patients who do not tolerate nitroprusside. A prolonged infusion of amrinone may produce sustained improvement, whereas the effectiveness of dobutamine tends to decrease over time.[45] Because they work via different cellular mechanisms, amrinone and dobutamine may occasionally be combined to produce additive improvement in left ventricular performance.[46]

Amrinone is a bipyridine derivative with potent vasodilator and inotropic properties. The increase in myocardial cyclic AMP prompted by PDE-III inhibition increases peak developed tension, maximal rate of tension development, and maximal rate of relaxation.[47] Intravenous amrinone given to patients with heart failure results in a marked increase in cardiac output and a modest reduction in left ventricular filling pressure. Its hemodynamic profile is similar to that of dobutamine,[48] but the improvement may occur with less myocardial oxygen demand. This diminished oxygen demand is probably due to the potent peripheral vasodilator effect of amrinone, which contributes to improved left ventricular performance with little or no oxygen expenditure.[49] As expected of any agent that increases cellular cyclic AMP concentration, amrinone enhances atrioventricular (AV) nodal conduction[50] and has the potential to produce ventricular arrhythmias. Heart rate and blood pressure are not greatly affected by conventional doses of amrinone, but high doses can produce tachycardia and hypotension.

Therapy should be initiated with a 0.75 mg/kg bolus given slowly over two to three minutes, and maintained at 5 to 10 μg/kg/min, with titration of the infusion according to the patient's clinical and hemodynamic response. The total daily dose, including boluses, should not exceed 10 mg/kg. Invasive hemodynamic monitoring is required during administration of amrinone. Like other preload-reducing agents, it may produce no change or even a reduction in cardiac output in patients with normal or low left ventricular filling pressure and should be used with great care in this setting.[51]

ORAL INOTROPIC AGENTS

Commercial and clinical development of the newer oral inotropic agents has been slow and sometimes disappointing. Yet, as heart transplantation becomes more common, there appears to be a definite need to develop such therapy to help bridge the gap between severely decompensated heart failure and the uncertain timing of the availability of a new heart for transplantation.

An additional impetus to the development of synthetic oral inotropic drugs are the three million patients in the United States with heart failure and 250,000 new cases that are diagnosed each year. Digitalis use is limited by specific and well-known toxic effects that occur after a modest increase in inotropic response. The new inotropic agents are much more potent and generate considerably more positive contractile forces before toxic effects ensue, but it is not certain whether the new, more potent oral inotropic agents will be widely applied as therapy for patients with heart failure. There is a growing concern that agents producing markedly increased contractile forces may be detrimental; however, definitive support for this concept is lacking.

Digitalis

Digitalis is the only oral inotropic agent approved by the Food and Drug Administration for use in patients with congestive heart failure. A detailed discussion of its use is presented in Chapter 7.

Phospho-diesterase Inhibitors

Milrinone: Milrinone is a new and potent bipyridine derivative.[52] Like amrinone and other PDE-III inhibitors, it has both vasodilator and positive inotropic properties. It is better tolerated than amrinone, and can be given intravenously or orally. Milrinone is about 15 times more potent than amrinone on a per milligram basis.

Compared with dobutamine, intravenous milrinone decreases left ventricular filling pressure to a greater extent, while both drugs increase cardiac output to the same degree.[53] Milrinone reduces arterial pressure when used intravenously in patients with heart failure.[53] This may limit its use in severely ill patients. As with amrinone, there is less myocardial oxygen demand with milrinone compared with β-adrenergic agonists, presumably because of its important vasodilator property.

Oral milrinone[54] and amrinone[55] reportedly increase maximal exercise capacity in patients with heart failure. Milrinone improved maximal oxygen consumption (from 9.0 ± 1.9 to 11.6 ± 2.5 mL/kg/min) after four weeks of therapy in an open study of 11 patients.[54] A subsequent placebo-controlled trial failed to confirm this observation, but the number of patients studied was too small to permit firm conclusions.[56] In a placebo-controlled trial, intravenous milrinone acutely improved peak oxygen consumption (12.4 ± 0.7 vs 10.8 ± 0.6 mL/kg/min) and anaerobic threshold.[57] Of interest, withdrawal of chronic milrinone therapy can precipitate hemodynamic deterioration.[54,58] Chronic oral milrinone therapy appears to improve functional status in some patients with advanced heart failure,[3,59] but fluid retention frequently develops, requiring increased doses of diuretics. The results of a multicenter, randomized, placebo-controlled trial of oral milrinone will be of great importance in determining the eventual utility of this agent.

Dose ranges for both the intravenous and oral forms of milrinone are not well defined. Typically, milrinone is given intravenously as a 25-μg/kg bolus over one minute, with subsequent infusion rates of 100 to 400 μg/min resulting in systemic drug levels of 100 to 400 ng/mL. Oral therapy is begun at 5 to 7.5 mg every four to six hours, with an average daily dose of 50 mg. Milrinone has a half-life of approximately two hours; it is excreted by the kidney and should be used in reduced amounts in patients with renal impairment.

Enoximone (MDL 17,043) and Piroximone (MDL 19,205): The inotropic properties of the imidazoles, for example, enoximone[60] and piroximone,[61] have been known since at least 1973.[62] Both agents are PDE-III inhibitors. They have important vasodilator and inotropic properties and exert hemodynamic effects that are similar to those of dobutamine. Piroximone is five to ten times more potent than enoximone on a per milligram basis.

Intravenous preparations of enoximone and piroximone produce substantial short-term improvement in cardiac output and reduction in left ventricular filling pressure. Results of long-term clinical trials with the oral agents have been disappointing, with side effects and apparent tolerance playing a major limiting role.[63,64] Occasionally patients do, however, clinically respond to oral piroximone and demonstrate sustained improvement. More clinical experience with these agents is needed in the context of a controlled, randomized trial.

Other Phosphodiesterase Inhibitors: New PDE-III inhibitors have been developed in recent years (see Table 8-1). All of them appear to produce short-term beneficial hemodynamic responses, but have either failed to demonstrate long-term efficacy or lack data regarding long-term efficacy. More experience with these drugs will be required in order to define their role in the clinical treatment of heart failure.

Dopamine Analogs

Levodopa: Levodopa, which is pharmacologically inert, is converted to dopamine via aromatic amino acid decarboxylase after ingestion. It has been successfully used to treat patients with congestive heart failure.[65] Dopamine acts directly on myocardial β_1-adrenergic receptors to increase myocardial contractility. Some of the hemodynamic improvement observed with levodopa may also be due to activation of vascular DA_1-receptors (which subserve vasodilation in specific vascular beds) and presynaptic neuronal DA_2-receptors (which subserve inhibition of norepinephrine release).[66]

The principal side effects (nausea and vomiting) can be avoided by starting at a low dose of 250 mg four times a day and gradually increasing the dose to 1.5 to 2 g four times a day over five to seven days. Pyridoxine 50 mg/d is given with the levodopa as a cofactor required for the action of aromatic amino acid decarboxylase.

Ibopamine: Ibopamine is a diisobutyric ester of epinine. Following ingestion, ibopamine is hydrolyzed by plasma esterases to epinine, which has agonist activity at the DA_1-receptor. Oral administration of ibopamine 150 mg to patients with congestive heart failure increases cardiac index and stroke volume by 30% and modestly reduces left ventricular filling pressure.[67] Pulmonary capillary wedge pressure may transiently increase but then falls slightly below the control value. Chronic administration is associated with a decline in plasma norepinephrine levels, but no long-term benefits, as measured by hemodynamic response or exercise tolerance, have been described.[68] A long-term multicenter trial is currently in progress.

Dopexamine: Dopexamine is DA_1- and β_2-receptor agonist. It does not stimulate α-adrenergic receptors.[69] It therefore has primarily vasodilator properties, but may have direct inotropic activity. There have been few clinical studies conducted with this agent.

Miscellaneous The ideal positive inotropic agent may be one that primarily sensitizes contractile proteins to calcium. This is because the failing myocardium demonstrates an abnormality in cyclic AMP production.[70] The cardiac effects of most clinically available positive inotropic agents (ie, dobutamine, dopamine, norepinephrine, amrinone, enoximone, piroximone, pimobendan, and milrinone) are mediated through mechanisms that depend on the generation of the cyclic nucleotide (cyclic AMP) for the production of a positive inotropic effect. Therefore, it is possible that each of these agents will lose effectiveness as heart failure progresses. They may be destined to serve as short-term or temporary measures, useful until cyclic AMP can no longer be adequately restored in the failing myocardium.

Agents that may sensitize contractile proteins to Ca^{2+} include ARL 115 BS,[71] OPC-8212,[72] DPI 201-106,[73] and pimobendan. These agents are poorly understood and likely have alternative mechanisms involving the sodium channel and PDE-III inhibition. Some are characterized by very modest positive inotropic effects, but they may prove to be safer long term than currently available phosphodiesterase inhibitor agents.

PRACTICAL CONSIDERATIONS IN THE MANAGEMENT OF PATIENTS WITH INOTROPIC AGENTS Optimal management of patients with congestive heart failure requires an understanding of the etiology of heart failure and the basic underlying disturbed hemodynamic profile. It also requires knowledge of the site and mechanism of action of the various drugs used to treat the condition.

Patients with advanced heart failure and hypoperfusion at rest generally should be evaluated with invasive hemodynamic monitoring to characterize their hemodynamic profile. Some of these patients are volume responsive, but most already have markedly elevated filling pressure or fail to improve forward flow with further increase in preload. Hemodynamic monitoring is essential to accurately assess preload (pulmonary capillary wedge pressure) and is necessary to understand the relationship between preload and cardiac output in the individual patient.

Patients require inotropic therapy when restoration of blood pressure becomes a major immediate goal. It is our practice to restore blood pressure with high-dose dopamine ($>$ 3 μg/kg/min) in such patients, providing that left ventricular filling pressure is adequate. Mechanical lesions such as valvular heart disease or ruptured septum are generally treated surgically once the patient is stabilized. When perfusion pressure is adequately restored, addition of nitroprusside is often useful to control elevated filling pressure and to promote a further increase in cardiac output. The goal is to titrate the positive inotropic effect of the dopamine and the vasodilator effect of nitroprusside. Comparison of dopamine and dobutamine in patients with shock suggests that dobutamine does not sufficiently raise the cardiac output to maintain adequate blood pressure (Fig. 8-5).[26] However, the use of dopamine in this setting may substantially raise left ventricular filling pressure. It is often necessary, therefore, to add nitroprusside to dopamine in order to control preload once blood pressure is restored.

For patients with acutely decompensated heart failure (pulmonary edema), nitroprusside alone is most useful when systemic pressure is not excessively low. For patients who demonstrate worsening heart failure but maintain a reasonable blood pressure, either nitroprusside or dobutamine may be used. Nitroprusside tends to reduce filling pressure further than dobutamine, but occasionally will lower blood pressure to unacceptable levels. Dobutamine, being a direct positive inotropic agent, raises myocardial oxygen consumption more than nitroprusside and tends to produce a greater increase in heart rate at higher doses ($>$ 7.5 μg/kg/min) than does nitroprusside. The choice between dobutamine and nitroprusside in the nonhypotensive patient with severe heart failure will depend on the patient's left ventricular filling pressure, heart rate, and blood pressure. No universal recommendation can be made.

It is not always clear when intravenous inotropic therapy is indicated in the less acute stages of heart failure. The threshold for starting such therapy varies widely among physicians. Patients who are uncomfortable at rest with dyspnea or evidence of poor perfusion (eg, oliguria, cool and moist skin) should generally be considered for intravenous therapy because, in many cases, dramatic relief can be provided for a short period of time (24 to 72 hours). Such decisions obviously must take into account the total patient profile. In some cases, when it is clear from the history and physical examination that the cardiac output is low and the left ventricular filling pressure is high, invasive monitoring is not necessary. If dyspnea and tachypnea dominate the picture and systolic blood pressure is greater than 90 mm Hg, dramatic clinical improvement is usually observed with intravenous nitroprusside instituted at a dosage of 10 to 15 μg/min and titrated upward while monitoring blood pressure. If systolic blood pressure falls below 90 mm Hg with nitroprusside, dopamine (3 to 4 μg/kg/min) should be added to augment cardiac contractile state (β_1-activity) and elevate blood pressure (α_1-activity). An alternative approach in the patient with systolic blood pressure greater than 90 mm Hg is to infuse dobutamine (5 to 10 μg/kg/min) as needed to improve the clinical state. This therapy usually reduces dyspnea and tachypnea, improves blood flow to the brain and the extremities, and improves urine

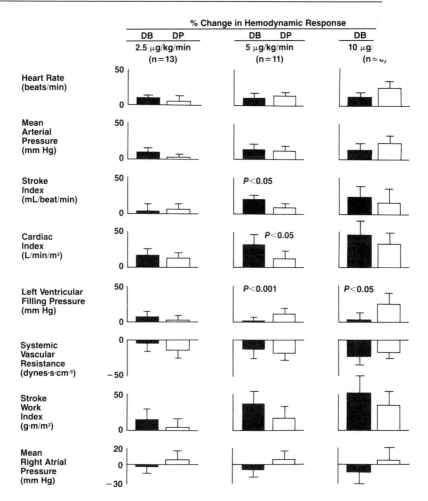

Fig. 8-5. Percent change in response to dobutamine (DB) and dopamine (DP) at three different dosages in patients with cardiogenic shock. Although both drugs increase cardiac output, dopamine increases left ventricular filling pressure significantly more than dobutamine at equivalent dosages. (Adapted from Francis et al[26] with permission.)

flow, all of which can be monitored clinically.

Invasive hemodynamic monitoring facilitates documentation of clinical efficacy, but it is not always necessary. It may, in some cases, simply prolong the patient's discomfort while awaiting urgent intravenous therapy. In general, the importance of invasive monitoring increases with advancing illness of the patient. Invasive monitoring becomes mandatory when there is attendant hypotension (systolic blood pressure < 90 mm Hg) or if there is serious doubt as to the left ventricular filling pressure. It is often prudent to begin therapy with dopamine for hypotension or nitroprusside for pulmonary edema before catheters for invasive monitoring are inserted, particularly when a prolonged procedure is anticipated. Patients with chronic severe heart failure often have large, dilated right ventricles, making passage of even a flow-directed catheter challenging in certain instances. Peripheral vasoconstriction may be intense, making arterial cannulation difficult. When systolic blood pressure is less than 70 mm Hg by cuff or palpation, insertion of an arterial cannula should be quickly performed, as the directly measured arterial pressure may markedly differ from that obtained using more indirect measurements.

Occasionally, therapy is limited by tachycardia. This is particularly true of dopamine and dobutamine at higher doses ($>$ 7 μg/kg/min), but seems to be less of a problem with the newer non-β-agonists. Any of the inotropic agents may increase myocardial oxygen demand to the point of inducing angina. This must be guarded against in patients with underlying coronary artery disease. Ventricular rhythm disturbances may occur, necessitating a reduction in dosage or change to a different agent. Left ventricular filling pressure may fail to diminish and may actually increase with higher doses of dopamine ($>$ 3 μg/kg/min), requiring addition of a vasodilator such as nitroprusside. Amrinone causes less oxygen demand than dobutamine or dopamine for an equivalent amount of positive inotropy, and should be considered as alternative or additive therapy. Increasing the dose of a loop diuretic is frequently useful. In this situation, it is, therefore, not unusual to taper the dose of the drug or even add or delete therapies when attempting to optimize treatment.

Once therapy is instituted and a favorable response by the patient is noted, intravenous therapy may be continued for 24 to 48 hours. At this point, an attempt can be made to wean the patient from therapy and consider the need for either oral inotropic or oral vasodilator therapy. When changing to oral therapy, invasive hemodynamic monitoring should be available. This will permit construction of a cardiac function curve and facilitate assessment of optimal left ventricular filling pressure (ie, left ventricular filling pressure that promotes the greatest cardiac output). These data clearly help to tailor oral therapy to the patient's hemodynamic status. It is currently premature to speculate as to which oral agent or type of oral agent (eg, inotropic or vasodilator) is best when converting to chronic maintenance therapy. Nor is it possible to comment on the ideal way in which to make the change, as this will vary substantially according to the preference of the physician. A flow diagram summarizing the treatment of decompensated heart failure is shown in Figure 8-6.

CONCLUSION   The benefits of long-term inotropic therapy are obvious. Improved functional class, exercise performance, and renal function are among the expected endpoints. Improved patient longevity is desired, but as yet this has not been demonstrated. Patients receiving chronic inotropic therapy are frequently monitored by repeat catheterization and exercise testing to document long-term efficacy.

Noninvasive techniques such as radionuclide left ventriculography, echocardiography, and chest x-ray appear to be too insensitive to measure chronic efficacy. It is hoped that tolerance to these drugs will not occur, although tolerance might be expected, to some extent, during the use of drugs that work by stimulating β-receptors. As we gain more experience with the newer agents, dosage requirements are likely to change, and special advantages and disadvantages with certain therapies or combinations of therapies may emerge.

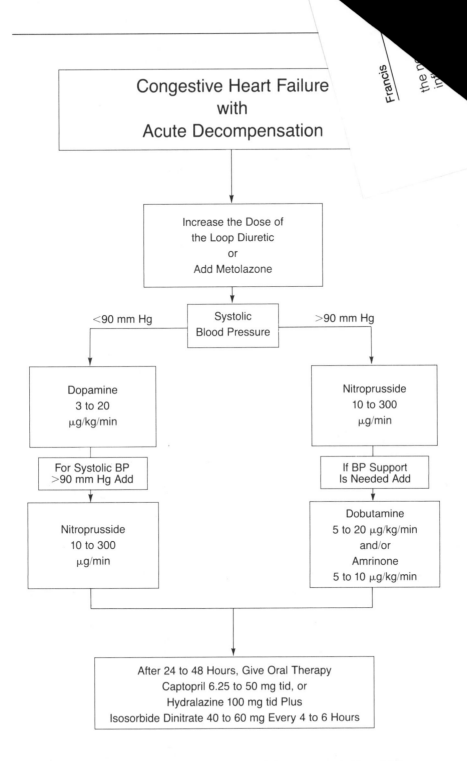

Fig. 8-6. Flow diagram summarizing treatment of decompensated heart failure.

Many questions remain to be answered. Although all of the new oral agents are effective in acutely stimulating the failing heart, their influence on the long-term outcome of severe heart failure remains to be determined. Perhaps no agent will influence the natural course of a class IV patient, yet this is the type of patient on whom most of these agents are being tested. Whether there is an earlier stage during which myocardial dysfunction can be reversed is an important question that is, as yet, unanswered. It is disturbing that a progressive downhill clinical course is observed in some patients despite both initial and sustained hemodynamic benefits from drug therapy. Whether or not chronic vasodilator therapy is preferable to inotropic therapy in advanced heart failure is uncertain. Perhaps a combination of vasodilator and inotropic therapy will ultimately emerge as superior to either type of agent used alone. Despite these uncertainties, palliation of symptoms can now be achieved with a wide variety of inotropic agents.

ACKNOWLEDG-MENTS The assistance of the Heart Failure Study Group at the University of Minnesota, particularly Susan Ziesche, is gratefully acknowledged. The secretarial assistance of Sandy Thiesse is gratefully appreciated.

REFERENCES

1. Captopril Multicenter Study Group: A placebo trial of captopril in refractory congestive heart failure. *J Am Coll Cardiol* 1983;2:755-763.
2. Cohn JN, Archibald DG, Ziesche S, et al: Effect of vasodilator therapy on mortality in chronic congestive heart failure: Results of a Veterans Administration Cooperative Study. *N Engl J Med* 1986;314:1547-1552.
3. Baim DS, Colucci WS, Monrad ES, et al: Survival of patients with severe congestive heart failure treated with oral milrinone. *J Am Coll Cardiol* 1986;7:661-670.
4. Katz AM: A new inotropic drug: Its promise and a caution (editorial). *N Engl J Med* 1978;299:1409-1410.
5. LeJemtel TH, Sonnenblick EH: Should the failing heart be stimulated (editorial)? *N Engl J Med* 1984;310:1384-1385.
6. Colucci WS, Alexander RW, Williams GH, et al: Decreased lymphocyte beta-adrenergic-receptor density in patients with heart failure and tolerance to the beta-adrenergic agonist pirbuterol. *N Engl J Med* 1981;305:185-190.
7. DiBianco R, Shabetai R, Silverman BD, et al: Oral amrinone for the treatment of chronic congestive heart failure: Results of a multicenter randomized double-blind and placebo-controlled withdrawal study. *J Am Coll Cardiol* 1984;4:855-866.
8. Massie B, Bourassa M, DiBianco R, et al: Long-term oral administration of amrinone for congestive heart failure: Lack of efficacy in a multi-center controlled trial. *Circulation* 1985;71:963-971.
9. Colucci WS, Wright RF, Braunwald E: New positive inotropic agents in the treatment of congestive heart failure. *N Engl J Med* 1986;314:290-299, 349-358.
10. Tsien RW: Cyclic AMP and contractile activity in heart. *Adv Cyclic Nucleotide Res* 1977;8:363-420.
11. Katz AM: Role of the contractile proteins and sarcoplasmic reticulum in the response of the heart to catecholamines: A historical review. *Adv Cyclic Nucleotide Res* 1979;11:303-343.
12. Scholz H: Inotropic drugs and their mechanisms. *J Am Coll Cardiol* 1984;4:389-397.

13. Goldberg LI, Hsieh Y-Y, Resnekov L: Newer catecholamines for treatment of heart failure and shock: An update on dopamine and first look at dobutamine. *Prog Cardiovasc Dis* 1977;19:327-340.
14. Sonnenblick EH, Frishman WH, LeJemtel T: Dobutamine: A new synthetic cardioactive sympathetic amine. *N Engl J Med* 1979;300:17-22.
15. Reuter H, Scholz H: The regulation of calcium conductance of cardiac muscle by adrenaline. *J Physiol* 1977;264:49-62.
16. Reuter H: Calcium channel modulation by neurotransmitters, enzymes and drugs. *Nature* 1983;301:569-574.
17. Goldberg LI: Dopamine: Clinical uses of an endogenous catecholamine. *N Engl J Med* 1974;291:707-710.
18. Goldberg LI: Cardiovascular and renal actions of dopamine: Potential clinical applications. *Pharmacol Rev* 1972;24:1-29.
19. Goldberg LI, Wolkman PH, Kohli JD: A comparison of the vascular dopamine receptor with other dopamine receptors. *Annu Rev Pharmacol Toxicol* 1978;18:57-79.
20. Goldberg LI, McDonald RH, Zimmerman AM: Sodium diuresis produced by dopamine in patients with congestive heart failure. *N Engl J Med* 1963;269:1060-1064.
21. McDonald RH Jr, Goldberg LI, McNay JL, et al: Effects of dopamine in man: Augmentation of sodium excretion, glomerular filtration rate and renal plasma flow. *J Clin Invest* 1964;43:1116-1124.
22. Goldberg LI, Talley RC, McNay JL: The potential role of dopamine in the treatment of shock. *Prog Cardiovasc Dis* 1969;12:40-51.
23. Loeb HS, Winslow EBJ, Rahimtoola SH, et al: Acute hemodynamic effects of dopamine in patients with shock. *Circulation* 1971;44:163-173.
24. Leier CV, Heban PT, Huss P, et al: Comparative systemic and regional hemodynamic effects of dopamine and dobutamine in patients with cardiomyopathic heart failure. *Circulation* 1978;58:466-475.
25. Loeb HS, Bredakis J, Gunnar RM: Superiority of dobutamine over dopamine for augmentation of cardiac output in patients with chronic low output cardiac failure. *Circulation* 1977;55:375-381.
26. Francis GS, Sharma B, Hodges M: Comparative hemodynamic effects of dopamine and dobutamine in patients with acute cardiogenic circulatory collapse. *Am Heart J* 1982;103:995-1000.
27. Miller RR, Awan NA, Joye JE, et al: Combined dopamine and nitroprusside therapy in congestive heart failure: Greater augmentation of cardiac performance by addition of inotropic stimulation to afterload reduction. *Circulation* 1977;55:881-884.
28. Stemple DR, Kleiman JH, Harrison DC: Combined nitroprusside-dopamine therapy in severe chronic congestive heart failure: Dose-related hemodynamic advantages over single drug infusions. *Am J Cardiol* 1978;42:267-275.
29. Maskin CS, Ocken S, Chadwick B, et al: Comparative systemic and renal effects of dopamine and angiotensin-converting enzyme inhibition with enalaprilat in patients with heart failure. *Circulation* 1985;72:846-852.
30. Crea F, Chierchia S, Kaski JC, et al: Provocation of coronary spasm by dopamine in patients with active variant angina pectoris. *Circulation* 1986;74:262-269.
31. Ruffolo RR Jr, Spradlin TA, Pollock GD, et al: Alpha and beta adrenergic effects of the stereoisomers of dobutamine. *J Pharmacol Exp Ther* 1981;219:447-452.
32. Richard C, Ricome JL, Rimailho A, et al: Combined hemodynamic effects of dopamine and dobutamine in cardiogenic shock. *Circulation* 1983;67:620-626.
33. Berkowitz C, McKeever L, Croke RP, et al: Comparative responses to dobutamine and nitroprusside in patients with chronic low output cardiac failure. *Circulation* 1977;56:918-924.
34. Weinstein JS, Baim DS: The effects of acute dobutamine administration on myocardial metabolism and energetics. *Heart Failure* 1986;1:110-116.
35. Mikulic E, Cohn JN, Franciosa JA: Comparative hemodynamic effects of inotropic and vasodilator drugs in severe heart failure. *Circulation* 1977;56:528-533.

36. Leier CV, Unverferth DV: Dobutamine. *Ann Intern Med* 1983;99:490-496.
37. Unverferth DV, Blanford M, Kates RE, et al: Tolerance to dobutamine after a 72 hour continuous infusion. *Am J Med* 1980;69:262-266.
38. Applefeld MM, Neuman KA, Grove WR, et al: Intermittent, continuous outpatient dobutamine infusion in the management of congestive heart failure. *Am J Cardiol* 1983;51:455-458.
39. Unverferth DV, Magorien RD, Altschuld R, et al: The hemodynamic and metabolic advantages gained by a three-day infusion of dobutamine in patients with congestive cardiomyopathy. *Am Heart J* 1983;106:29-34.
40. Liang C-S, Sherman LG, Doherty JU, et al: Sustained improvement of cardiac function in patients with congestive heart failure after short-term infusion of dobutamine. *Circulation* 1984;69:113-119.
41. Unverferth DV, Magorian RD, Lewis RB, et al: Long-term benefit of dobutamine in patients with congestive cardiomyopathy. *Am Heart J* 1980;100:622-630.
42. Berger M, McSherry CK: Outpatient dobutamine infusion using a totally implantable infusion pump for refractory congestive heart failure. *Chest* 1985;88:295-296.
43. Unverferth DV, Leier CV, Magorien RD, et al: Improvement of human myocardial mitochondria after dobutamine: A quantitative ultrastructural study. *J Pharmacol Exp Ther* 1980;215:527-532.
44. Krell MJ, Kline EM, Bates ER, et al: Intermittent, ambulatory dobutamine infusions in patients with severe congestive heart failure. *Am Heart J* 1986;112:787-791.
45. Klein NA, Siskind SJ, Frishman WH, et al: Hemodynamic comparison of intravenous amrinone and dobutamine in patients with chronic congestive heart failure. *Am J Cardiol* 1981;48:170-175.
46. Gage J, Rutman H, Lucido D, et al: Additive effects of dobutamine and amrinone on myocardial contractility and ventricular performance in patients with severe heart failure. *Circulation* 1986;74:367-373.
47. Endoh M, Yamashita S, Taira N: Positive inotropic effect of amrinone in relation to cyclic nucleotide metabolism in canine ventricular muscle. *J Pharmacol Exp Ther* 1982;221:775-783.
48. Benotti JR, McCue JE, Alpert JS: Comparative vasoactive therapy for heart failure. *Am J Cardiol* 1985;56:19B-24B
49. Baim DS: Effects of amrinone on myocardial energetics in severe congestive heart failure. *Am J Cardiol* 1985;56:16B-18B.
50. Goldstein RA, Gray EL, Dougherty AA, et al: Electrophysiologic effects of amrinone. *Am J Cardiol* 1985;56:25B-28B.
51. Firth BG, Ratner A, Grassman ED, et al: Assessment of the inotropic and vasodilator effects of amrinone versus isoproterenol. *Am J Cardiol* 1984;54:1331-1336.
52. Alousi AA, Canter JM, Montenaro MJ, et al: Cardiotonic activity of milrinone, a new and potent cardiac bipyridine, on the normal and failing heart of experimental animals. *J Cardiovasc Pharmacol* 1983;5:792-803.
53. Grose R, Strain J, Greenberg M, et al: Systemic and coronary effects in congestive heart failure. *J Am Coll Cardiol* 1986;7:1107-1113.
54. Maskin CS, Sinoway L, Chadwick B, et al: Sustained hemodynamic and clinical effects of a new cardiotonic agent, WIN 47203, in patients with severe congestive heart failure. *Circulation* 1983;67:1065-1070.
55. Weber KT, Andrews V, Janicki JS, et al: Amrinone and exercise performance in patients with chronic heart failure. *Am J Cardiol* 1981;48:164-169.
56. Likoff MJ, Weber KT, Andrews V, et al: Milrinone in the treatment of chronic cardiac failure: A controlled trial. *Am Heart J* 1985;110:1035-1042.
57. White HD, Ribeiro JP, Hartley LH, et al: Immediate effects of milrinone on metabolic sympathetic response to exercise in severe congestive heart failure. *Am J Cardiol* 1985;56:93-98.
58. Sinoway LS, Maskin CS, Chadwick B, et al: Long-term therapy with a new cardiotonic agent, WIN 47203: Drug dependent improvement in cardiac performance and progression of the underlying disease. *J Am Coll Cardiol* 1983;2:327-331.

59. Simonton CA, Chatterjee K, Cody RJ, et al: Milrinone in congestive heart failure: Acute and chronic hemodynamic and clinical evaluation. *J Am Coll Cardiol* 1985;6:453-459.
60. Kariya T, Wille LJ, Dage RC: Biochemical studies on the mechanism of cardiotonic activity of MDL 17,043. *J Cardiovasc Pharmacol* 1982;4:509-514.
61. Cheng HC, Kariya T, Gleason EM, et al: Studies on the mechanism of the positive inotropic effect of piroximone in cat papillary muscle. *J Cardiovasc Pharmacol* 1985;7:747-752.
62. Knope R, Moe GK, Saunders J, et al: Myocardial effects of imidazole. *J Pharmacol Exp Ther* 1973;185:29-34.
63. Shah PK, Amin DK, Hulse S, et al: Inotropic therapy for refractory congestive heart failure with oral fenoximone (MDL 17,043): Poor long-term results despite early hemodynamic and clinical improvement. *Circulation* 1985;71:326-331.
64. Petein M, Levine TB, Cohn JN: Hemodynamic effects of a new inotropic agent, piroximone (MDL 19,025), in patients with chronic heart failure. *J Am Coll Cardiol* 1984;4:364-371.
65. Rajfer SI, Anton AH, Rossen JD, et al: Beneficial hemodynamic effects of oral levodopa in heart failure: Relation to the generation of dopamine. *N Engl J Med* 1984;310:1357-1362.
66. Goldberg LI, Rajfer SI: Dopamine receptors: Applications in clinical cardiology. *Circulation* 1985;72:245-248.
67. Dei Cas L, Bolognesi R, Cucchini F, et al: Hemodynamic effects of ibopamine in patients with idiopathic congestive cardiomyopthy. *J Cardiovasc Pharmacol* 1983;5:249-253.
68. Rajfer SI, Rossen JD, Douglass FL, et al: Effects of long-term therapy with oral ibopamine on resting hemodynamics and exercise capacity in patients with heart failure: Relationship to the generation of N-methyldopa and to plasma norepinephrine levels. *Circulation* 1986;73:740-748.
69. Brown RA, Dixon J, Farmer JB, et al: Dopexamine: A novel agonist of peripheral dopamine receptors and β-adrenoceptors. *Br J Pharmacol* 1985;85:599-608.
70. Feldman MC, Copelas L, Gwathmey JK, et al: Deficient production of cyclic AMP: Pharmacologic evidence of an important cause of contractile dysfunction in patients with end-stage heart failure. *Circulation* 1987;75:331-339.
71. Solaro RJ, Ruegg JC: Stimulation of Ca^{++} binding and ATPase activity of dog cardiac myofibrils by ARL 115BS, a novel cardiotonic agent. *Circ Res* 1982;51:290-294.
72. Asanoi H, Sasayama S, Iuchi K, et al: Acute hemodynamic effects of a new inotropic agent (OPC-8212) in patients with congestive heart failure. *J Am Coll Cardiol* 1987;9:865-871.
73. Herzig JW, Quast U: Increase in Ca^{++} sensitivity of myocardial contractile structures by DPI 201-106. *J Mol Cell Cardiol* 1984;16(suppl 3):6.

KANU CHATTERJEE, MB, FRCP

9

Vasodilator Therapy for Heart Failure

Vasodilator therapy has gained widespread acceptance in the management of heart failure. A large number of vasodilator agents with different mechanisms of action have undergone clinical evaluation and have been used in the treatment of both acute and chronic heart failure resulting from coronary artery disease, primary myocardial disease, and valvular heart disease. The effects of vasodilator therapy on cardiac function, symptomatic status, and prognosis of patients with heart failure have been extensively investigated, and the results suggest that vasodilator drugs are important therapeutic adjuncts in the management of heart failure. In this chapter, the rationale for vasodilator therapy and the relative advantages and disadvantages of various vasodilator agents are reviewed.

RATIONALE FOR VASODILATOR THERAPY   Heart failure may result from myocardial disease, valvular heart disease, or endomyocardial or pericardial disease. Depressed myocardial function resulting from the consequences of atherosclerotic coronary artery disease or primary myocardial disease is, however, a more frequent cause of heart failure. A number of functional derangements are observed in these patients including decreased ventricular contractility and pump function. In patients with congestive cardiomyopathy, the ratio of end-systolic stress to end-systolic volume, an index of contractile function, is lower than that of normal controls, indicating reduced contractile function.[1] When compared with normal controls, left ventricular systolic stress is considerably higher in patients with dilated cardiomyopathy, while ejection fraction and normalized ejection rate are lower. Decreased ejection fraction is not only due to decreased contractility but also due to elevated systolic wall stress (ie, afterload). Increased wall stress in patients with dilated cardiomyopathy primarily results from a marked increase in ventricular volume, as intraventricular pressure and wall thickness may not change significantly in many patients. Thus not infrequently there is an excessive increase in ventricular preload and afterload. Increased end-diastolic volume is associated with increased ventricular diastolic pressures resulting in increased systemic and pulmonary venous pressures—the hemodynamic determinants of congestive symptoms.

Increased afterload decreases ventricular stroke volume, as an inverse relationship exists between the stroke output and afterload. Reduction in preload has the potential to relieve congestive symptoms, while a reduction in afterload can relieve symptoms due to low cardiac output.

Although arterial pressure and systemic vascular resistance do not precisely define left ventricular afterload, they contribute to the total left ventricular outflow resistance. In many patients with heart failure, mean arterial pressure remains in the normal range despite a lower cardiac output.[2] Maintenance of arterial pressure in the presence of low cardiac output results from increased systemic vascular resistance. Calculated aortic input impedance also may be higher in patients with heart failure.[3] These alterations in peripheral vascular dynamics cause further impairment of cardiac performance in patients with heart failure, as the failing ventricle is more sensitive to alterations in outflow resistance.[4] Even a modest increase in systemic vascular resistance may cause a substantial decrease in cardiac output. This is followed by the development of a vicious circle characterized by low cardiac output and elevated systemic vascular resistance, with the latter causing a further decrease in cardiac output.[5] Conversely, reduction of systemic vascular resistance is associated with increased cardiac output due to decreased left ventricular outflow resistance.

Although peripheral vascular tone is elevated, the mechanisms responsible for this response may not be similar in all patients. An understanding of the different mechanisms contributing to vasoconstriction has important implications regarding the mechanisms of vasodilation of various vasodilator agents. The reader is referred to Chapters 3 and 4 for this discussion.

The rationale for vasodilator therapy is to decrease arterial and venous tone in order to improve abnormal systemic hemodynamics and cardiac performance. A reduction in arterial tone is associated with increased stroke volume and cardiac output, while a reduction in peripheral venous tone results in decreased systemic and pulmonary venous pressures, probably due to decreased venous return to the heart and reduction in intracardiac volumes. The rationale for the use of vasodilator agents with predominantly venodilating properties is to decrease systemic and pulmonary venous pressures, while that of the predominant arteriolar dilators is to increase cardiac output.

Myocardial Ischemia Besides a reduction of systemic resistance and intracardiac volumes, vasodilators have the potential to decrease segmental myocardial ischemia, which can contribute to improving left ventricular function.[6-8] Most vasodilators do not cause any significant change in heart rate when administered for heart failure. However, with captopril and nitroprusside, heart rate may decline. Arterial pressure may also decrease, usually accompanied by some reduction in left ventricular diastolic volume, particularly with vasodilator drugs that have venodilating properties (eg, nitrates and captopril). Myocardial oxygen demand tends to decrease during vasodilator therapy because most vasodilators do not possess any direct positive inotropic effects. Furthermore, a number of vasodilator agents (eg, nitrates) can potentially increase collateral coronary blood flow to the relatively ischemic myocardium. Thus, during vasodilator therapy, segmental myocardial ischemia can decrease, either because of decreased myocardial oxygen demand, increased myocardial perfusion, or both. Any of these responses may improve left ventricular function; therefore, vasodilator therapy is particularly attractive in the treatment of heart failure due to ischemic heart disease.

Ventricular Diastolic Compliance   In patients with severe left ventricular failure associated with dilated ventricular chambers and pulmonary arterial hypertension, vasodilator therapy may be associated with an acute increase in left ventricular diastolic compliance, which can contribute toward improving left ventricular function.[9] The improved diastolic compliance may result from the interaction of right and left ventricles in a confined pericardial space.[9,10] In this situation, the pericardium, being a very stiff structure, tends to maintain a constant overall cardiac volume at high filling pressures. A vasodilator that reduces right heart pressures will also reduce the end-diastolic volume of the right ventricle and allow for a larger left ventricle at the same left ventricular diastolic pressure. Thus, agents that lower right-sided pressures will tend to produce an apparent increase in compliance of the left ventricle.

MECHANISMS OF VASO-DILATATION   There are a number of mechanisms by which different vasodilator agents cause vasodilation, with a subsequent reduction of systemic vascular tone.[11,12] Vasodilator agents such as hydralazine, nitrates, and nitroprusside cause direct smooth muscle relaxation of the peripheral vascular bed. Other agents cause vasodilation by decreasing or inhibiting the vasoconstricting effects mediated by the sympathetic adrenergic nervous system. Clonidine decreases peripheral sympathetic outflow by stimulating the α-adrenergic receptors located in the central nervous system. Drugs like phentolamine or prazosin cause vasodilation by peripheral α-adrenergic receptor blockade. Ganglionic blocking agents, trimethaphan or hexamethonium, also cause vasodilation and have been used for the treatment of heart failure. Stimulation of β_2-receptors with salbutamol and pirbuterol is associated with peripheral vasodilation and decreased systemic vascular resistance. Drugs like nifedipine, diltiazem, and verapamil decrease systemic vascular resistance and arterial pressure by inhibiting the inward calcium current to the smooth muscles of the peripheral vascular beds. Prostacyclin and prostaglandin E increase cyclic adenosine monophosphate (AMP) levels in the smooth muscle of the vascular bed and cause vasodilation. Saralasin is a competitive antagonist of angiotensin-II. Captopril, enalapril, and teprotide decrease the production of angiotensin-II from angiotensin-I by inhibiting angiotensin converting enzyme. Attenuation or inhibition of the effects of angiotensin-II is associated with arteriolar dilation, reduction of systemic vascular resistance, and a fall in arterial pressure.[12]

It should be emphasized that many of these vasodilator drugs possess additional pharmacologic properties that might contribute to peripheral vasodilation. For example, although phentolamine is an α-adrenergic blocking agent, it also directly relaxes the smooth muscle of arteries and veins.[13] There is also evidence that phentolamine possesses β-adrenergic stimulating effects that may contribute to peripheral vasodilation.[14] Similarly, captopril, in addition to decreasing the vasoconstricting effects of angiotensin-II, inhibits the degradation of bradykinin and causes increased synthesis of vasodilator prostaglandins.

The major hemodynamic effects of these vasodilator drugs appear to be related to their principal site of action on the peripheral vascular bed, regardless of their mechanism of action (Table 9-1). Vasodilators that principally dilate systemic veins consistently decrease systemic and pulmonary venous pressures. They increase the capacitance of these vessels and effectively redistribute circulating blood volume. The peripheral pooling of blood decreases ventricular filling pressures by reducing intracardiac volumes, thereby relieving pulmonary and systemic venous congestion.

The effects of a predominant venodilator drug on cardiac performance are dependent on the initial level of left ventricular filling pressure. In the setting of high filling pressure, a reduction in filling pressure will occur along the flat portion of the ventricular function curve (Fig. 9-1). Therefore,

Table 9-1. The principal hemodynamic effects of vasodilators used to treat heart failure

Vasodilator	Heart Rate	Blood Pressure	Cardiac Output	Systemic and Pulmonary Venous Pressures
Nitroglycerin and nitrates	— or ↑	↓ or —	— or ↑ (slight)	↓
Hydralazine	— or ↑	↓ or —	↑	— or ↓ (slight)
Minoxidil	— or ↑	↓ or —	↑	— or ↓ (slight)
Prazosin	— or ↑	↓	↑	↓
Captopril and enalapril	— or ↓	↓	↑	↓
Nifedipine	↑ or —	↓	↑	— or ↓
Diltiazem	—	↓ or —	↑	↓ or —
Hydralazine and nitrates	—	— or ↓	↑	↓

↑ = increase; ↓ = decrease; — = no change.

no decrease in stroke volume may result. Indeed, there may be an increase in stroke volume. In contrast, with a normal filling pressure, a reduction will tend to lower stroke volume as the ventricle moves down the ascending limb of its curve. In order to maintain cardiac output under these circumstances, there may be a compensatory increase in heart rate.

Vasodilator agents that primarily decrease arteriolar tone will decrease systemic vascular resistance, increase stroke volume and cardiac output, and produce little or no change in systemic and pulmonary venous pressures. Drugs with a balanced effect on arteriolar and venous beds not only decrease systemic vascular resistance and increase cardiac output, but also decrease systemic and pulmonary venous pressures. With these agents, the net increase in stroke volume is necessarily less than that expected from their arteriolar dilating effect, because of the concomitant reduction of filling pressure related to venodilation.

Fig. 9-1. Left ventricular function curves plotting stroke volume as a function of left ventricular filling pressure. Administration of a vasodilator decreases aortic impedance and shifts the curve up and to the left. Note that if a vasodilator is given to a patient with an initial filling pressure of 20 mm Hg, the reduction in filling pressure would be accompanied by an increase in stroke volume (A). However, if a vasodilator is given at a filling pressure of 10 mm Hg, there would be a decrease in stroke volume (B). Thus, the net effects of a vasodilator on stroke volume are dependent on the initial level of left ventricular filling pressure. (Adapted from K Chatterjee, WW Parmley, The role of vasodilator therapy in heart failure, *Prog Cardiovasc Dis* 1977;19:301-325.)

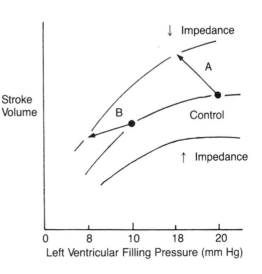

HEMODYNAMIC AND CLINICAL APPLICATIONS

Sodium Nitroprusside

Sodium nitroprusside causes relaxation of both the arteriolar resistance and the venous capacitance beds by a direct action of the free nitroprusside radical on vascular smooth muscle. A balanced effect on these vascular beds results in hemodynamic effects characterized by a significant reduction of systemic vascular resistance, an increase in cardiac output and stroke volume, and a concomitant decrease in systemic and pulmonary venous pressures. Systemic and pulmonary arterial pressures tend to decrease, while heart rate tends to remain unchanged.[15,16] Renal hemodynamics and function may be variably affected by nitroprusside, depending on whether or not heart failure and low cardiac output coexist. In heart failure, renal blood flow increases due to decreased renal vascular resistance, provided a marked fall in arterial pressure does not occur.[17] In patients with congestive heart failure, sodium nitroprusside increases renal blood flow and increases sodium and potassium excretion without any change in the glomerular filtration rate.[18] However, marked reduction in arterial pressure may decrease glomerular filtration rate and sodium excretion, and increase plasma renin activity.[19]

The effects of sodium nitroprusside on coronary hemodynamics are varied. An increase in coronary blood flow due to a primary decrease in coronary vascular resistance has been reported.[20,21] In contrast, a decrease in coronary blood flow along with decreased myocardial oxygen demand has also been observed.[22,23] These findings suggest that changes in coronary blood flow are likely to be determined not only by changes in coronary vascular resistance but also by changes in the determinants of myocardial oxygen demand. However, primary coronary vasodilation does occur as the coronary venous oxygen saturation tends to increase and myocardial oxygen extraction decreases.[5,21] The effects of sodium nitroprusside on the extent of myocardial ischemia and injury in the presence of acute myocardial infarction are also divergent: both a reduction and an increase in the extent of myocardial injury have been reported.[24]

The influence of sodium nitroprusside therapy on left ventricular function is largely determined by the initial level of left ventricular function. Table 9-2 demonstrates this in patients with acute myocardial infarction. Group I patients who were not in clinical heart failure had left ventricular filling pressure of 15 mm Hg or less. Patients in group II with moderate left ventricular failure had initial left ventricular filling pressure greater than 15 mm Hg, and left ventricular stroke work index exceeding 20 g·m/m². Group III patients had pulmonary edema, and more than 50% had features of cardiogenic shock. Initial left ventricular filling pressure in all patients was elevated (> 15 mm Hg), and left ventricular stroke work index was markedly reduced (< 20 g·m/m²). During sodium nitroprusside infusion, systemic and pulmonary arterial pressure, left ventricular filling pressure, and right atrial pressure decreased in all groups. However, cardiac index and stroke work index increased only in group II and group III patients (ie, in those who had initial left ventricular filling pressure higher than 15 mm Hg). In patients with normal left ventricular filling pressure, stroke work index decreased along with a further decline in left ventricular filling pressure, indicating no improvement in left ventricular function. The magnitude of increase in cardiac index and stroke work index was comparatively greater in group III patients with severely depressed cardiac function. It is essential, therefore, to determine the initial hemodynamics in order to identify the subsets of patients likely to benefit from sodium nitroprusside therapy.

Changes in regional myocardial function and the extent of myocardial injury during sodium nitroprusside therapy in patients with acute myocardial infarction have been the subject of a number of investigations, with conflicting results. In some studies an increase of infarct size was reported, while in others a reduction has been observed.[25-27] The influence of this therapy on the mortality of patients with acute myocardial infarction has been evaluated in both randomized studies and in uncontrolled studies[28-30]; again, conflicting results have emerged. Some studies demonstrated favorable prognosis, and others detected no beneficial effects. In patients with severe pump failure, the hospital mortality with sodium nitroprusside therapy appears to be lower than expected with conventional therapy. However, the long-term prognosis still remains unfavorable. At present, the routine use of sodium nitroprusside therapy in patients with an acute myocardial infarction is not recommended. It should be reserved for the treatment of pump failure complicating myocardial infarction.

It is important to note that potential hazards do exist with sodium nitroprusside use in patients with acute myocardial infarction. Reduction of arterial pressure may compromise myocardial perfusion and enhance existing myocardial ischemia. The purpose of sodium nitroprusside therapy in heart failure is to improve left ventricular function by decreasing systemic vascular resistance. This beneficial effect can be achieved without a significant reduction in arterial pressure if the increase in cardiac output is proportional to the decrease in systemic vascular resistance. It is apparent that hemodynamic monitoring is essential not only to identify the subset of patients likely to benefit from nitroprusside therapy but also to evaluate the therapeutic response.

Vasodilator Therapy

Table 9-2. Hemodynamic effects of nitroprusside in patients with acute myocardial infarction*

Hemodynamic Variable	Group I (n = 6)		Group II (n = 9)		Group III (n = 12)	
	C	NP	C	NP	C	NP
Heart rate (beats/min)	89.0 ± 7.1	96.7 ± 8.6	91.3 ± 4.2	94.7 ± 3.4	100.2 ± 4.0	100.5 ± 4.8
Mean arterial pressure (mm Hg)	91.0 ± 2.6	85.8 ± 3.9	100.6 ± 4.5	87.7 ± 4.1	82.4 ± 2.2	76.2 ± 2.8†
Mean pulmonary arterial pressure (mm Hg)	16.5 ± 1.7	11.3 ± 1.0†	31.8 ± 1.6	23.0 ± 2.0†	37.0 ± 1.5	24.7 ± 1.4
Mean right atrial pressure (mm Hg)	5.2 ± 1.4	2.8 ± 1.2	10.4 ± 1.5	7.2 ± 1.4†	12.8 ± 1.4	8.5 ± 1.3†
Left ventricular filling pressure (mm Hg)	11.1 ± 4.6	6.3 ± 1.1†	23.6 ± 1.0	15.2 ± 1.5†	29.0 ± 1.6	18.7 ± 1.8†
Cardiac index (L/min/m²)	2.9 ± 0.2	2.9 ± 0.2	2.6 ± 0.1	3.1 ± 0.2†	1.8 ± 0.1	2.2 ± 0.1†
Stroke work index (g·m/m²)	38.8 ± 7.6	34.5 ± 6.2	33.6 ± 2.9	34.2 ± 1.8	13.8 ± 1.1	17.6 ± 1.5†
Systemic vascular resistance (dynes·s·cm⁻⁵)	1383 ± 148	1321 ± 119	1577 ± 141	1231 ± 146	1908 ± 260	1431 ± 137†
Pulmonary vascular resistance (dynes·s·cm⁻⁵)	6.4 ± 12	77 ± 19	148 ± 32	84 ± 21†	234 ± 28	114 ± 14†

*Mean ± SEM; see text for description of groups.
†P < 0.05 nitroprusside versus control.
C = control; NP = nitroprusside.
Adapted from K Chatterjee, WW Parmley, W Ganz, et al, Hemodynamic and metabolic responses to vasodilator therapy in acute myocardial infarction, *Circulation* 1973;48:1183-1193, by permission of the American Heart Association, Inc.

Sodium nitroprusside decreases regurgitant volume and increases forward stroke volume in patients with mitral or aortic regurgitation. Decreased regurgitant volume is associated with decreased left ventricular end-diastolic volume and pressure, and pulmonary venous pressure.

The hemodynamic effects of sodium nitroprusside are promptly reversed with discontinuation of infusion. Clinical use is restricted to the treatment of acute heart failure complicating myocardial infarction, postoperative heart failure, acute severe mitral or aortic regurgitation, or short-term therapy for severe chronic failure before the initiation of nonparenteral vasodilator therapy.

Hypotension is the major and most frequent undesirable effect of sodium nitroprusside therapy. If marked hypotension occurs, therapy should be discontinued and a vasopressor agent administered to reverse hypotension. Other rare complications include decreased arterial oxygen tension, cyanide toxicity, thiocyanate toxicity, hypothyroidism, methemoglobinemia, lactic acidosis, vitamin B_{12} deficiency, inhibition of platelet function, and gastrointestinal symptoms.

Phentolamine Phentolamine is an α-adrenergic blocking agent with a prominent direct relaxing effect on vascular smooth muscle and β-adrenergic stimulating properties. Thus, phentolamine has the potential to improve left ventricular function, not only by decreasing left ventricular outflow resistance but also by enhancing contractility. An immediate and significant reversal of the insulin suppression that occurs in heart failure is observed after phentolamine administration. Although this can potentially improve myocardial metabolism, the significance of this pharmacologic effect is unclear.[31]

Phentolamine can be administered by intravenous and oral routes, although the latter route is rarely used for the management of heart failure. The onset of hemodynamic effects is observed within five minutes of intravenous administration; these effects are quickly reversed within minutes of discontinuing therapy. Intravenous phentolamine therapy is indicated for the treatment of acute heart failure or before the initiation of nonparenteral vasodilator therapy in patients with severe chronic congestive heart failure.

The hemodynamic effects of phentolamine are similar to those of sodium nitroprusside. Arterial pressure, systemic vascular resistance, pulmonary capillary wedge pressure, right atrial pressure, and pulmonary artery pressure decline, while cardiac output and stroke volume increase. In contrast to sodium nitroprusside, phentolamine tends to increase heart rate, even in patients with heart failure. The changes in left ventricular function accompanying phentolamine administration are influenced by the initial level of left ventricular filling pressure. In patients with high initial left ventricular filling pressure, stroke volume and cardiac output increase along with a decrease in filling pressure, indicating improved left ventricular function. In the presence of normal filling pressure, stroke volume infrequently increases, even though left ventricular filling pressure decreases.

Gould et al[32] reported that phentolamine may decrease coronary vascular resistance and increase coronary blood flow. In patients with acute myocardial infarction, the effects of phentolamine on coronary blood flow and myocardial oxygen consumption appear to be related to the changes in myocardial oxygen demand. In most patients, arterial pressure significantly decreases and heart rate increases. However, the systolic blood pressure–heart rate product (an index of myocardial oxygen demand), coronary blood flow, and myocardial oxygen consumption usually remain unchanged.[12] Thus, improved cardiac function occurs after phentolamine administration, with little or no increase in metabolic cost.

The major complication associated with phentolamine therapy is hypotension, requiring cautious dosage titration. Thus, in normotensive patients with heart failure, the initial dose of intravenous phentolamine should be low (0.1 mg/min). Changes in arterial pressure, systemic vascular resistance, cardiac output, and left ventricular filling pressure should be monitored as the dose is increased by 0.1 mg/min every ten minutes. In most patients, the beneficial hemodynamic effects are observed with a 1- to 2-mg/min infusion of phentolamine. Palpitation and gastrointestinal symptoms are occasionally seen, and angina can be precipitated. A decrease in arterial oxygen saturation with phentolamine is less than that seen with nitroprusside and nitrates.

Trimethaphan   Trimethaphan is a ganglion blocking agent that has been used in a limited number of patients with acute myocardial infarction.[33] After intravenous administration, pulmonary capillary wedge pressure usually decreases without any significant change in cardiac output. Arterial pressure and heart rate also decrease. The hemodynamic effects of trimethaphan in these patients are similar to those seen with nitroglycerin. Because of the potential for development of tachyphylaxis, trimethaphan is rarely used for the treatment of heart failure.

Nitroglycerin   Nitroglycerin and other organic nitrates relax vascular
and Nitrates   smooth muscle of the venous capacitance bed, with a lesser effect on the arterial resistance bed. Nitrates have a greater effect on large than on small arteries and arterioles. Their action is relatively selective, with vasodilation occurring in the pulmonary and coronary circulations, and vasoconstriction in splanchnic beds. Renal blood flow falls if mean arterial pressure decreases.[34] Nitroglycerin dilates the large epicardial coronary arteries (conductance vessels) with little or no effect on the small intramyocardial arteries and arterioles.[35]

The mechanisms of vasodilation by nitroglycerin or nitrates are not entirely clear. However, it has been suggested that vasodilation is, in part, mediated by increasing the production of prostaglandin (PG) I_2 and PGE_2. In studies of cultured human cells, nitroglycerin has stimulated the production of prostacyclin.[36] The cardiovascular effects of nitroglycerin are also attenuated by indomethacin.[37]

Nitroglycerin, whether administered sublingually, topically, or intravenously, tends to produce qualitatively similar hemodynamic effects in patients with acute or chronic heart failure.[38,39] Reduction in pulmonary capillary wedge and right atrial pressures is the most consistent effect. A modest decrease in arterial pressure usually occurs, and pulmonary artery pressure and pulmonary vascular resistance tend to decrease in the majority of patients. Variable changes in systemic vascular resistance, cardiac output, and stroke volume are observed. In patients with normal left ventricular filling pressure or in those in whom it falls to a very low level, cardiac output and stroke volume tend to decrease and systemic vascular resistance may not change. In the presence of elevated left ventricular filling pressure, cardiac output and stroke volume either remain unchanged or increase slightly.

The hemodynamic effects of sublingual, oral, or chewable isosorbide dinitrate are similar to those of nitroglycerin. Systemic and pulmonary venous pressures significantly decrease, together with a modest increase or no change in cardiac output.[40,41] Very large oral doses of isosorbide dinitrate have been reported to considerably increase cardiac output in some patients with chronic heart failure.[42]

Nitroglycerin and organic nitrates have been used for the treatment of pump failure complicating myocardial infarction. Nitroglycerin is most effective in patients with mild or moderate left ventricular failure with elevated pulmonary capillary wedge pressure and adequate or slightly decreased cardiac output. Nitrates do not significantly increase cardiac output in patients with a markedly reduced cardiac output and are less effective than sodium nitroprusside in this subset of patients.

Nitroglycerin and isosorbide dinitrate have been used to decrease the extent of myocardial ischemia and infarct size in patients with acute myocardial infarction. Nitroglycerin has been shown to decrease the extent of myocardial injury.[26] An increase in transmyocardial blood flow and subendocardial flow to the ischemic myocardial segments has been reported in experimental myocardial infarction. In a limited number of patients with acute myocardial infarction, intravenous nitroglycerin decreased infarct size calculated from creatine phosphokinase (CPK) and CPK-MB activity curves,[43] but this has not been confirmed by others.[44] Prospective randomized trials reported inconclusive evidence for the benefit of routine use of intravenous nitroglycerin in patients with acute myocardial infarction.[43] An early administration of nitroglycerin was found to decrease early and late mortality in one trial.[43] In another study,[45] there was no difference in the total mortality and the subsequent rates of complications between nitroglycerin-treated patients and placebo-treated patients. However, in patients receiving nitroglycerin within ten hours of onset of symptoms, there was a beneficial trend, although this was not statistically significant. In another study,[43] oral isosorbide dinitrate was used in a controlled, randomized trial of 498 patients with acute myocardial infarction. Overall mortality was 11.6% among the treated group, compared with 11.3% among the control group, demonstrating no benefit from active treatment. However, when a subgroup of 248 patients receiving treatment within eight hours of the onset of symptoms was compared with controls in a retrospective analysis, the isosorbide dinitrate group had a mortality of 8.3%, compared with 17.2% among the controls ($P < 0.05$). It must be emphasized that trends suggesting benefit from early intervention and nitroglycerin are based on retrospective subgroup analysis. Thus, routine use of nitroglycerin cannot be recommended to decrease infarct size or mortality of patients with acute myocardial infarction. The use of nitroglycerin should be considered for treatment of pump failure or postinfarction angina.

Nitroglycerin and nitrates have been used for the long-term management of patients with chronic left ventricular failure (Table 9-3).[46] Isosorbide dinitrate given orally improves exercise tolerance in patients with chronic heart failure. Short-acting nitrate preparations used sublingually are not practical in the chronic management of congestive heart failure. The effect of sublingual nitroglycerin occurs within two minutes and lasts for 20 to 30 minutes. Oral nitrates are more frequently used for chronic treatment of heart failure due to their longer duration of action. These agents can be administered as oral, sublingual, or chewable preparations. Administration of nitroglycerin by any of these preparations produces similar hemodynamic effects but different durations of action. For example, the duration of action of isosorbide dinitrate is up to three hours after administration of sublingual or chewable forms, and approximately four to six hours by oral administration. Pentaerythritol tetranitrate is another long-acting nitrate with a duration of action of four to six hours and can usually be administered orally.[47] The duration of action of topical nitroglycerin is three to six hours and can be as long as eight hours.[48] Olivari and colleagues[49,50] reported that the transdermal patch (20 to 40 cm^2) sustained its effects for 24 hours in a limited number of severe heart failure patients (New York Heart Association [NYHA] class III

Table 9-3. Nitrate preparations, dosage, and duration of action

Preparation	Dose	Duration of Action (h)
Isosorbide dinitrate Sublingual	2.5-10 mg every 2-4 h	1.5-3
Oral	20-80 mg every 4-6 h	4-6
Chewable	5-10 mg every 2-4 h	2-3
Nitroglycerin Oral	6.5-19.5 mg every 4-6 h	4
2% ointment	0.5-2 inches (6.5-25 mg) every 4-6 h	3-6
Transdermal*	20-40 cm^2 every 24 h	24
Pentaerythritol tetranitrate	40 mg every 4-6 h	4-6

*From Olivari and Cohn.[50]
Table adapted from Abrams[46] with permission.

and IV). However, the transdermal patch may not produce a sustained and prolonged decrease in pulmonary and systemic venous pressures even when large doses are used. Presumably this is due to the development of tolerance.

Nitrates produce beneficial hemodynamic effects in patients with mitral and aortic regurgitation; regurgitant volumes decrease along with a decrease in left ventricular filling pressure. Pulmonary artery and pulmonary capillary wedge pressures decrease, but forward stroke volume and cardiac output may not increase.[51] Nitrates can be used to decrease symptoms of pulmonary venous congestion in patients with mitral stenosis, although care must be taken not to lower left ventricular end-diastolic volume excessively, because cardiac output might decrease.

Headache is the most common side effect of nitrate therapy. It is most prominent during initial exposure and usually resolves with chronic treatment. In patients with right ventricular infarctions, nitroglycerin should not be used without concomitant fluid administration; otherwise, severe hypotension and shocklike syndrome may be precipitated. In some patients with acute myocardial infarction, extreme bradycardia and hypotension may occur, which can be reversed by intravenous atropine. Postural dizziness and weakness occur less frequently in patients with heart failure. Methemoglobinemia, although extremely rare, has been reported during long-term treatment with larger doses of nitrates.[52] The major clinical problem appears to be a fairly rapid development of tolerance.[53,54] Although pulmonary and systemic venous pressures initially decrease, these changes are attenuated within six to eight hours of continual administration of nitroglycerin. Cross tolerance to isosorbide dinitrate was also observed. It has been suggested that a 12-hour drug-free interval is sufficient to maintain responsiveness to nitroglycerin.[54]

Hydralazine   Hydralazine is a direct-acting vasodilator that causes smooth muscle relaxation, primarily of the precapillary resistance vessels.[55,56] Hydralazine-induced vasodilation is relatively selective. Renal and limb blood flow increase without any significant change in hepatic blood flow.[57] In the absence of obstructive coronary disease, coronary vascular resistance decreases and coronary blood flow increases.[58] In patients with ischemic heart failure, however, changes in coronary blood flow and myocardial oxygen consumption appear to be dependent on changes in the determinants of myocardial oxygen demand. A variable effect on rate-pressure product occurs following hydralazine administration—increases in some and decreases in others.[59,60]

Hydralazine is rapidly and nearly completely absorbed from the gastrointestinal tract. The bioavailability of hydralazine correlates with the acetylator phenotype and is greater for slow than for fast acetylators. Bioavailability ranges from 26% to 55% of an identical intravenous dose, indicating that significant first-pass hepatic biotransformation occurs. The onset of action after an oral dose is 20 to 30 minutes. Peak serum concentration is attained within 30 minutes to two hours and is higher in slow acetylators. The drug is approximately 90% protein bound. The main metabolic products are the triazolo compounds resulting from N-acetylation and the hydrazones. Hydrazones possess activity equal to that of hydralazine; however, little is known about their pharmacokinetics or clinical importance. Unchanged hydralazine, ranging from 1.5% to 14% of an administered dose, is excreted in the urine.

Hydralazine is predominantly an arteriolar dilator with little effect on the venous capacitance bed. The hemodynamic effects of hydralazine are characterized by a marked increase in cardiac index and stroke volume index, and a substantial fall in systemic vascular resistance (Table 9-4). Arterial pressure either remains unchanged or decreases slightly. There is also little or no decrease in systemic or pulmonary venous pressure.[61-64] Unlike the experience in hypertensive patients, reflex tachycardia usually does not occur. Pulmonary vascular resistance decreases in the majority of patients, although the magnitude of decrease is much smaller than with predominant venodilators.

Hydralazine, particularly in combination with nitrates, is useful for the long-term management of chronic heart failure. Beneficial hemodynamic and clinical effects are reported in patients with both ischemic and primary cardiomyopathy. Hydralazine improves left ventricular function not only at rest, but also during exercise.[65,66] Although exercise tolerance may not increase after short-term therapy, improvement is usually seen with chronic treatment. Sustained beneficial hemodynamic and clinical effects have been observed,[62,67] but in some patients tolerance may develop to the beneficial effects of hydralazine therapy.[68]

Table 9-4. Hemodynamic effects* of oral hydralazine in ten patients with refractory heart failure

Hemodynamic Variable	Control	Hydralazine	P Value
Heart rate (beats/min)	90 ± 6.9	90 ± 5.8	NS
Arterial pressure (mm Hg)	89 ± 4.5	89 ± 4.0	NS
Pulmonary arterial pressure (mm Hg)	37 ± 3.4	38 ± 3.1	NS
Left ventricular filling pressure (mm Hg)	24 ± 2	23 ± 2.1	NS
Cardiac index (L/min/m²)	1.99 ± 0.15	3.39 ± 0.29	< 0.001
Stroke volume index (mL/m²)	23 ± 3	38 ± 3.5	< 0.001
Stroke work index (g·m/m²)	23 ± 2.4	36 ± 3.7	< 0.001
Systemic vascular resistance (dynes·s·cm⁻⁵)	1748 ± 129	998 ± 115	< 0.001
Pulmonary vascular resistance (dynes·s·cm⁻⁵)	328 ± 54	203 ± 32	< 0.001

*Mean ± SEM.
NS = not significant.
Adapted from K Chatterjee, WW Parmley, The role of vasodilator therapy in heart failure, *Prog Cardiovasc Dis* 1977;19:301-325.

Hydralazine also produces beneficial hemodynamic and clinical effects in patients with chronic mitral and aortic regurgitation.[69] A marked increase in forward stroke volume and cardiac output with a concomitant decrease in regurgitant volume is usually seen. However, total stroke volume does not change significantly. Thus, hydralazine causes redistribution of left ventricular stroke volume in mitral regurgitation; more blood is pumped forward into the aorta and less backward toward the left atrium. In patients with mitral regurgitation, pulmonary capillary wedge pressure decreases along with a decrease in magnitude of the regurgitant V wave. Hydralazine has been successfully used in a limited number of patients with mild to moderate aortic stenosis.[70] However, vasodilators should not be used in patients with severe aortic stenosis who have fixed cardiac output because hypotension and syncope may occur. Hydralazine has been used to decrease pulmonary vascular resistance in patients with cor pulmonale and precapillary pulmonary hypertension, including primary hypertension.[71] The clinical and hemodynamic responses, however, are unpredictable,[72] and severe adverse effects may occur in these patients.[73] Thus, hydralazine therapy should be initiated cautiously and with hemodynamic monitoring in patients with precapillary pulmonary hypertension.

The usual dose of oral hydralazine for the treatment of chronic heart failure is 200 to 400 mg daily. Larger doses (800 to 1,200 mg daily) are required for some patients. However, the incidence of adverse effects increases with larger doses. The most serious side effect of hydralazine is drug-induced lupus syndrome,[74,75] which is seen in 15% to 20% of patients receiving daily doses of 400 mg or more. A genetic deficiency in the hepatic enzyme *N*-acetyltransferase, which inactivates hydralazine, is a risk factor for the development of this side effect.[76] Some patients with severe coronary artery disease develop angina during hydralazine therapy.[68,77] Increased diuretic dosage or addition of antialdosterone agents is required to avoid the fluid retention and weight gain that occur in some patients during chronic therapy. Gastrointestinal symptoms (nausea and anorexia) are also frequently experienced. Polyneuropathy due to pyridoxine deficiency has been reported.[78-80] Other infrequent side effects include an acute febrile illness[74] and a syndrome of flushing, sweating, and urticaria, which may be secondary to hydralazine-induced inhibition of histamine.[81]

Minoxidil   Minoxidil is a potent direct-acting smooth muscle relaxant. It predominantly affects the arteriolar resistance vessels, with a slight effect on the venous capacitance vessels.[82] In hypertensive patients, reflex stimulation of renin and norepinephrine is observed in response to a fall in blood pressure.[83] The pharmacokinetics of this drug in humans have not been entirely elucidated, and information is based mostly on animal studies.[83,84]

Minoxidil is completely (95%) absorbed after an oral dose, appearing in plasma within 30 minutes and reaching a peak concentration in one hour. The elimination half-life is about four hours. Approximately 10% of a dose of minoxidil is excreted unchanged in the urine. The usual dosage of minoxidil in the management of chronic heart failure ranges from 10 to 20 mg twice daily.

The hemodynamic effects of minoxidil are similar to those of hydralazine.[82,85,86] Cardiac index, stroke volume index, and stroke work index increase, accompanied by a decrease in systemic vascular resistance. No significant change in systemic and pulmonary venous pressures occurs (Table 9-5).[86] In general, heart rate and mean arterial pressure remain unchanged. In some patients with chronic congestive heart failure, marked hypotension and tachycardia are occasionally seen.

The clinical uses of minoxidil are similar to those of hydralazine. The most common side effect is hypertrichosis. The major clinical problem for chronic minoxidil therapy, however, is fluid retention and weight gain, occurring in almost 100% of patients with heart failure. In some patients, fluid retention can be prevented by increasing the dose of diuretics.[86]

Prazosin   Prazosin is a quinazoline derivative that selectively blocks postsynaptic (α_1) receptors in the walls of the blood vessels, leading to vasodilation.[87] Prazosin also inhibits phosphodiesterase,[88] which causes smooth muscle relaxation and interferes with norepinephrine synthesis, although the significance of this action remains unclear. Vasodilation associated with prazosin is relatively selective. Limb vascular resistance decreases and limb blood flow increases. Hepatic blood flow increases with lower doses and does not change with higher doses. Prazosin therapy does not influence renal vascular resistance or renal blood flow. The effects of prazosin on coronary hemodynamics are variable. In some patients with ischemic heart failure, coronary blood flow and myocardial oxygen consumption decrease along with reduction

Table 9-5. Mean hemodynamic effects of increasing single doses of minoxidil

Variable	Control	10 mg	15 mg	20 mg	25 mg	30 mg
Number of patients	11	11	9	9	9	7
Heart rate (beats/min)	91 ± 15	97 ± 26	92 ± 18	97 ± 18	95 ± 18	91 ± 20
Mean arterial pressure (mm Hg)	84 ± 7	86 ± 10	79 ± 11	82 ± 12	82 ± 12	80 ± 10
Pulmonary capillary wedge pressure (mm Hg)	24 ± 8	23 ± 12	23 ± 10	21 ± 7	22 ± 8	22 ± 8
Right atrial pressure (mm Hg)	13 ± 6	12 ± 7	11 ± 5	11 ± 6	13 ± 6	12 ± 7
Cardiac index (L/min/m²)	1.9 ± 0.5	2.7 ± 0.6 ($P < 0.01$)	2.8 ± 0.8 ($P < 0.025$)	3.1 ± 0.6 ($P < 0.005$)	3.0 ± 0.8 ($P < 0.005$)	3.2 ± 0.8 ($P < 0.005$)
Stroke volume index (mL/m²)	21.9 ± 6.9	30.5 ± 10.3 ($P < 0.05$)	31.7 ± 11.0	33.3 ± 8.1	32.9 ± 10.1	35.3 ± 9.0 ($P < 0.05$)
Stroke work index (g·m/m²)	23.6 ± 11.9	33.4 ± 16.2	31.8 ± 13.5	36.3 ± 13.9	35.8 ± 15.3	37.6 ± 13.5
Systemic vascular resistance (dynes·s·cm⁻⁵)	1691 ± 558	1164 ± 211 ($P < 0.001$)	1090 ± 367 ($P < 0.001$)	982 ± 133 ($P < 0.001$)	1022 ± 235 ($P < 0.001$)	885 ± 233 ($P < 0.001$)
Pulmonary vascular resistance (dynes·s·cm⁻⁵)	259 ± 143	193 ± 121	213 ± 92	199 ± 105	196 ± 112	180 ± 77

Adapted from McKay et al[86] with permission.

in the determinants of myocardial oxygen demand; in others, coronary blood flow and myocardial oxygen consumption tend to increase despite a decrease in myocardial oxygen demand.[59,60] The mechanism for this divergent response is not clear. It cannot be excluded that there is a primary decrease of the coronary vascular resistance due to α-adrenergic receptor blockade and, therefore, an increase in coronary blood flow despite a decreased myocardial oxygen demand.

Prazosin is rapidly absorbed from the gastrointestinal tract.[89-91] Oral bioavailability ranges from 44% to 70% and is not influenced by congestive heart failure.[89] Approximately 6% of the drug is excreted unchanged in the urine. The majority of the drug is excreted in the feces, and it is highly protein bound (92% to 97%). The mean elimination half-life is 2.5 hours and is slightly prolonged in patients with heart failure. The hemodynamic effects last approximately six hours. Patients with renal failure have increased plasma levels with a prolonged elimination half-life, decreased plasma protein binding, and an increase in the free fraction of prazosin.

Prazosin produces a balanced effect on precapillary resistance and postcapillary venous capacitance vessels, resulting in increases in cardiac output and stroke volume as systemic vascular resistance and arterial pressure decrease. Pulmonary and systemic venous pressures and pulmonary artery pressure decrease as a result of venodilation (Table 9-6).[92] Pulmonary vascular resistance also declines in most patients.[64,93] In patients with heart failure, prazosin improves left ventricular function during exercise,[94,95] and exercise tolerance and duration are increased.[96,97]

Table 9-6. Prazosin multidose hemodynamic evaluation* in 12 patients

Hemodynamic Variable	Control	Dose1†	Dose 5†
Cardiac index (L/min/m²)	2.3 ± 0.2	2.7 ± 0.2‡	2.4 ± 0.2
Heart rate (beats/min)	86 ± 4	85 ± 4	80 ± 2‡
Mean arterial pressure (mm Hg)	91 ± 4	80 ± 4§	82 ± 4§
Systemic vascular resistance (dynes·s·cm⁻⁵)	1568 ± 128	1269 ± 108‡	1423 ± 128
Pulmonary capillary wedge pressure (mm Hg)	26 ± 3	19 ± 2§	21 ± 2‡
Right atrial pressure (mm Hg)	14 ± 2	10 ± 1‡	10 ± 1
Stroke work index (g·m/m²)	28 ± 5	34 ± 5‡	28 ± 3
Stoke volume index (mL/m²)	27 ± 3	33 ± 3‡	29 ± 3

*Mean ± SEM.
†Data obtained 2 hours after the respective dose. Each dose was 5 mg.
‡$P < 0.05$.
§$P < 0.01$ compared with control.
Reprinted with permission from Chatterjee K, Ports T, Parmley WW: Use of vasodilators in heart failure, in Donso E: *Advances and Controversies in Cardiology*, Thieme Medical Publishers, Inc., New York, ©1981.

Although a number of studies demonstrated sustained hemodynamic and clinical effects in patients with chronic heart failure,[94,97-103] attenuation of the beneficial hemodynamic effects with chronic therapy has also been observed.[104-106] During chronic therapy, cardiac output and systemic vascular resistance may return to the pretreatment level, even though lower left ventricular filling pressure is still observed. The mechanism for the attenuation of prazosin's hemodynamic effects remains unclear. Plasma norepinephrine has been shown to be increased following chronic therapy.[107] This may result in peripheral vasoconstriction, which counteracts the effect of prazosin. Sodium retention due to aldosterone stimulation has also been postulated to account for attenuation of effects. The addition of antialdosterone agents can potentially prevent attenuation of the hemodynamic effects.[103]

The attenuation of some of the beneficial hemodynamic effects of prazosin during long-term treatment appears to be related to initial plasma renin activity and neurohumoral changes during therapy. In patients with lower initial renin activity, prazosin caused a decrease in plasma epinephrine and arginine vasopressin; in patients with higher initial plasma renin activity, there was an increase in plasma norepinephrine, and plasma renin activity and aldosterone levels remained high.[108] Prazosin increased water excretion and decreased minimal urinary osmolality in patients with lower renin but had no effect in patients with higher renin.[108]

The usual dose of prazosin for treating congestive heart failure ranges from 3 to 5 mg three or four times daily. Serious side effects are uncommon. When prazosin has been used to treat hypertension, marked hypotension has occurred after the first dose, but this effect can be minimized when therapy is initiated with a smaller dose. This effect has not been associated with the use of prazosin in heart failure; however, caution should be observed. Gastrointestinal symptoms are seen in a few patients, and palpitations, drowsiness, depression, and nervousness are infrequent. Sexual dysfunction is rare.

Long-term prognosis of patients with severe chronic heart failure is not favorably influenced by prazosin therapy, and one-year survival remains between 50% and 60%.[103] Prazosin also does not appear to improve prognosis of patients with moderately severe heart failure. In the Veterans Administration Cooperative Study,[109] the cumulative mortality rates at two years and three years in the group treated with digitalis and diuretics were 34.3% and 46.9%, respectively, and there was no reduction in mortality with the addition of prazosin. Left ventricular ejection fraction also remained unchanged in the prazosin-treated group. As long-term clinical benefit also occurs infrequently, prazosin should not be considered as the vasodilator of choice for treatment of chronic heart failure.

Trimazosin   Trimazosin is also a quinazoline derivative with a mechanism of action and hemodynamic response similar to those of prazosin.[38,110-112] Experience with trimazosin in treating patients with congestive heart failure is limited.

Following administration of trimazosin to patients with heart failure, cardiac output and stroke volume increase, and systemic and pulmonary venous pressures and pulmonary arterial pressures decrease. Systemic and pulmonary vascular resistances are also reduced; heart rate and mean arterial pressure remain unchanged. These hemodynamic effects persist during chronic therapy.[111] During maintenance trimazosin therapy, exercise tolerance and maximum oxygen consumption increase.[112,113] Trimazosin has produced improvements in patients with heart failure after doses ranging from 25 to 100 mg three times daily.[111] The advantage of this drug over other vasodilators and its potential adverse reactions after chronic treatment require further study.[114]

Converting-Enzyme Inhibitors — The angiotensin converting-enzyme inhibitors captopril and enalapril show promise for the long-term management of chronic heart failure. They produce similar hemodynamic effects, which are like those of the α_1-blocking agents prazosin and trimazosin.

In patients with heart failure, substantial increases in cardiac output and stroke volume occur along with significant decreases in right atrial and pulmonary capillary wedge pressures.[115] Mean arterial pressure, systemic vascular resistance, and pulmonary artery pressures decline, while heart rate and pulmonary vascular resistance usually do not change. These beneficial hemodynamic effects are accompanied by clinical improvement in the majority of patients with heart failure (see Chap. 10).

Enalapril improved survival in patients with severe chronic heart failure.[116] In this double-blind study, patients in New York Heart Association functional class IV (approximately 57% with coronary artery disease) were randomly assigned to receive either placebo (n = 126) or enalapril (n = 127). Some of the patients in the control group continued taking other vasodilators. The mortality was reduced by 40% at six months and by 31% at one year in the enalapril-treated group, and there were also a significant improvement in the clinical status and reduction in heart size. Hypotension and deterioration in renal function were observed more frequently in the enalapril-treated group.

Calcium Antagonists — Calcium antagonists selectively inhibit the slow inward calcium current through the calcium channel in both smooth muscle and myocardium and decrease availability of calcium to the contractile elements in both tissues. As a result, calcium antagonists exert peripheral vasodilating and negative inotropic effects. Peripheral vasodilatation is the rationale for their use in the treatment of heart failure. The contractile mechanism in smooth muscle is regulated by calcium ions that interact with calmodulin to form the calcium-calmodulin complex, which then stimulates myosin light chain kinase to phosphorylate the myosin light chains for the interaction of actin and myosin. Decreased availability of calcium ions following the use of calcium antagonists retards these effects of calcium ions and is associated with peripheral vasodilatation. Some calcium antagonists (verapamil and diltiazem) exert their inhibitory effects on nodal tissues and decrease sinus rate and atrioventricular nodal conduction. It is not known why different calcium antagonists have different effects on nodal and vascular tissues. Verapamil, a papaverine derivative, and diltiazem, a benzothiazepine compound, interact with similar but different binding sites. Nifedipine, a dihydropyridine, binds to a different site and has little effect on nodal tissues.

The negative inotropic effects of calcium antagonists are usually offset by peripheral vasodilatation, which decreases left ventricular resistance and improves cardiac performance. The calcium antagonists with more potent vasodilating effects have greater potential to improve cardiac function in patients with heart failure. Dihydropyridine derivatives, nifedipine and felodipine are potent vasodilators and have been used for treatment of heart failure.[117-119] Their hemodynamic effects are characterized by a substantial decrease in systemic vascular resistance and arterial pressure, along with increased stroke volume and cardiac output. Pulmonary capillary wedge, right atrial, and left ventricular diastolic pressures remain unchanged or are slightly decreased. Nifedipine improves left ventricular distensibility in patients with elevated left ventricular end-diastolic pressure. This may contribute to the reduction of left ventricular diastolic pressure in some patients. Nifedipine has been combined with nitroglycerin to enhance its hemodynamic effects.[120]

Nifedipine decreases coronary vascular resistance in patients with congestive heart failure at rest and during exercise.[121] Coronary blood flow increases but myocardial oxygen consumption does not change as myocardial oxygen extraction declines. Thus, improved cardiac performance is not associated with increased metabolic cost. In general, nifedipine does not cause any significant change in glomerular filtration rate in patients with congestive heart failure.[122] In some patients, nifedipine can cause deterioration of renal function, particularly if significant hypotension occurs.[123] Nifedipine is also a less effective arterial vasodilator than hydralazine. Furthermore, nifedipine does not appear to improve exercise tolerance even when systemic hemodynamics improve. Changes in exercise capacity were compared during nifedipine and captopril therapy in a prospective crossover trial.[124] Although captopril consistently increased exercise tolerance, there was no change in exercise capacity during nifedipine therapy.

Verapamil is not well tolerated by patients with overt failure. Diltiazem tends to increase cardiac output and stroke volume with a modest decrease in pulmonary capillary wedge pressure. However, experience with diltiazem is limited. Similarly, there is limited experience with felodipine in the long-term management of chronic heart failure. Furthermore, some patients may develop hypotension and low cardiac output even with dihydropyridines (nifedipine), and these adverse responses cannot be predicted from the clinical features and initial hemodynamics.[118] Thus, calcium antagonists are not ideal vasodilator drugs for treatment of heart failure and should chiefly be considered for use in patients with mild to moderate heart failure associated with angina or hypertension.

Calcium antagonists occasionally decrease pulmonary vascular resistance in patients with precapillary pulmonary hypertension[125]; however, adverse responses such as systemic hypotension and decreased cardiac output may also occur so that treatment should not be initiated without hemodynamic monitoring. The side effects of calcium antagonists include hypotension, headache, dizziness, constipation, edema, and renal failure.

Other Vasodilators
Exogenous prostaglandins produce peripheral vasodilatation and have the potential to improve cardiac performance in patients with heart failure. However, both PGE_2 and the PGI_2 analog CL115,347 are active when administered orally, intravenously, or transdermally and have produced beneficial hemodynamic effects in a limited number of patients.[126] Intravenous prostacyclin also effectively decreases pulmonary artery pressure and pulmonary vascular resistance in some patients with precapillary pulmonary hypertension.

Labetalol, an agent with α- and β-antagonist properties, decreases systemic vascular resistance and arterial pressure. Its hemodynamic effects have not been adequately evaluated in patients with heart failure.

Indoramin is an α_1-blocking agent and its hemodynamic effects are expected to be similar to those of prazosin.

The β_2-receptor agonists (salbutamol, pirbuterol) cause peripheral vasodilation and have been used to treat heart failure. These agents also produce some positive inotropic effect. Their long-term effects, however, have not been adequately evaluated. Furthermore, rapid attenuation of clinical response and ventricular arrhythmias may occur.

New dopaminergic agents bromocriptine, fenoldopam, and dopexamine are vasodilators without significant inotropic effect. These agents produce beneficial systemic hemodynamic effects in patients with heart failure; however, long-term studies are required to determine their sustained benefit and lack of undesirable side effects.

Atrial natriuretic peptide (ANP) or factor (ANF) is secreted by atrial myocytes in response to atrial distension. The endogenous level is significantly elevated in patients with heart failure.[127] ANP acts on vascular cells to produce vasodilatory cyclic guanosine monophosphate (GMP).[128] Synthetic human ANP possesses expected natriuretic, diuretic, and vaso-dilatory properties. Infusion of atrial peptides in patients with heart failure causes a substantial increase in cardiac output and a decrease in systemic vascular resistance and pulmonary capillary wedge pressure.[129] However, natriuresis and diuresis may not occur. Furthermore, delayed hypotension has been observed. Thus, without further studies, the role of ANP in the management of heart failure remains uncertain.

COMBINATION THERAPY The hemodynamic abnormalities in patients with heart failure are variable. In some patients, decreased cardiac output and elevated systemic vascular resistance are not associated with marked elevation of pulmonary or systemic venous pressures. In others, marked elevation of pulmonary venous pressure is the major hemodynamic abnormality in the presence of an adequate cardiac output. In most patients with advanced heart failure, not only is the cardiac output low, but pulmonary venous pressure is elevated. The hemodynamic objectives of therapy in these patients are to increase cardiac output and to decrease systemic and pulmonary venous pressures. These objectives can be fulfilled through the use of vasodilators with balanced effects on arterial and venous beds. Alternatively, a venodilator (eg, nitrates) to decrease pulmonary venous pressure and an arteriolar dilator (eg, hy-dralazine) to increase cardiac output can be combined to achieve similar hemodynamic effects. It should be remembered that significant differences exist among the effects of some of these vasodilator drugs on regional circulation and function, which might be relevant during long-term vasodilator treatment (Table 9-7).

Hydralazine and nitrates administered in combination have shown clinical effectiveness during long-term management of severe chronic congestive heart failure.[77] This combination also improved hemodynamics and symptoms during exercise.[65]

Table 9-7. Differences in the effects of vasodilators on regional circulation

Vasodilator	Limb Blood Flow	Hepatic Blood Flow	Renal Blood Flow	Coronary Blood Flow	Myocardial Oxygen Consumption
Captopril	↑	—	↑	↓	↓
Hydralazine	↑	↑	↑	↑ or ↓	↑ or ↓
Prazosin	↑	↑ (with smaller doses)	—	↑ or ↓	↑ or ↓
Nitrates	—	—	—	↓	↓

↑ = increase; ↓ = decrease; — = no change.

The individual and combined hemodynamic effects of nitrates and hydralazine in patients with chronic congestive heart failure are summarized in Table 9-8.[130] Nitrates produce a significant reduction in right atrial and pulmonary capillary wedge pressure and a modest decrease in pulmonary artery pressure. Systemic vascular resistance and cardiac output do not change. Hydralazine alone produces a marked increase in cardiac output along with a decrease in systemic vascular resistance, but right atrial and pulmonary capillary wedge pressure remain unchanged. The combination of hydralazine and nitrates causes a substantial increase in cardiac output and a reduction of systemic and pulmonary venous pressures. No significant change in heart rate or blood pressure is noted with the use of these vasodilator agents, either alone or in combination. Minoxidil and nitrates can also be combined to obtain similar hemodynamic effects.[82]

Table 9-8. Hemodynamic results of individual and combined vasodilator therapy

Hemodynamic Variable	Control	Nitrates	Hydralazine	Combined
Number of patients	12	8	11	12
Heart rate (beats/min)	80 ± 5	74 ± 5	84 ± 5	85 ± 5
Mean arterial pressure (mm Hg)	87 ± 4	84 ±6	83 ± 3	85 ± 4
Mean right atrial pressure (mm Hg)	14 ± 2	10 ± 2*	14 ± 2	9 ± 2†
Mean pulmonary artery pressure (mm Hg)	38 ± 4	30 ± 3*	39 ± 3	32 ± 3
Mean pulmonary capillary wedge pressure (mm Hg)	28 ± 1	17 ± 1†	25 ± 2	18 ± 1†
Cardiac index (L/min/m²)	2.1 ± 0.1	2.1 ± 0.1	3.2 ± 0.3	3.3 ± 0.3
Stroke volume index (mL/m²)	27 ± 2	28 ± 2	39 ± 3†	39 ± 3†
Stroke work index (g•m/m²)	25 ± 2	28 ± 3	38 ± 3	42 ± 3†
Systemic vascular resistance (dynes•s•cm⁻⁵)	1690 ± 150	1710 ± 160	1030 ± 110	1110 ± 110†
Pulmonary vascular resistance (dynes•s•cm⁻⁵)	310 ± 50	300 ± 60	170 ± 40	200 ± 40

*Change from control $P < 0.01$.
†Change from control $P < 0.001$.
From Chatterjee K, Brundage BH, Ports TA: Nonparenteral vasodilator therapy for chronic congestive heart failure. *Compr Ther* 1979;5(11):48-55. With permission of The Laux Co Inc.

In patients with severe chronic heart failure (NYHA class IV), combination therapy with hydralazine and nitrates does not improve prognosis, and one-year survival is still only 50% to 60%. Patients who derive marked clinical and hemodynamic improvement during the initiation of treatment appear to do better than those who do not experience clinical improvement and those who show modest or no improvement in left ventricular function. The combination of hydralazine (300 mg/d) and isosorbide dinitrate (160 mg/d) appears to improve the prognosis of patients with mild to moderately severe congestive heart failure. In the Veterans Administration Cooperative Study,[109] the cumulative mortality rate at two years was 25.6% in the hydralazine–isosorbide dinitrate group and 34.3% in the placebo group (ie, digoxin and diuretics). At three years, the respective mortality rates were 36.2% versus 46.9%. With hydralazine-nitrate therapy, there was 38%, 25%, and 23% reduction in the cumulative mortality rates at one, two, and three years, respectively. There was also a substantial increase in left ventricular ejection fraction with hydralazine-nitrate therapy.

Comparative crossover hemodynamic studies of captopril, prazosin, and hydralazine in patients with chronic heart failure suggest that the magnitude of increase in cardiac output with hydralazine is relatively greater than that seen with prazosin or captopril. Thus, potential exists for cautious use of combination therapy with prazosin or captopril and hydralazine when there is an inadequate increase in cardiac output with prazosin or captopril alone. The hemodynamic effects of combined captopril and hydralazine therapy have been evaluated in a small number of patients with severe chronic heart failure.[131] Captopril alone decreased pulmonary capillary wedge pressure by an average of 30%. The addition of hydralazine was not associated with any further decrease in pulmonary venous pressure. Cardiac output increased by 17% with captopril alone and increased to 65% over baseline following the addition of hydralazine to the captopril regimen, which suggests that vasodilators with different mechanisms of action can be combined to achieve hemodynamic advantages. However, long-term studies are required to evaluate the clinical effectiveness and potential hazards of combination therapy.

CONCLUSION Reduction of left ventricular outflow resistance in order to increase cardiac output and to improve left ventricular function is the principal rationale for vasodilator therapy in heart failure. Decreased intracardiac volumes and pressures produced by vasodilator drugs with predominantly venodilating effects are also useful in relieving congestive symptoms of heart failure. Although vasodilation can be mediated by different mechanisms, the systemic hemodynamic effects of these drugs are qualitatively similar. However, quantitative differences in their hemodynamic effects and their effects on regional circulation exist. These differences in systemic and regional hemodynamic effects should be considered when the physician elects to use a vasodilator agent for the treatment of heart failure.

Of all the vasodilators currently available, the combination of hydralazine and nitrates or angiotensin converting-enzyme inhibitors appears to produce sustained benefit in patients with chronic congestive heart failure. In patients with severe heart failure with marked abnormalities of neuroendocrine function, angiotensin converting-enzyme inhibitors may provide some advantage over other vasodilators, because the neuroendocrine dysfunction frequently improves. Angiotensin converting-enzyme inhibitors may also improve prognosis of these patients. However, further comparative studies will be needed to establish the relative advantages of hydralazine-nitrate and angiotensin converting-enzyme inhibitors.

REFERENCES

1. Gaasch WH, Zile MR: Evaluation of myocardial function in cardiomyopathic states. *Prog Cardiovasc Dis* 1984;27:115.
2. Chatterjee K, Viquerat CE, Daly P: Neurohumoral abnormalities in heart failure. *Heart Failure* 1985;1:69-83.
3. Pepine CJ, Nichols WW, Conti CR: Aortic input impedance in heart failure. *Circulation* 1978;58:460-465.
4. Cohn JN: Vasodilator therapy for heart failure: The influence of impedance on left ventricular performance. *Circulation* 1973;48:5-8.
5. Parmley WW, Chatterjee K: Vasodilator therapy. *Curr Prob Cardiol* 1978;2:8-75.
6. Banka VS, Bodenheimer MM, Shah R, et al: Intervention ventriculography: Comparative value of nitroglycerin, post-extrasystolic potentiation and nitroglycerin plus post-extrasystolic potentiation. *Circulation* 1976;53:632-637.
7. Klausner SC, Ratshin RA, Tybert JV: The similarity of changes in segmental contraction patterns induced by post-extrasystolic potentiation and nitroglycerin. *Circulation* 1976;54:615-623.
8. McAnulty JH, Hattenhauer MT, Rosch J: Improvement in left ventricular wall motion following nitroglycerin. *Circulation* 1975;51:140-145.
9. Parmley WW, Chuck L, Chatterjee K, et al: Acute changes in the diastolic pressure volume relationship of the left ventricle. *Eur J Cardiol* 1976;4(suppl):105.
10. Alderman EL, Glantz SA: Acute hemodynamic interventions shift the diastolic pressure-volume curve in man. *Circulation* 1976;54:662-671.
11. Chatterjee K, Parmley WW: The role of vasodilator therapy in heart failure. *Prog Cardiovasc Dis* 1977;19:301-325.
12. Chatterjee K: Vasodilation in heart failure, in Ledingham JGG, Warrell DA, Weatherall DJ (eds): *Oxford Textbook of Medicine.* Oxford, England, Oxford University Press, 1982, chap 12.4.
13. Zelis R, Mason DT, Braunwald E: A comparison of the effects of vasodilator stimuli on peripheral resistance vessels in normal subjects and in patients with congestive heart failure. *J Clin Invest* 1968;47:960-970.
14. Zahir M, Gould L: Phentolamine and beta-adrenergic receptors. *J Clin Pharmacol* 1971;11:197-203.
15. Chatterjee K, Ports TA, Parmley WW: Nitroprusside: Its clinical pharmacology and application in acute heart failure, in Gould L, Land B, Reddy CVR (eds): *Vasodilator Therapy for Cardiac Disorders.* Mt Kisco, NY, Futura Publishing Co, 1979, chap 3.
16. Franciosa JA, Cuiha NH, Limas CJ, et al: Improved left ventricular function during nitroprusside infusion in acute myocardial infarction. *Lancet* 1972;1:640-647.
17. Bastrow R, Kaloyanides GJ: Effect of sodium nitroprusside on function in isolated intact dog kidney. *J Pharmacol Exp Ther* 1972;181:244-249.
18. Cogan JS, Humphreys MH, Carson CJ, et al: Afterload reduction increases renal blood flow and maintains glomerular filtration rate in patients with congestive heart failure. *Clin Res* 1979;27:3A.
19. Kaneky Y, Ikeda T, Takeda T, et al: Renin release during acute reduction of arterial pressure in normotensive subjects and patients with renal vascular hypertension. *J Clin Invest* 1967;46:705-716.
20. Cohn JN, Franciosa JA, Notargiacomo A: Nitroprusside and dobutamine effect on myocardial oxygen supply/demand in experimental myocardial infarction. *Circulation* 1974;103(suppl 3):49-50.
21. Powers ER, Reison DS, Berke A, et al: The effect of nitroprusside on coronary and systemic hemodynamics in patients with severe congestive heart failure. *Circulation* 1982;66(suppl 2):211.
22. Chatterjee K, Parmley WW, Ganz W, et al: Hemodynamic and metabolic responses to vasodilator therapy in acute myocardial infarction. *Circulation* 1973;48:1183-1193.

23. Chatterjee K, Parmley WW: Vasodilator therapy in chronic heart failure. *Annu Rev Pharmacol Toxicol* 1980;22:475-512.

24. Chatterjee K, Brundage BH, Ports TA: Nonparenteral vasodilator therapy for chronic congestive heart failure. *Comp Ther* 1979;5(11):48-55.

25. Awan NA, Miller RR, Vera Z, et al: Reduction of ST segment elevation with infusion of nitroprusside in patients with acute myocardial infarction. *Am J Cardiol* 1976;38:435-447.

26. Chiariello M, Gold HK, Leinbach RC, et al: Comparison between the effects of nitroprusside and nitroglycerin on ischemic injury during acute myocardial infarction. *Circulation* 1976;54:766-773.

27. Gold HK, Chiariello M, Leinbach RC: Deleterious effects of nitroprusside on myocardial injury during acute myocardial infarction. *Herz* 1976;1:161-166.

28. Chatterjee K, Swan HJ, Kaushik VS, et al: Effects of vasodilator therapy for severe pump failure in acute myocardial infarction on short-term and late prognosis. *Circulation* 1976;53:979.

29. Cohn JN, Franciosa JA, Francis GS, et al: Effect of short-term infusion of sodium nitroprusside on mortality rate in acute myocardial infarction complicated by left ventricular failure: Results of a Veterans Administration Cooperative Study. *N Engl J Med* 1982;306:1129-1135.

30. Durrer JD, Lie KI, VanCabelle FSL, et al: Effect of sodium nitroprusside on mortality in acute myocardial infarction. *N Engl J Med* 1982;306:1121-1128.

31. Gould L, Reddy CVR: Phentolamine in acute heart failure, in Gould L, Land B, Reddy CVR (eds): *Vasodilator Therapy for Cardiac Disorders*. Mt Kisco, NY, Futura Publishing Co, 1979, chap 4.

32. Gould L, Reddy CVR, Blatt CJ, et al: Phentolamine effects on coronary blood flow in humans with recent myocardial infarction. *Br Heart J* 1975;37:647.

33. Shell WE, Sobel BE: Protection of jeopardized ischemic myocardium by reduction of ventricular afterload. *N Engl J Med* 1974;291:481-486.

34. Winbury MM: Redistribution of left ventricular blood flow produced by nitroglycerin. *Circ Res* 1971; 1(suppl 1):140-147.

35. Feldman RC, Pepine C, Conti R: Magnitude of dilatation of large and small coronary arteries by nitroglycerin. *Circulation* 1981;64:324-332.

36. Levine RI, Weksler BB, Jaffe EA, et al: Nitroglycerin stimulates production of prostacyclin by cultured human endothelial cells. *J Clin Invest* 1981;67:762-769.

37. Morcillo E, Pitt B, Reid P: Attenuation of the cardiovascular effects of nitroglycerin by indomethacin. *Am J Cardiol* 1978;41:367.

38. Franciosa JA, Cohn JN: Sustained hemodynamic effects of nitrates without tolerance in heart failure. *Circulation* 1978;58(suppl 2):28.

39. Taylor WR, Forrester J, Magnusson P, et al: The hemodynamic effects of nitroglycerin ointment in congestive heart failure. *Am J Cardiol* 1976;38:469-473.

40. Chatterjee K, Massie B, Rubin S, et al: Long-term outpatient vasodilator therapy of congestive heart failure. *Am J Med* 1978;65:134-144.

41. Gray R, Chatterjee K, Vyden JK, et al: Hemodynamic and metabolic effects of isosorbide dinitrate in chronic congestive heart failure. *Am Heart J* 1975;90:346-351.

42. Packer M, Meller J, Medina N, et al: Equivalent hemodynamic effects of intravenous nitroprusside and high oral doses of oral isosorbide dinitrate in severe heart failure. *Circulation* 1979;59, 60: 531-539.

43. Rapaport E: Early and late interventions in acute myocardial infarction. *Primary Cardiol* 1985;11(11):11.

44. Bowen WG, Branconi JM, Goldstein RA, et al: A randomized prospective study of the effects of intravenous nitroglycerin in patients during myocardial infarction. *Circulation* 1979;59(suppl 2):170.

45. Flaherty JT, Becker LC, Bulkely BH, et al: A randomized prospective trial of intravenous nitroglycerin in patients with acute myocardial infarction. *Circulation* 1983;68:576-588.

46. Abrams J: Pharmacology for long-acting nitrates and their usefulness in the treatment of chronic congestive heart failure, in Gould L, Land B, Reddy CVR (eds): *Vasodilator Therapy for Cardiac Disorders.* Mt Kisco, NY, Futura Publishing Co, 1979, pp 129-167.

47. Klein RC, Amsterdam EA, Pratt C, et al: Sustained reduction of elevated left ventricular filling pressure in cardiac failure by oral long-acting nitrate therapy. *Clin Res* 1978;26:243A.

48. Armstrong PW, Armstrong JA, Marks GS: Pharmacokinetic-hemodynamic studies of nitroglycerin ointment in congestive heart failure. *Am J Cardiol* 1980;46:670-676.

49. Olivari MT, Carlyle PF, Levine TB, et al: Hemodynamic and humoral response to transdermal nitroglycerin in congestive heart failure. *Clin Res* 1982;30:548.

50. Olivari MT, Cohn JN: Cutaneous administration of nitroglycerin: A review. *Pharmacotherapy* 1983;3:149-157.

51. Sniderman AD, Marpole DG, Palmer WH, et al: Response of the left ventricle to nitroglycerin in patients with and without mitral regurgitation. *Br Heart J* 1974;36:357-361.

52. Nickelson M: Vasodilators, in Goodman LS, Gilman AG (eds): *The Pharmacologic Basis of Therapeutics.* New York, Macmillan and Company, 1975, p 733.

53. Elkayam U, Kulick D, McIntosh N, et al: Incidence of early tolerance to continuous intravenous nitroglycerin infusion in patients with coronary artery disease and heart failure (abstract). *J Am Coll Cardiol* 1987;9(suppl A):103A.

54. Packer M, Kessler PD, Lee WH, et al: Does the intermittent administration of nitroglycerin prevent the development of hemodynamic tolerance in patients with severe heart failure (abstract)? *J Am Coll Cardiol* 1987;9(suppl A):103A.

55. Freis ED, Rose JC, Higgins TF, et al: The hemodynamic effects of hypotensive drugs in man: IV. 1-Hydrazinophthalazine. *Circulation* 1953;8:199-204.

56. Koch-Weser J: Hydralazine. *N Engl J Med* 1976;295:320-323.

57. Leier CV, Magorien RD, Desch CE, et al: Hydralazine and isosorbide dinitrate: Comparative central and regional hemodynamic effects when administered alone or in combination. *Circulation* 1981;63:102-109.

58. Magorien RD, Brown GP, Unverferth DV, et al: Effects of hydralazine on coronary blood flow and myocardial energetics in congestive heart failure. *Circulation* 1982;65:528-533.

59. Chatterjee K, Rouleau JL: Hemodynamic and metabolic effects of vasodilators, nitrates, hydralazine, prazosin and captopril in chronic ischemic heart failure. *Acta Med Scand* 1981;651:295-303.

60. Rouleau JL, Chatterjee K, Benge W, et al: Alterations in left ventricular function and coronary hemodynamics with captopril, hydralazine and prazosin in chronic ischemic heart failure: A comparative study. *Circulation* 1982;65:671-678.

61. Chatterjee K, Parmley WW, Massie B, et al: Oral hydralazine therapy for chronic refractory heart failure. *Circulation* 1976;54:879-883.

62. Fitchett D, Neto J, Oakley C, et al: Hydralazine in the management of left ventricular failure. *Am J Cardiol* 1979;44:303-309.

63. Franciosa JA, Pierpont G, Cohn JN: Hemodynamic improvement after oral hydralazine in left ventricular failure. *Ann Intern Med* 1977;86:388-393.

64. Mehta J, Iacona M, Pepine C, et al: Comparative hemodynamic effects of nitroprusside, prazosin and hydralazine in refractory heart failure. *Am J Cardiol* 1978;41:418.

65. Franciosa JA, Cohn JN: Immediate effects of hydralazine-isosorbide dinitrate combination on exercise capacity and exercise hemodynamics in patients with left ventricular failure. *Circulation* 1979;50:1085-1091.

66. Rubin SA, Chatterjee K, Ports TA, et al: Influence of short-term oral hydralazine therapy on exercise hemodynamics in patients with severe chronic heart failure. *Am J Cardiol* 1979;44:1183-1189.

67. Chatterjee K, Ports T, Brundage B, et al: Oral hydralazine in chronic heart failure: Sustained beneficial hemodynamic effects. *Ann Intern Med* 1980;92:600-604.

68. Packer M, Meller J, Medina N, et al: Hemodynamic characterization of tolerance to long-term hydralazine therapy in severe chronic heart failure. *N Engl J Med* 1982;306:57-62.

69. Greenberg BH, Massie BM: Beneficial effects of afterload reduction therapy in patients with congestive heart failure and moderate aortic stenosis. *Circulation* 1981;61:1212-1216.

70. Greenberg BH, Massie BM, Brundage BH, et al: Beneficial effects of hydralazine in severe mitral regurgitation. *Circulation* 1978;58:273-279.

71. Rubin LJ, Peter RH: Oral hydralazine for primary pulmonary hypertension. *N Engl J Med* 1980;302:69-73.

72. McKay C, Chatterjee K, Raff GL, et al: Comparative hemodynamic and clinical responses to Isuprel, diazoxide, and hydralazine in severe precapillary pulmonary hypertension. *Am J Cardiol* 1981;47:422.

73. Packer M, Greenberg B, Massie B, et al: Deleterious effects of hydralazine in patients with pulmonary hypertension. *N Engl J Med* 1982;306:1328-1331.

74. Perry HM Jr, Tan FM, Carmody S, et al: Relationship of acetyl transferase activity to antinuclear antibodies and toxic symptoms in hypertensive patients treated with hydralazine. *J Lab Clin Med* 1970;76:114-117.

75. Perry H: Late toxicity to hydralazine resembling systemic lupus erythematosus or rheumatoid arthritis. *Am J Med* 1973;54:56-72.

76. Talseth T: Serum concentrations of hydralazine in man after a single dose and at steady state. *Eur J Clin Pharmacol* 1976;10:183-187.

77. Massie B, Ports T, Chatterjee K, et al: Long-term vasodilator treatment for congestive heart failure: Clinical response and its related hemodynamic measurements. *Circulation* 1981;63:269-278.

78. Kirkendall WM, Page EB: Polyneuritis occurring during hydralazine therapy. *JAMA* 1958;167:427-432.

79. Pierpont GL, Brown DC, Franciosa JA, et al: Effect of hydralazine on renal function in patients with congestive heart failure. *Circulation* 1980;61:323-327.

80. Raskin NH, Rishman RA: Pyrodoxine-deficiency neuropathy due to hydralazine. *N Engl J Med* 1965;273:1182-1185.

81. Morrow JD, Schroeder HA, Perry HM Jr: Studies on the control of hypertension by hyphex: II. Toxic reaction and side effects. *Circulation* 1953;8:829-839.

82. Chatterjee K, Drew D, Parmley WW, et al: Combination vasodilator therapy for severe chronic congestive heart failure. *Ann Intern Med* 1976;85:467-470.

83. Pettinger W: Minoxidil and the treatment of severe hypertension. *N Engl J Med* 1980;303:922-926.

84. Ducharme D, Freyburger W, Graham B, et al: Pharmacologic properties in minoxidil: A new hypotensive agent. *J Pharmacol Exp Ther* 1973;184:662-670.

85. Franciosa JA, Cohn JN: Effects of minoxidil on hemodynamics of patients with congestive heart failure. *Circulation* 1981;63:652-657.

86. McKay CR, Chatterjee K, Ports TA, et al: Minoxidil therapy in chronic congestive heart failure: Acute plus long-term hemodynamic and clinical study. *Am Heart J* 1982;104:575-580.

87. Brogden RN, Heel RC, Speight TM, et al: Prazosin: A review of its pharmacological properties and therapeutic efficacy in hypertension. *Drugs* 1977;14:163-167.

88. Constantine JW: Analysis of the hypotensive action of prazosin, in Cotton DWK (ed): *Prazosin: Evaluation of a New Antihypertensive Agent.* Amsterdam, Excerpta Medica, 1974, pp 16-36.

89. Baughman R, Arnold S, Benet L, et al: Altered prazosin pharmacokinetics in congestive heart failure. *Eur J Clin Pharmacol* 1980;17:425-428.

90. Graham RM, Pettinger WA: Prazosin. *N Engl J Med* 1979;300:232-236.

91. Rubin R, Blaschke T: Clinical pharmacology of prazosin: I. Cardiovascular, catecholamine and endocrine changes following a single dose. *Br J Clin Pharmacol* 1980;10:23-32.

92. Chatterjee K, Ports T, Parmley WW: Use of vasodilators in heart failure, in Donso E (ed): *Advances and Controversies in Cardiology*. New York, Thieme Medical Publishers Inc, 1981, pp 13-186.

93. Miller RR, Awan NA, Maxwell KS, et al: Sustained reduction of cardiac impedance and preload in congestive heart failure with the antihypertensive vasodilator prazosin. *N Engl J Med* 1977;297:303-307.

94. Goldman SA, Johnson II, Escala E, et al: Improved exercise ejection fraction with long-term prazosin therapy in patients with heart failure. *Am J Med* 1980;68:36-42.

95. Rubin SA, Chatterjee K, Gelberg HJ, et al: Paradox of improved exercise but not resting hemodynamics with short-term prazosin in chronic heart failure. *Am J Cardiol* 1979;43:810-815.

96. Aronow WS, Lurie M, Turbow M, et al: Effect of prazosin versus placebo on chronic left ventricular heart failure. *Circulation* 1979;59:344-349.

97. Colucci WS, Wynne J, Holman B, et al: Long-term therapy of heart failure with prazosin: A randomized double-blind trial. *Am J Cardiol* 1980;45:337-344.

98. Awan NA, Miller RR, DeMaria AN, et al: Efficacy of ambulatory systemic vasodilator therapy with oral prazosin in chronic refractory heart failure. *Circulation* 1977;56:346-354.

99. Awan NA, Miller RR, Maxwell KS: Development of systemic vasodilator tolerance to prazosin with chronic use of the agent in ambulatory therapy of severe congestive heart failure. *Am J Cardiol* 1978;41:367.

100. Awan NA, Lee G, DeMaria AN, et al: Ambulatory prazosin treatment of chronic congestive heart failure: Development of late tolerance reversible by higher dosage and interrupted substitution therapy. *Am Heart J* 1981;101:541-547.

101. Bertel O, Burkart F, Buhler F: Sustained effect of chronic prazosin treatment in severe congestive heart failure. *Am Heart J* 1981;101:529-533.

102. Feldman RC, Ball RM, Winchester MA, et al: Beneficial hemodynamic response to chronic prazosin therapy in congestive heart failure. *Am Heart J* 1981;101:534-540.

103. Rouleau JL, Warnica J, Burgess J: Prazosin and congestive heart failure: Short- and long-term therapy. *Am J Med* 1981;71:147-152.

104. Arnold S, Williams R, Ports TA, et al: Attenuation of prazosin effect on cardiac output in chronic heart failure. *Ann Intern Med* 1979;91:345-349.

105. Elkayam U, LeJemtel T, Mathur M, et al: Marked early attenuation of hemodynamic effects of oral prazosin therapy in chronic heart failure. *Am J Cardiol* 1980;43:403.

106. Packer M, Meller J, Gorlin R, et al: Hemodynamic and clinical tachyphylaxis to prazosin-mediated afterload reduction in severe chronic congestive heart failure. *Circulation* 1979;59:531-539.

107. Colucci WS, Williams G, Braunwald E: Increased plasma norepinephrine during prazosin treatment for severe congestive heart failure. *Ann Intern Med* 1980;93:452-453.

108. Mettauer B, Rouleau JL, Bichet D, et al: Differential long-term intrarenal and neurohormonal effects of captopril and prazosin in patients with congestive heart failure: Importance of initial plasma renin activity. *Circulation* 1986;73:492-502.

109. Cohn JN, Archibald DG, Ziesche S, et al: Effect of vasodilator therapy on mortality in chronic congestive heart failure: Results of a Veterans Administration Cooperative Study. *N Engl J Med* 1986;314:1547-1552.

110. Awan NA, Hermanovich J, Whitcomb C, et al: Cardio-circulatory effects on afterload reduction with oral trimazosin in severe chronic heart failure. *Am J Cardiol* 1979;44:126-131.

111. Ports TA, Chatterjee K, Wilkinson P, et al: Beneficial hemodynamic effects of a new oral vasodilator, trimazosin, in chronic heart failure (abstract). *Clin Res* 1980;28:13A .

112. Weber KT, Kinasewitz GT, West JS, et al: Long-term vasodilator therapy with trimazosin in chronic cardiac failure. *N Engl J Med* 1980;303:242-250.

113. Aronow WS, Greenfield PS, Alimadadian H, et al: Effect of vasodilator trimazosin versus placebo on exercise performance in chronic left ventricular failure. *Am J Cardiol* 1977;30:789-793.

114. Mason DE, Awan NA, Hermanovich J: Comparison of cardiocirculatory actions of the oral systemic vasodilators trimazosin and prazosin: Demonstration of similar efficacy in therapy of severe heart failure. *Am J Cardiol* 1979;43:403.

115. DiCarlo L Jr, Chatterjee K, Swedberg K, et al: MK-421: A new angiotensin converting enzyme inhibitor in chronic heart failure; Acute and chronic hemodynamic response (abstract). *Circulation* 1982;66(suppl 2):209.

116. CONSENSUS Trial Study Group: Effects of enalapril on mortality in severe congestive heart failure: Results of the Cooperative North Scandinavian Enalapril Survival Study (CONSENSUS). *N Engl J Med* 1987;316:1429-1435.

117. Colucci WS, Fifer MA, Lorell BH, et al: Calcium channel blockers in congestive heart failure: Theoretic considerations and clinical experience. *Am J Med* 1985;78(suppl 2B):9-17.

118. Elkayam U, Weber L, Torkan B, et al: Acute hemodynamic effect of oral nifedipine in severe chronic congestive heart failure. *Am J Cardiol* 1983;52:1041-1045.

119. Timmis AD, Jewitt DE: Studies with felodipine in congestive heart failure. *Drugs* 1985;29(suppl 2):66-75.

120. Kubo SH, Fox SC, Prida XE, et al: Combined hemodynamic effects of nifedipine and nitroglycerin in congestive heart failure. *Am Heart J* 1985;110:1032-1034.

121. Magorien RD, Leier CV, Kolibash AJ, et al: Beneficial effects of nifedipine on rest and exercise myocardial energetics in patients with congestive heart failure. *Circulation* 1984;70:884-890.

122. Elkayam U, Weber L, Campese VM, et al: Renal hemodynamic effects of vasodilation with nifedipine and hydralazine in patients with heart failure. *J Am Coll Cardiol* 1984;4:1261-1267.

123. Diamond JR, Cheung JY, Fang TL: Nifedipine-induced renal dysfunction: Alterations in renal function. *Am J Med* 1984;77:905-909.

124. Agostoni PG, DeCesare N, Doria E, et al: Afterload reduction: A comparison of captopril and nifedipine in dilated cardiomyopathy. *Br Heart J* 1986;55:391-399.

125. Rich S, Ganz R, Levy PS: Comparative actions of hydralazine, nifedipine and amrinone in primary pulmonary hypertension. *Am J Cardiol* 1983;52:1104-1107.

126. Dzau VJ, Swartz SL, Creager MA: The role of prostaglandins in the pathophysiology of and therapy for congestive heart failure. *Heart Failure* 1986;2:6-13.

127. Cody RJ: The potential role of atrial natriuretic factor in the pathophysiology of congestive heart failure. *Heart Failure* 1987;2:258-263.

128. Garcia R, Thibault M, Cantin M, et al: Effect of purified atrial natriuretic factor on rat and rabbit vascular strips and vascular beds. *Am J Physiol* 1984;247: R34-R39.

129. Crozier IG, Ikram H, Gomez HJ, et al: Hemodynamic effects of atrial peptide infusion in heart failure. *Lancet* 1986;2:1242-1245.

130. Massie B, Chatterjee K, Werner J, et al: Hemodynamic advantage of combined administration of hydralazine orally and nitrates non-parenterally in the vasodilator therapy of chronic heart failure. *Am J Cardiol* 1977;40:794-801.

131. Massie B, Packer M, Kramer B, et al: Hemodynamic and clinical responses to combined captopril-hydralazine therapy. *Circulation* 1982;66(suppl 2):210.

WILLIAM W. PARMLEY, MD

10

Angiotensin Converting-Enzyme Inhibitors in the Treatment of Heart Failure

Although a number of vasodilator drugs are commonly used in the management of patients with both acute and chronic heart failure, captopril is the first angiotensin converting-enzyme (ACE) inhibitor formally approved for the treatment of severe chronic heart failure. The results of controlled and uncontrolled studies of its use for the treatment of severe chronic heart failure are indicative of the importance of its mechanism of action. It is now clear that stimulation of the renin-angiotensin-aldosterone system is an important pathophysiologic component of the syndrome of severe chronic heart failure in many patients. ACE inhibitors, therefore, fill an important need by counteracting the adverse effects contributed by this system. In this chapter, some of these aspects of the pathophysiology of heart failure (Table 10-1) as they apply to the use of captopril and other ACE inhibitors in managing this condition are reviewed.

Table 10-1. Pathophysiologic changes in heart failure

Hemodynamic

↑ Preload (↑ right and left atrial filling pressures)
↑ Afterload (↑ systemic vascular resistance)
↑ Heart rate
↓ Myocardial contractility

Neurohumoral

↑ Sympathetic tone and circulating catecholamines
↑ Arginine vasopressin levels
↑ Activity of the renin-angiotensin-aldosterone system
↓ Baroreceptor reflex activity

227

HEMO-DYNAMIC CHANGES IN HEART FAILURE Characteristic hemodynamic changes occur in chronic congestive heart failure and set the stage for various therapeutic interventions. First, heart rate is usually increased because of higher levels of circulating catecholamines and increased sympathetic tone to the sinoatrial node. This is an important compensatory mechanism for maintaining cardiac output, because stroke volume becomes relatively fixed with severe depression of ventricular function (see Chap. 2). In order to maintain cardiac output, therefore, an increase in heart rate is mandatory. Second, the preload or ventricular filling pressures are increased because the ability of the heart to eject blood is reduced. A concomitant increase in blood volume due to retention of salt and water by the kidneys occurs and sets the stage for diuretic therapy and/or venodilator therapy, both of which reduce the filling pressures of the right and left ventricles. Third, a rise in afterload, as manifested by increases in aortic impedance and systemic vascular resistance, occurs despite a decrease in arterial pressure, reflecting the inability of the heart to eject a normal stroke volume. Finally, the intrinsic contractile state of the myocardium is usually depressed in severe chronic heart failure,[1] and provides the rationale for the use of positive inotropic agents (see Chaps. 7 and 8) such as digitalis and catecholamines, which can improve the depressed contractility of the failing myocardium. Therefore, amelioration or attenuation of the above four hemodynamic factors is an important goal in improving the signs and symptoms of congestive heart failure.

CONTRIBUTION OF NEURO-HUMORAL FACTORS TO HEMODYNAMIC DERANGE-MENTS Important neurohumoral influences are involved in these pathophysiologic alterations. Increased sympathetic tone and circulating catecholamines are observed, which are, in part, responsible for the increased arteriolar constriction or systemic vascular resistance.[2] Teleologically, this mechanism appears to be compensatory. With a decrease in cardiac output, an increase in arteriolar tone is necessary to maintain the arterial pressure perfusing vital organs. However, as part of a vicious cycle, it further increases the impedance to left ventricular ejection and reduces cardiac output. Overall, cardiac output is frequently lower and arteriolar resistance higher than is optimal for the patient (see Chap. 4).

Antidiuretic hormone may also contribute to the hemodynamic profile of heart failure.[3] Vasopressin, a potent smooth muscle vasoconstrictor, is elevated in heart failure, potentially adding to the excessive increase in systemic vascular resistance in these patients.

Activation of the renin-angiotensin-aldosterone system is one of the most important neurohumoral derangements that can occur in heart failure[3] (see Chap. 3). Decreased perfusion pressure, adrenergic stimulation, and/or reduced sodium intake stimulate the juxtaglomerular apparatus to release renin. Renin converts angiotensinogen to angiotensin-I, an inactive decapeptide. Angiotensin-I is then altered by converting enzyme to angiotensin-II, a potent vasoconstrictor. In addition to its direct vasoconstricting effect, angiotensin-II facilitates sympathetic outflow and also provides feedback to the adrenal gland to promote the release of aldosterone. Although both potassium and angiotensin-II have been suggested as major regulators of aldosterone secretion, studies in patients receiving captopril suggest that angiotensin-II is far more important than potassium in regulating the release of aldosterone.[4] In turn, aldosterone promotes the absorption of salt and water, which further increases the volume of the circulatory system. Angiotensin-II may also affect receptor sites in the central nervous system and the kidney, although the precise role of these sites is not clear.

In congestive heart failure, the renin-angiotensin-aldosterone system is generally activated because there are increased levels of these hormones (see Chap. 4). Measurements of plasma renin activity on three successive days are relatively constant in patients with heart failure, and they tend to correlate inversely with serum sodium levels. A consistent correlation between baseline plasma renin activity and systemic vascular resistance does not exist in patients with heart failure. However, the greatest decrease in mean arterial pressure tends to be seen in patients with the highest plasma renin activity.[5] Based on this evidence, the renin-angiotensin-aldosterone system can significantly contribute to the hemodynamics seen with severe heart failure. Blockade of this system with an ACE inhibitor should return the altered hemodynamics toward normal and improve cardiac function and symptoms.

The relative contribution of angiotensin-II, sympathetic tone, and arginine vasopressin to vasoconstriction in patients with heart failure was evaluated by giving antagonists to all three neurohumoral systems in ten patients with congestive heart failure.[6] The relative importance in rank order was α-vasoconstriction > angiotensin-II > arginine vasopressin. Riegger and Kochsiek[7] studied the relationship between captopril therapy and elevated arginine vasopressin (ADH) levels. ADH levels were not lowered during acute therapy, but did normalize during chronic therapy.

Acute Hemodynamic Effects   The important therapeutic hemodynamic effects of captopril in patients with chronic congestive heart failure are well documented. In general, the same effects were noted in all of the acute studies.[8-18] Following captopril administration, a drop in mean arterial pressure ranging from 7% to 25% occurs with no change or a slight fall in heart rate. A substantial fall in systemic vascular resistance (20% to 45%), with a moderate increase in cardiac output (25% to 30%), is seen. There are also striking reductions in pulmonary capillary wedge pressure (25% to 50%), pulmonary artery pressure (15% to 30%), and right atrial pressure (25% to 45%). These hemodynamic effects begin in about 30 minutes. Maximum responses occur between 60 and 90 minutes and are maintained for three to eight hours. Maximum hemodynamic effects are usually seen with single doses of 25 mg or less, but increasing the dose may result in prolonged action.

Captopril has the ability to reverse the major hemodynamic abnormalities associated with symptoms of heart failure such as an elevation in pulmonary capillary wedge pressure, which causes dyspnea, and a low cardiac output, which produces fatigue or weakness. The drop in blood pressure that it produces, however, may be deleterious in patients with severe heart failure who have baseline hypotension. Reduced perfusion pressure of the coronary arteries or the brain may lead to symptoms and signs of ischemia and/or dizziness. Fortunately, the prevalence of these potential side effects appears to be minimal, and even relatively low blood pressures are well tolerated in these patients with severe chronic heart failure.

The typical acute hemodynamic response is illustrated in a study by Ader et al.[8] In ten patients with severe heart failure, increasing doses of captopril were administered during invasive hemodynamic monitoring. The time course of the response to captopril 25 mg is shown in Figures 10-1 and 10-2. The fall in mean arterial pressure was greatest 1.5 hours after administration. Mean arterial pressure approached control between six and eight hours (Fig. 10-1). The fall in systemic vascular resistance exhibited a

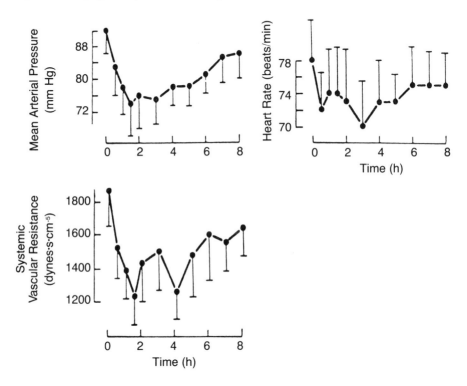

Fig. 10-1. Time course of the hemodynamic effects of a single dose of captopril 25 mg in ten patients with severe chronic heart failure; mean ± SD. (Data from a study reported by Ader et al.[8])

similar time course. Despite the fall in mean arterial pressure, there was a slight reduction in resting heart rate. Although not all studies have shown a fall in heart rate, there is no evidence of a significant reflex tachycardia. Figure 10-2 illustrates the moderate increase in cardiac output seen with captopril, together with a striking reduction in pulmonary capillary wedge pressure. The same time course is evident in the response of these hemodynamic parameters.

Similar changes in hemodynamics occur after a 25-, 50-, or 100-mg dose of captopril. Figure 10-3 shows the percentage changes

230

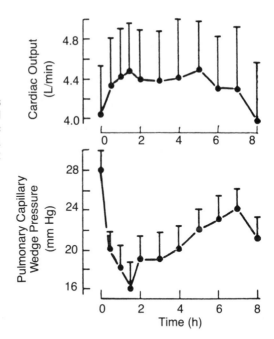

Fig. 10-2. Hemodynamic effects of a single 25-mg dose of captopril in ten patients with severe chronic heart failure; mean ± SD. (Data from a study reported by Ader et al.[8])

from control in each of the hemodynamic variables. Maximum changes after captopril 25 mg were cardiac output, +28%; stroke volume index, +49%; stroke work index, +26%; systemic vascular resistance, −41%; mean arterial pressure, −23%; heart rate, −4%; pulmonary capillary wedge pressure, −46%; and right atrial pressure, −27%. It is of interest that despite a reduction in mean arterial pressure, there was no reflex tachycardia. On the contrary, heart rate actually decreased slightly. This presumably reflects a withdrawal of sympathetic tone together with the blunted baroreceptor reflex seen in congestive heart failure. The time course of action was basically the same at all three doses. Effects were observed about 30 minutes after administration, with a maximum effect at about 1.5 hours. Some degree of residual hypotension was still observed as long as six hours after a single dose.

There was no significant relationship between the initial systemic vascular resistance and the wide range of control plasma renin values. There was, however, a significant relationship between the increase in cardiac output and the control systemic vascular resistance values. Patients with the highest initial systemic vascular resistance had the greatest increase in cardiac output. This finding is not unique to captopril; it also occurs with the other vasodilator drugs.

Some differences between short- and long-acting ACE inhibitors should be noted. The onset of action of captopril is faster, but its action is less prolonged. In a comparative study using high fixed doses of each drug, enalapril resulted in prolonged and symptomatic hypotension.[19] Other differences include a slightly different side effect profile.[20] In addition, captopril increases prostaglandin production.[21,22]

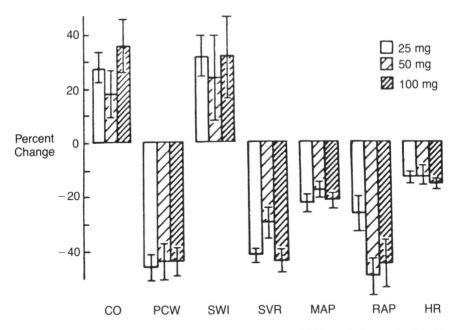

Fig. 10-3. Hemodynamic effects of captopril 25, 50, and 100 mg in ten patients with class III or IV heart failure. Peak effects for each dose are plotted as percent of control. Note that the response is essentially the same at all three dose levels. (CO = cardiac output; PCW = pulmonary capillary wedge pressure; SWI = stroke work index; SVR = systemic vascular resistance; MAP = mean arterial pressure; RAP = right atrial pressure; HR = heart rate.) (Reprinted from R Ader, K Chatterjee, T Ports, et al, Immediate and sustained hemodynamic and clinical improvement in chronic heart failure by an oral angiotensin-converting enzyme inhibitor, *Circulation* 1980;61:931-937, by permission of the American Heart Association, Inc.)

Overall, similar hemodynamic effects are produced by both short- and long-acting ACE inhibitors. The shorter-acting captopril produces less prolonged and symptomatic hypotension in susceptible patients, compared with the longer-acting agents.

Effects in Ischemic Heart Disease
Mortality is extremely high in patients with severe congestive heart failure. The majority of these patients suffer from severe coronary artery disease with one or more myocardial infarctions. Such patients have high mortality secondary to ischemic episodes, serious arrhythmias, and/or repeat myocardial infarctions. In a study of 56 patients treated primarily with hydralazine and nitrates, the mortality rate was approximately 50% in 15 months. A large percentage of these patients died suddenly, suggesting serious cardiac arrhythmias. Therefore, the effects of vasodilators on coronary blood flow, myocardial oxygen consumption, and arrhythmias may be particularly important in patients with severe heart failure secondary to coronary artery disease.[23]

In patients with chronic left ventricular failure, myocardial oxygen extraction and consumption and coronary sinus blood flow were measured before and after captopril therapy. In general, the rate-pressure product, coronary blood flow, and myocardial oxygen consumption significantly decreased after captopril administration. Myocardial lactate production occurred in one patient, despite decreased myocardial oxygen consumption. These findings suggest that captopril reduces the determinants of myocardial oxygen demand.[24]

The effects of hydralazine, prazosin, and captopril on coronary hemodynamics and lactate metabolism have been compared in patients with severe coronary artery disease. Captopril consistently lowered the heart rate–blood pressure product and also lowered coronary blood flow and myocardial oxygen consumption. This was accompanied by an increase in cardiac output and a reduction in pulmonary capillary wedge pressure. Thus, the beneficial hemodynamic effects of captopril were obtained at a lower oxygen cost. Prazosin also lowered the heart rate–blood pressure product, although some patients showed an increase in myocardial oxygen consumption. Hydralazine altered coronary sinus blood flow and myocardial oxygen consumption in general proportion to changes in the heart rate–blood pressure product, with some patients showing a slight increase in myocardial oxygen consumption. All three drugs produced somewhat similar effects on cardiac output and pulmonary capillary wedge pressure, although hydralazine produced the largest increase in cardiac output, and prazosin produced the greatest reduction in pulmonary capillary wedge pressure. In each of the three patient groups, lactate production was demonstrated in one or two patients, despite the lack of evidence of overt ischemia, as manifested by electrocardiographic changes or angina pectoris.[25]

These data suggest that despite beneficial hemodynamic effects, all vasodilators have the propensity for producing ischemia in some patients who have severe heart failure due to coronary artery disease. Captopril, however, produced the most consistent reduction in myocardial oxygen consumption of the three drugs, suggesting a potentially beneficial effect in reducing ischemia.

Effects on Renal and Other Vascular Beds Acute administration of captopril to patients with heart failure usually decreases renal vascular resistance and increases renal blood flow.[11,13] An increase in sodium excretion and potassium retention accompanies these changes. Improvement or maintenance of renal function following captopril administration depends on the reduction in mean arterial pressure.[26] Correlation between the change in blood pressure and creatinine clearance has been demonstrated, suggesting that it is critical to avoid a profound reduction in blood pressure in order to prevent deterioration of renal function following captopril administration. In long-term studies in patients with severe heart failure, captopril produced a sustained improvement in renal function[27] (Fig. 10-4).

When the effects of captopril on renal function in patients with heart failure were compared with those of hydralazine and prazosin, similar qualitative effects were noted. However, captopril had a tendency to decrease creatinine clearance and sodium excretion, probably reflecting a greater effect of captopril on blood pressure reduction.[28]

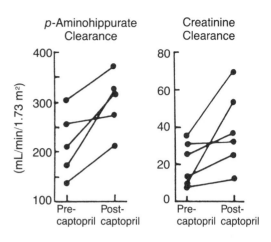

Fig. 10-4. Influence of therapy with captopril on renal plasma flow and glomerular filtration rate, assessed as the clearances of p-amino-hippurate and creatinine in six patients with severe heart failure. (Adapted from Dzau et al.[27] Reprinted, by permission of *The New England Journal of Medicine*, 302;1373-1379, 1980.)

In 16 patients with heart failure who were given captopril, effective renal plasma flow increased in 10, was unchanged in 4, and decreased in 2. Mean arterial pressure fell to 54 and 47 mm Hg in the latter 2 patients.[29] Thus, excessive lowering of arterial pressure appears to play an important role in decreasing renal function. Although glomerular filtration rate is preserved by angiotensin-II-mediated efferent arteriolar vasoconstriction in experimental low-output states, this is true only if blood pressure is relatively preserved.[30] In patients with stable congestive heart failure, captopril enhanced renal blood flow, despite a reduction in arterial pressure.[31] In another double-blind study of the effects of captopril on renal function in patients with heart failure there was a slight decline in renal function, which was felt to be due to both the drop in blood pressure and loss of the compensatory effects of angiotensin-II within the kidney.[32] It is of interest that the best long-term response to captopril therapy occurs in patients with preserved renal function.[33]

Even though captopril lowers blood pressure in patients with severe heart failure, it does not reduce cerebral blood flow.[34] In one study, it actually improved cerebral blood flow.[35]

MECHANISM OF ACTION The acute beneficial hemodynamic effects of captopril are well documented; however, the precise mechanism for these actions is not totally clear. The reduction in systemic vascular resistance, which results in an increase in cardiac output, is probably not completely explained by the reduced vasoconstrictive effects of angiotensin-II. Because there is also a reduction in serum catecholamines and sympathetic tone, a reduction in catecholamines and lowered angiotensin-II are both probably responsible for the reduction in peripheral vascular resistance. In general, there has only been a modest correlation between plasma renin activity and a decrease in systemic vascular resistance.[8,12,13] Similarly, there is no consistent relationship between elevated plasma renin activity and the severity of heart failure.[36] Further studies will be required to determine the relative importance of reductions in plasma norepinephrine[4] and angiotensin-II in patients with heart failure.

Captopril may also reduce the inactivation of bradykinin or act via the prostaglandin system to contribute to the lowering of systemic vascular resistance.[37,38] In addition, the reduction of aldosterone and concomitant sodium retention may contribute to its action. There is also evidence that captopril increases the production of vasodilating prostaglandins, which may contribute to its unloading effects.[21,22]

A reduction in pulmonary capillary wedge pressure suggests that there is peripheral venodilatation of some magnitude, which redistributes blood away from the chest. This mechanism of action is presumed to be similar to the effects of nitroglycerin, the prototype venodilator. It has been reported, however, that angiotensin-II has no direct effects on venous tone.[39] Thus, it is unlikely that a reduction in angiotensin-II levels is directly responsible for the peripheral venodilatation. Because norepinephrine levels are markedly elevated in heart failure, and are reduced following captopril administration, catecholamines probably play the most important role in mediating venoconstriction. However, a reduction in plasma norepinephrine levels (20% to 30%) correlated only weakly with a reduction in venous pressure.[40] Variable effects on different venous beds may help to explain this lack of correlation and our current inability to define the precise mechanism mediating the fall in right and left atrial pressures. The reduction in blood pressure itself must contribute to the fall in filling pressure enhancing ventricular emptying. This relationship between blood pressure and pulmonary capillary wedge pressure has been previously demonstrated for other vasodilators.

SHORT-ACTING VERSUS LONG-ACTING ACE INHIBITORS Since the introduction of captopril for the management of congestive heart failure, a number of other longer-acting ACE inhibitors have followed. These include enalapril,[41,42] lisinopril,[43] and ramipril.[44] In general, these longer-acting ACE inhibitors have the same general hemodynamic effects as the shorter-acting captopril. For example, enalapril's acute hemodynamic effects[45-47] consist of lowering pulmonary capillary wedge pressure and increasing cardiac output. Sustained beneficial hemodynamic effects are seen for up to four months.[48-50] Placebo-controlled trials have also shown clinical benefit compared with placebo.[51-53] Enalapril and ramipril are prodrugs that are converted to their active metabolites enalaprilat and ramiprilat. Intravenous administration of enalaprilat[54] produced the characteristic hemodynamic effects of the oral ACE inhibitors.

CHRONIC CLINICAL USE Captopril has been evaluated in a large number of patients with heart failure refractory to digitalis and diuretics and, occasionally, vasodilator therapy. Most evaluated patients were in New York Heart Association functional class III or IV. A few were in class I and II. In all follow-up studies, which ranged from six months to more than three years, the initial hemodynamic effects were sustained during chronic treatment. In these chronic studies, 80% to 85% of patients responded to captopril, with significant improvements in cardiac function, relief of symptoms, subjective and objective evidence of functional capacity improvement, and increase in exercise tolerance. The results of a controlled trial comparing captopril with placebo confirmed the beneficial effects that were observed in uncontrolled studies.[55]

Beneficial Long-Term Effects

The hemodynamic improvements seen after acute administration of captopril are sustained during long-term treatment. Increases in cardiac output or cardiac index, stroke volume, and stroke work index and reductions in systemic vascular resistance and pulmonary capillary wedge pressure have been maintained for more than three years in some cases.[8,9,14,27,55-68]

In mild heart failure, captopril improved exercise tolerance and New York Heart Association classification, compared with the response in placebo-treated patients.[58] Digitalis was maintained; diuretics were withdrawn. No differences in survival curves were seen after six months. In a double-blind controlled trial, captopril provided long-term benefits in 14 patients with heart failure, including a reduction in complex ventricular ectopy.[64] In patients with low-renin congestive heart failure, reactive hyperreninemia distinguished the responders to captopril from the nonresponders.[66]

A cooperative multicenter study evaluated the hemodynamic response to captopril in 124 patients. About 80% of patients showed sustained hemodynamic and clinical improvement at eight weeks. There was no evidence of tachyphylaxis to captopril.[69]

Improvements in left ventricular ejection fraction have ranged from 20% to 120%.[27,70,71] The greatest improvements occur in patients with the poorest baseline cardiac function.[27] Reductions in left ventricular end-diastolic dimension are reported,[70] and a reduction in the cardiothoracic ratio is observed.[14]

Improvements in exercise tolerance time occur within one week of captopril administration. Increases range from 33% to 88%. Progressive improvement has been observed over 12 months. However, after one year, a modest deterioration in mean exercise time was noted in some patients, presumably reflecting deterioration due to the disease.[72] An increase in estimated total body oxygen consumption accompanied improvements in exercise performance in some patients.[9]

Consistent improvement or stabilization in the New York Heart Association functional classification with captopril therapy is a common observation. Approximately 85% of treated patients experience improvement in functional classification.[9,13,14,27,56,70] Approximately 60% of patients improve by one functional class and 25% by two classes. Approximately 1.5% show deterioration, and the remainder show no change.[72]

Additional benefits of captopril therapy include reduction in body weight associated with diuresis and natriuresis.[27,73] It should be noted that clinical improvement may occur in the absence of these findings.[74] Improved renal function, correction of hyponatremia, and normalization of pretreatment hypokalemia have also followed captopril therapy for heart failure.[72] As an additional benefit, a reduction in the number of days of hospitalization to 10% of pretreatment values was reported by Dzau et al.[27]

In a double-blind, placebo-controlled trial conducted over 12 weeks in patients with less severe heart failure (mean New York Heart Association functional classification 2.8), the beneficial effects of captopril were confirmed.[55] Exercise tolerance time and New York Heart Association functional classification improved significantly by comparison with placebo-treated patients.

State of
Well-Being
One of the most interesting phenomena related to the use of ACE inhibitors in congestive heart failure is the feeling of relative well-being among the treated patients. Angiotensin-II facilitates sympathetic outflow; therefore, administration of captopril has been consistently associated with a reduction in plasma catecholamine levels. This reduction may, in part, lead to an enhanced feeling of well-being, because high plasma catecholamines are often associated with anxiety and may not be well tolerated.

Although it is far more difficult to judge changes in subjective feeling than it is to judge objective performance (eg, on an exercise test), general experience with captopril suggests that subjective improvement achieved by these patients may have clinical significance. Further studies will be required to elucidate the specific cause or causes of this phenomenon. Nevertheless, it appears to be a useful property of the drug, because a major goal in the therapy of congestive heart failure is to improve symptoms.

ACE Inhibitors
and Other
Drugs
The effects of captopril have been compared with those of hydralazine in an eight-week crossover study.[75] Both drugs produced similar improvements in New York Heart Association functional classification, exercise tolerance, and ejection fraction. Deterioration occurred in 40% of the captopril responders and in 63% of the hydralazine-treated patients. A predictor of chronic response to captopril was 25% or greater reduction in pulmonary capillary wedge pressure following treatment.

The neurohumoral effects of nitroprusside were evaluated in patients with severe congestive heart failure and in normal subjects. There was reflex activation of both the sympathetic nervous system and the renin-angiotensin system in the normals. In heart failure patients, plasma renin concentrations rose but plasma norepinephrine was unchanged. This dissociation in neurohumoral responses has relevance to the potential added beneficial effects of captopril when given to patients already taking other potent vasodilators.[76]

The acute hemodynamic effects of captopril qualitatively resemble those seen with prazosin and are characterized by a balanced effect on preload and afterload. Increases in cardiac output and stroke work index, and reductions in pulmonary capillary wedge pressure, systemic vascular resistance, heart rate, and mean arterial pressure are similar following short-term use of each drug.[25,77,78] However, the magnitude of change is often more pronounced after captopril.[79] In a double-blind study comparing prazosin and captopril, only captopril produced long-term clinical and hemodynamic benefit.[59] In another comparative study, prazosin produced striking acute changes, but no long-term benefit. Captopril produced modest acute benefits, but sustained long-term benefit.[80] Activation of the renin-angiotensin system does not fully explain the long-term tolerance to prazosin.[81]

It should be noted that tolerance to the initial beneficial effects of both hydralazine and prazosin has been observed in patients with heart failure[82-84] (see Chap. 9). In contrast, the incidence of tolerance to the effects of captopril is rare in published reports. This may be explained in part by the mechanism of action of captopril. Presumably, the reduction in effects of hydralazine and prazosin is related, in part, to stimulation of the renin-angiotensin-aldosterone system with subsequent fluid retention. Increasing doses of diuretics or administration of spironolactone successfully overcome tolerance in many patients.[85]

Because captopril inhibits the renin-angiotensin-aldosterone system, this mechanism for tolerance is negated. In support of this, many patients treated with captopril can have their diuretic dosage reduced. If stimulation of the renin-angiotensin-aldosterone system is the mechanism for tolerance to vasodilators in some patients, then a rationale exists for cautiously combining captopril with vasodilators.

Captopril and hydralazine produce similar effects on afterload. However, the increases in cardiac output and heart rate with hydralazine are often greater than with captopril, while the effects on pulmonary capillary wedge pressure, right atrial pressure, and pulmonary artery pressure are much less than those seen with captopril. This probably reflects the predominant arteriolar dilator effect of hydralazine.[25,75] The addition of hydralazine to captopril enhances cardiac output without further lowering blood pressure.[86] This may be a distinct advantage in some patients with heart failure.

Because of questions raised about the safety and efficacy of long-term digoxin therapy among patients with congestive heart failure who have a sinus rhythm, captopril would seem to be an interesting alternative drug. In patients with mild to moderate heart failure, captopril and digoxin were equally effective in improving exercise tolerance and cardiac function.[87] Captopril causes an increase in serum digoxin levels by reducing the renal clearance of the drug. In one report of 20 patients with congestive heart failure, none developed evidence of digoxin toxicity during combined treatment.[88]

Effects of ACE Inhibition Therapy on Mortality The overall effects of vasodilators on mortality have been difficult to determine. Two long-term follow-up studies revealed the high mortality of patients with class IV heart failure[23,89]: approximately 50% of patients die within 15 months. Many patients discontinued their medications because of side effects. In the multicenter Veterans Administration Cooperative Trial, patients with less severe heart failure were randomized to treatment with placebo, prazosin, hydralazine, and/or isosorbide dinitrate in addition to digitalis and diuretics. The group randomized to hydralazine and isosorbide dinitrate had a significant reduction in mortality.[90] An important question is whether this effect is restricted to the drugs used or is a more general justification of the use of vasodilators. Tachyphylaxis is a problem with prazosin[91]; therefore, it is not surprising that prazosin did not show long-term benefit. A subsequent Veterans Administration Cooperative Trial is under way to compare an ACE inhibitor with the combination of hydralazine and isosorbide dinitrate.

ACE inhibitors seem well suited to prolong life in patients with congestive heart failure.[92] In patients with a low serum sodium, there is evidence that captopril may prolong life.[93] No prolongation of life was seen in patients with a normal serum sodium. In a review of studies with ACE inhibitors, there is suggestive evidence of prolonged life with ACE inhibition.[94] This has led the National Institutes of Health to use an ACE inhibitor in its long-term trial in patients with impaired left ventricular function (SOLVD). Very recently, a placebo-controlled trial with enalapril showed a 31% reduction in mortality in patients with severe congestive heart failure. There was no reduction in the relative incidence of sudden death.[95]

CONSIDERA-TIONS FOR CLINICAL USE OF CAPTOPRIL

Indications for Captopril in the Management of Chronic Heart Failure

Based on our present understanding of chronic congestive heart failure, it appears that the decrease in myocardial contractility that inevitably occurs is essentially irreversible. This leads to increased loading conditions that compound the circulatory problem. Increased preload is associated with dyspnea and venous congestion, while the increased afterload reduces cardiac output. Thus, our primary goals in treating heart failure are to correct these adverse loading conditions and improve symptoms. Captopril is especially attractive as a therapeutic agent for the following reasons: (1) It produces both arteriolar dilatation and venodilatation. (2) It blocks the renin-angiotensin-aldosterone system, an important factor in the adverse pathophysiologic sequence of events that occurs in heart failure. (3) Its side effects are relatively benign. (4) Its effects with positive inotropic agents and diuretics are additive.

Results with captopril convincingly demonstrate that it can produce beneficial hemodynamic effects in patients with congestive heart failure who respond poorly to digitalis and diuretics. These appear to be sustained long-term effects and are associated with an improvement in exercise tolerance and clinical class. It is reasonable, therefore, to consider the use of captopril in all patients who do not respond to conventional medical therapy.

There appears to be little relationship between the acute response to captopril and the chronic response.[96] Thus, acute hemodynamic monitoring is not necessarily helpful in identifying patients who will benefit in the long run. Captopril has especially pronounced effects in patients who have a low serum sodium, a group of patients who are generally more ill than those with a normal serum sodium.

The ability of captopril to correct dilutional hyponatremia in patients with congestive heart failure suggests a role for the renin-angiotensin-aldosterone system in producing this syndrome.[65] Data also suggest that furosemide is necessary to promote diuresis and correct hyponatremia in heart failure patients treated with captopril.[97] It is clear that the greatest response to captopril occurs in hyponatremia patients.[67] In general, therefore, captopril can be used in a wide variety of patients who have a spectrum of heart failure ranging from mild to severe.

Captopril is generally not a consideration in patients with myocardial infarction, but interesting experimental data suggest this as a possible future use. After a large myocardial infarction, the remaining normal myocardium is subject to increased wall stress as the heart dilates. "Unloading" the heart might reduce the stimulus for dilation and hypertrophy. In rats undergoing coronary ligation, captopril treatment reduced loading conditions, reduced end-diastolic pressure and volume, lessened hypertrophy, and prolonged life.[98] This benefit has not yet been tested in patients with myocardial infarction; however, the principle is of potential importance.

Pharmaco-kinetics   Approximately 70% to 75% of an oral dose of captopril is absorbed. The peak blood levels achieved within 1 to 1.5 hours correspond with the peak hemodynamic response.[99] Administration of captopril with a meal reduced absorption by 35% to 40%.[100]

Captopril is widely distributed throughout the body with a volume of distribution of 0.7 L/kg. Most studies indicate that it does not enter the central nervous system to a significant extent. Approximately 30% of captopril present in plasma is bound to plasma proteins.[100] In animal studies, captopril readily crosses the placenta. Very little drug is detected in breast milk of lactating women given captopril.[101]

Approximately 50% of a captopril dose is metabolized into inactive compounds. Both metabolites and active drug are excreted in the urine. The mean elimination half-life is two hours in patients with congestive heart failure.[99] In patients with impaired renal function, elimination of captopril may be prolonged, requiring a dosage adjustment.[102] Hemodialysis is effective in removing captopril.[103]

Combination with Inotropic Agents   In the management of congestive heart failure, vasodilator and inotropic drugs are usually synergistic. This occurs presumably because they work by different mechanisms. Inotropic agents increase the vigor of contraction, while vasodilator drugs reduce the work load. Thus, combination vasodilator and inotropic therapy has been effective in many patients with congestive heart failure. In one study of six patients taking captopril, increasing doses of dobutamine were infused to evaluate the potential synergistic effect. At low doses, there was a substantial increase in cardiac output, whereas myocardial oxygen consumption remained below control levels. At higher doses of dobutamine (10 and 20 μg/min), the rising cardiac output was accompanied by a pronounced increase in myocardial oxygen uptake, the appearance of chest pain, or multiple premature ventricular contractions. These data emphasize the synergistic effects of drugs and also point out the necessity for evaluating the effects of differing agents on myocardial oxygen demand, particularly in patients with severe coronary artery disease.[104]

Adverse Effects   Captopril is well tolerated by most patients treated for heart failure. A summary of adverse reactions reported at a frequency greater than 1% in clinical trials of captopril for treatment of heart failure is shown in Table 10-2. The more clinically relevant reactions are discussed here.

Cardiovascular Effects: The most common and significant effect following captopril administration is hypotension. Approximately half of the patients treated with captopril have a 20% fall in mean arterial blood pressure after the first dose (see Figs. 10-1 and 10-3), usually with a return to pretreatment levels during continued treatment.[8,27] This fall in blood pressure is rarely symptomatic. Predisposing factors to a symptomatic, precipitous fall in blood pressure following the initial dose of captopril include high renin,

Table 10-2. Summary of adverse reactions at a frequency greater than 1% in 498 patients with heart failure receiving captopril for up to 12 months

Primary Adverse Reaction	Incidence (%)	
Cardiovascular		
Dizziness	2.6	
Hypotension	23.7	
Asymptomatic		4.2
Orthostatic		2.0
Symptomatic		16.7
Renal insufficiency		0.8
Cutaneous	7.0	
Pruritus		2.4
Rash		3.0
Rash and pruritus		1.6
Gastrointestinal		
Abdominal discomfort*	1.6	
Anorexia	1.4	
Diarrhea	1.2	
Nausea	1.4	
Taste Alteration†	3.0	
Renal		
Renal insufficiency‡	2.6	

* Includes abdominal pain, "abdominal syndrome," and epigastric distress.
† Includes loss of taste.
‡ Includes renal failure, renal function impairment, renal toxicity, azotemia, and elevated BUN.
Adapted from JA Romankiewicz, RN Brogden, RC Heel, et al, Captopril: An update review of its pharmacologic properties and therapeutic efficacy in congestive heart failure, *Drugs* 1983;25:6-40, with permission.

low sodium, and aggressive diuresis with hypovolemia.[105,106] Therefore, it is important to note these factors prior to initiating administration of captopril. Initiating captopril at low doses (6.25 mg) minimizes this occurrence.[16,24]

Transient deterioration in renal function, which appears to be related to the fall in mean arterial pressure, has occurred in approximately 20% of patients treated with captopril for heart failure.[28] Improvement in indices of renal function has also been seen.[27]

Abrupt and temporary withdrawal of captopril does not result in sudden hemodynamic deterioration. Cessation of captopril in patients treated for 2.5 to 6 months resulted in abrupt increases of plasma angiotensin-II, norepinephrine, aldosterone, and mean arterial pressure. Despite these changes, cardiac output, pulmonary capillary wedge pressure, pulmonary artery pressure, and electrolyte balance were unaltered.[56,74] It is of considerable importance that there did not appear to be a rebound withdrawal phenomenon from acute cessation of captopril. In contrast, sustained withdrawal of captopril results in deterioration of hemodynamic status and symptoms, which responds to reinstitution of therapy.[27]

Skin Rash: The most common side effect associated with captopril involves the skin, occurring in 7% of patients treated for heart failure. These reactions are generally pruritic, erythematous, macular and papular eruptions of the trunk, face, and proximal extremities. They appear 1 to 31 weeks after initiation of captopril therapy, and occasionally are associated with diarrhea, fever, and generalized arthralgias. Some patients have peripheral leukocytosis or eosinophilia. In many cases, symptomatic skin eruptions resolve with continued captopril therapy or with a dose reduction.[107] Rarely, skin eruptions may include a pityriasis rosea–like pattern.[108] The reported incidence of skin rash with enalapril is 1.2%.[20]

Hematologic Effects: Neutropenia is potentially a more serious side effect of captopril. In one study, more than 6,000 patients treated as participants in clinical protocols, including patients with hypertension, were evaluated.[109] Captopril-induced neutropenia was identifed in 38 patients. The onset of neutropenia occurred between 1 and 12 weeks after initiation of therapy, and recovery after discontinuation of captopril usually occurred within 3 weeks. Of the 38 patients 22 had infections. There were five deaths, all in medically complex cases with severe renai failure. When the patients were stratified according to renal function, differences in the incidence of neutropenia arose. Captopril should be used with caution in patients with impaired renal function or serious autoimmune disease (particularly systemic lupus erythematosus) or those who are exposed to other drugs known to affect the white cells or immune response. These patients receiving captopril should have white blood cell counts performed at the initiation of therapy, at two-week intervals for the first three months of treatment, and periodically thereafter.*

Renal Insufficiency: The effects of captopril on renal function were discussed earlier in this chapter. Although ACE inhibition can directly improve renal blood flow, the hypotensive effects can worsen renal function.[11,28,29,31-33] The potential for the occurrence of this adverse effect must be considered, particularly in patients with preexisting renal insufficiency or those with an excessive drop in blood pressure.

Miscellaneous Effects: Although proteinuria has occurred in about 1.2% of hypertensive patients treated with captopril, it has not been a significant problem in studies of heart failure patients.[69] Patients receiving captopril should have estimates of urinary protein performed before therapy is initiated and periodically thereafter.*

Reversible taste alterations have occurred in about 3% of patients with heart failure who were treated with captopril. Included among these alterations are dysgeusia and hypogeusia.[16,110] The onset of taste alterations usually occurs within three months after initiating captopril. A higher incidence occurs in patients receiving higher doses and in whom renal disease or collagen vascular diseases are present. Return of taste generally occurs within two months, regardless of discontinuation of captopril.[72]

Although a slight increase in serum potassium may occur following captopril administration, hyperkalemia rarely develops.[4] The reduction in aldosterone is responsible for the increase in potassium. The increase is

*See WARNINGS section in the full prescribing information.

usually sufficient to eliminate the need for potassium supplements and/or potassium-sparing diuretics, which should be given only for documented hypokalemia.

In some instances severe life-threatening hyperkalemia has been reported, particularly when combination drug therapy has been used, such as an ACE inhibitor and potassium-retaining diuretics.[111]

Dose and Administration   When using many therapeutic agents in congestive heart failure, it is important to carefully titrate the dose of each drug so as to achieve an optimal effect without producing toxicity. In most cases, there is a dose-response relationship that causes an increasing effect with increasing doses. Many times it is useful to hospitalize the patient with severe heart failure and to place a balloon-tip catheter in the pulmonary artery to measure pressures and cardiac output. Under these circumstances, one can optimize the dose of diuretics, vasodilators, and inotropic agents.

With captopril, these considerations are slightly different. Because the drug acts to inhibit an enzyme, it follows that once the enzyme is inhibited, any increase in dose will have no further beneficial or, presumably, adverse effects. In most studies, approximately 90% of patients with severe heart failure show a response to a dose of 25 mg three times daily. For example, the effects of 25, 50, and 100 mg of captopril are illustrated in Figure 10-3. Note that all of these dose levels produced essentially the same hemodynamic response. However, total patient response necessitates individual dosage titration. In addition, this dosing plateau decreases the necessity for invasive hemodynamic monitoring in dosing titration. As a result, the majority of patients can be treated as ambulatory patients.

One potential problem with administering captopril is a profound lowering of blood pressure, particularly after the first dose. Because 12.5 mg is the lowest dose currently available, it is reasonable to break the tablet in half and begin with 6.25 mg three times daily in salt- and volume-depleted patients. One can then titrate the dosage to approximately 25 mg three times daily, according to individual patient response. One study (Fig. 10-5) demonstrated that this gradual incremental dosing tended to avoid the precipitous hypotension that could occur if 25 mg is given as the first dose.[24] When managing heart failure in ambulatory patients, it is recommended to give the first dose while the patient is in the office or clinic and under close medical supervision.

When employing captopril in the treatment of severe heart failure, digitalis and diuretic therapy should be continued. Vasodilators and inotropic agents may have synergistic effects; therefore, it is reasonable to consider continuation of digitalis in patients who require vasodilator therapy. Although there is considerable doubt about the efficacy of digitalis in patients with heart failure and sinus rhythm, recent studies suggest that moderate benefits can be expected from digitalis in the majority of patients treated with combination therapy. Future studies will be required to determine whether digitalis can be stopped in patients placed on vasodilators and whether other inotropic agents will be better in combination with vasodilator drugs such as captopril.

Fig. 10-5. Dose-response effect of captopril on mean arterial pressure (MAP) and diastolic arterial pressure (DAP) in 15 patients with severe chronic heart failure; mean ± SD. Zero values are control. Sequential doses of 2.5, 6.25, 12.5, and 25 mg of captopril were then administered. (Adapted from K Chatterjee, JL Rouleau, WW Parmley, Haemodynamic and myocardial metabolic effects of captopril in chronic heart failure, *Br Heart J* 1982;47:233-238, with permission.)

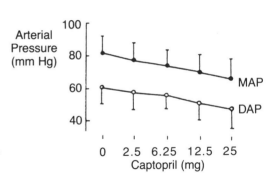

Mild potassium retention usually accompanies captopril therapy. Thus, it is important that potassium supplements or potassium-sparing diuretics be avoided. In addition, it is important to periodically check renal function, urinary protein, and white blood cell counts. In patients with severe renal disease, it may be reasonable to adjust dosage downward based on declining creatinine clearance.

CONCLUSION   During the development of chronic congestive heart failure, there is activation of a number of compensatory and reflex mechanisms, including the sympathetic and renin-angiotensin-aldosterone systems. Increased angiotensin-II levels increase sympathetic outflow, produce direct vasoconstriction, and increase aldosterone, which retains salt and water. These adverse effects on preload and afterload can be reduced by ACE inhibitors, which inhibit angiotensin converting enzyme and reduce circulating levels of angiotensin-II. Some of captopril's effects may possibly be mediated by the kinin, prostaglandin, and kallikrein systems.

In patients with severe chronic heart failure, the acute effects of ACE inhibitors include a reduction in arterial pressure, pulmonary capillary wedge pressure, systemic vascular resistance, and myocardial oxygen consumption. There is a moderate increase in cardiac output with little change in heart rate. Effects on renal function depend upon the fall in mean arterial pressure. Studies of chronic therapy show improved exercise tolerance and New York Heart Association functional classification with sustained improvement in hemodynamics. The major adverse cardiovascular effect is hypotension, which may lead to dizziness, ischemia, or decreased renal function. Other side effects include rash, taste alteration, proteinuria, and neutropenia.

Overall, ACE inhibitors are effective agents in treating congestive heart failure. Improved hemodynamics and symptoms can greatly enhance the quality of life for many patients, and evidence is emerging that life expectancy is also increased.

REFERENCES

1. Parmley WW, Wikman-Coffelt J: Myocardial hypertrophy and ischemia, in Parmley WW, Chatterjee K (eds): *Cardiology*. Philadelphia, JB Lippincott, 1987, chap 2.
2. Parmley WW: Principles of the management of congestive heart failure, in Parmley WW, Chatterjee K (eds): *Cardiology*. Philadelphia, JB Lippincott, 1987, chap 11.
3. Cohn JN, Levine TB, Francis GS, et al: Neurohumoral control mechanisms in congestive heart failure. *Am Heart J* 1981;102:509-514.
4. Nicholls MG, Espiner EA, Ikram H, et al: Angiotensin II is more potent than potassium in regulating aldosterone in cardiac failure: Evidence during captopril therapy. *J Clin Endocrinol Metab* 1981;52:1253-1256.
5. Cohn JN, Levine TB: Angiotensin-converting enzyme inhibition in congestive heart failure: The concept. *Am J Cardiol* 1982;49:1480-1483.
6. Creager MA, Faxon DP, Cutler SS, et al: Contribution of vasopressin to vasoconstriction in patients with congestive heart failure: Comparison with the renin-angiotensin system and the sympathetic nervous system. *J Am Coll Cardiol* 1986;7:758-765.
7. Riegger GA, Kochsiek K: Vasopressin, renin and norepinephrine levels before and after captopril administration in patients with congestive heart failure due to idiopathic dilated cardiomyopathy. *Am J Cardiol* 1986;58:300-303.
8. Ader R, Chatterjee K, Ports T, et al: Immediate and sustained hemodynamic and clinical improvement in chronic heart failure by an oral angiotensin-converting enzyme inhibitor. *Circulation* 1980;61:931-937.
9. Awan NA, Evenson MK, Needham KE, et al: Efficacy of oral angiotensin-converting enzyme inhibition with captopril therapy in severe chronic normotensive congestive heart failure. *Am Heart J* 1981;101:22-31.
10. Brivet F, Delfraissy JF, Guidicelli JF, et al: Immediate effects of captopril in acute left ventricular failure secondary to myocardial infarction. *Eur J Clin Invest* 1981;11:369-373.
11. Creager MA, Halperin JL, Bernard DB, et al: Acute regional circulatory and renal hemodynamic effects of converting-enzyme inhibition in patients with congestive heart failure. *Circulation* 1981;64:483-489.
12. Davis R, Ribner HS, Keung E, et al: Treatment of chronic congestive heart failure with captopril, an oral inhibitor of angiotensin-converting enzyme. *N Engl J Med* 1979;301:117-121.
13. Faxon DP, Halperin JL, Creager MA, et al: Angiotensin inhibition in severe heart failure: Acute central and limb hemodynamic effects of captopril with observations on sustained oral therapy. *Am Heart J* 1981;101:548-556.
14. Levine TB, Franciosa JA, Cohn JN: Acute and long-term response to an oral converting-enzyme inhibitor, captopril, in congestive heart failure. *Circulation* 1980;62:35-41.
15. Liebau G, Riegger AJG, Steiner H: Hemodynamic effects of captopril in patients with congestive heart failure and hypertension, in Brunner HR, Gross F (eds): *Recent Advances in Hypertension Therapy: Captopril*. Amsterdam, Excerpta Medica, 1980, p 76.
16. Sharpe DN, Coxon RJ, Douglas JE, et al: Low-dose captopril in chronic heart failure: Acute hemodynamic effects and long-term treatment. *Lancet* 1980;2:1154-1157.
17. Turini GA, Brunner HR, Ferguson RR, et al: Congestive heart failure in normotensive man: Haemodynamics, renin and angiotensin-II blockade. *Br Heart J* 1978;40:1134-1142.
18. Turini GA, Brunner HR, Gribic M, et al: Improvements of chronic congestive heart failure by oral captopril. *Lancet* 1979;1:1213-1215.

19. Packer M, Lee WH, Yushak M, et al: Comparison of captopril and enalapril in patients with severe chronic heart failure. *N Engl J Med* 1986;315:847-853.

20. Moncloa F, Sromovsky JA, Walker JF, et al: Enalapril in hypertension and congestive heart failure: Overall review of efficacy and safety (review). *Drugs* 1985;30:82-89.

21. Levine TB, Olivari MT, Cohn JN: Angiotensin converting enzyme inhibitors in congestive heart failure: Overview in comparison of captopril and enalapril. *Am J Med* 1986;81(suppl 4C):36-39.

22. Silberbauer K, Punzengruber C, Sinzinger H: Endogenous prostaglandin E_2 metabolite levels, renin-angiotensin system and catecholamines versus acute hemodynamic response to captopril in chronic congestive heart failure. *Cardiology* 1983;70:297-307.

23. Massie B, Ports T, Chatterjee K, et al: Long-term vasodilator therapy for heart failure: Clinical response and its relationship to hemodynamic measurements. *Circulation* 1981;63:269-278.

24. Chatterjee K, Rouleau JL, Parmley WW: Haemodynamic and myocardial metabolic effects of captopril in chronic heart failure. *Br Heart J* 1982;47:233-238.

25. Rouleau JL, Chatterjee K, Benge W, et al: Alterations in left ventricular function and coronary hemodynamics with captopril, hydralazine and prazosin in chronic ischemic heart failure: A comparative study. *Circulation* 1982;65:671-678.

26. Pierpont GL, Francis GS, Cohn JN: Effect of captopril on renal function in patients with congestive heart failure. *Br Heart J* 1981;46:522-527.

27. Dzau VJ, Colucci WS, Williams GH, et al: Sustained effectiveness of converting-enzyme inhibition in patients with severe congestive heart failure. *N Engl J Med* 1980;302:1373-1379.

28. Pierpont G, Cohn JN: Comparison of the renal effects of vasodilators used to treat congestive heart failure. *Cardiovasc Rev Rep* 1981;2:1199-1209.

29. Ribstein J, Mimran A: Acute renal effects of captopril in patients with congestive heart failure. *J Clin Hypertens* 1986;2:238-244.

30. Packer M, Lee WH, Kessler PD: Preservation of glomerular filtration rate in human heart failure by activation of the renin-angiotensin system. *Circulation* 1986;74:766-774.

31. LeJemtel TH, Maskin CS, Chadwick B: Effects of acute angiotensin converting enzyme inhibition on renal blood flow in patients with stable congestive heart failure. *Am J Med Sci* 1986;292:123-127.

32. Cleland JG, Dargie HJ, Gillen G, et al: Captopril in heart failure: A double-blind study of the effects on renal function. *J Cardiovasc Pharmacol* 1986:8:700-706.

33. Packer M, Lee WH, Medina N, et al: Influence of renal function on the hemodynamic and clinical responses to long-term prazosin therapy in patients with severe chronic heart failure. *J Am Coll Cardiol* 1986;7:671-680.

34. Paulson OB, Jarden JO, Vorsup S, et al: Effect of captopril on the cerebral circulation in chronic heart failure. *Eur J Clin Invest* 1986;16:124-132.

35. Rajagopalan B, Raine AEG, Cooper R, et al: Changes in cerebral blood flow in patients with severe congestive cardiac failure before and after captopril treatment. *Am J Med* 1984;76(suppl 5B):86-90.

36. Dzau VJ, Colucci WS, Hollenberg NK, et al: Relation of the renin-angiotensin-aldosterone system to clinical state in congestive heart failure. *Circulation* 1981;63:645-651.

37. Heel RC, Brogden RN, Speight TM, et al: Captopril: A preliminary review of its pharmacological properties and therapeutic efficacy. *Drugs* 1980;20:409-452.

38. Witzgall H, Hirsch F, Scherer B, et al: Acute hemodynamic and hormonal effects of captopril are diminished by indomethacin. *Clin Sci* 1982;62:611-615.

39. Rose JC, Kot PA, Cohn JN, et al: Comparison of the effects of angiotensin and norepinephrine on the pulmonary circulation, systemic arteries and veins and systemic vascular capacity in the dog. *Circulation* 1962;25:247-253.

40. Kubo S, Nishioka A, Nishimura H, et al: The renin-angiotensin-aldosterone system and catecholamines in chronic congestive heart failure: Effect of angiotensin I converting enzyme inhibitor SQ-14225 (captopril). *Jpn Circ J* 1980:44:427-437.
41. Todd PA, Heel RC: Enalapril: A review of its pharmacodynamic and pharmacokinetic properties, and therapeutic use in hypertension and congestive heart failure (review). *Drugs* 1986;3:198-248.
42. Gomez HJ, Cirillo VJ, Jones KH: The clinical pharmacology of enalapril. *J Hypertens* 1983;1:65-70.
43. Dickstein K, Aarsland T, Woie L, et al: Acute hemodynamic and hormonal effects of lisinopril (MK-521) in congestive heart failure. *Am Heart J* 1986;112:121-129.
44. Robertson JIS (ed): Ramipril: A new angiotensin converting enzyme inhibitor. *Am J Cardiol* 1987;59:1D-177D.
45. DiCarlo L, Chatterjee K, Parmley WW, et al: Enalapril: A new angiotensin-converting enzyme inhibitor in chronic heart failure: Acute and chronic hemodynamic evaluations. *J Am Coll Cardiol* 1983;2:865-871.
46. Duncman WB, Wilen M, Franciosa JA: Enalapril (MK-421), a new angiotensin-converting enzyme inhibitor: Acute and chronic effects in heart failure. *Chest* 1983;84:539-545.
47. Fitzpatrick D, Nicholls MG, Ikram H, et al: Hemodynamic, hormonal, and electrolyte effects of enalapril in heart failure. *Br Heart J* 1983;50:163-169.
48. Kromer EP, Riegger GA, Liebau G, et al: Effectiveness of converting enzyme inhibition (enalapril) for mild congestive heart failure. *Am J Cardiol* 1986;57:459-462.
49. Gomez HJ, Cirillo VJ, Davies RO, et al: Enalapril in congestive heart failure: Acute and chronic invasive hemodynamic evaluation. *Int J Cardiol* 1986;11:37-51.
50. Kjekshus JK, Syland E, Dickstein K, et al: Sustained hemodynamic effects of enalapril in left ventricular failure. *J Hypertens* 1983;1:143-145.
51. Remes J, Nikander P, Rehnberg S, et al: Enalapril in chronic heart failure: A double-blind placebo-controlled study. *Ann Clin Res* 1986;18:124-128.
52. McGrath BP, Arnolda L, Matthews PG, et al: Controlled trial of enalapril in congestive cardiac failure. *Br Heart J* 1985;54:405-414.
53. Cleland JG, Dargie HG, Ball SG, et al: Effects of enalapril in heart failure: A double-blind study of effects on exercise performance, renal function, hormones, and metabolic state. *Br Heart J* 1985;54:305-312.
54. DeMarco T, Daly PA, Liu M, et al: Enalaprilat, a new parenteral angiotensin-converting enzyme inhibitor: Rapid changes in systemic and coronary hemodynamics in humoral profile in chronic heart failure. *J Am Coll Cardiol* 1987;9:1124-1130.
55. Captopril Multicenter Study Group: A placebo trial of captopril in refractory chronic congestive heart failure. *J Am Coll Cardiol* 1983;2:755-763.
56. Fouad FM, Tarazi RC, Bravo EL, et al: Long-term control of congestive heart failure with captopril. *Am J Cardiol* 1982;49:1489-1496.
57. Mattioli G, Ricci S, Rigo R, et al: Effects of captopril in heart failure complicating acute myocardial infarction and persistence of acute hemodynamic effects in chronic heart failure after 3 years of treatment. *Postgrad Med J* 1986;62(suppl 1):164-166.
58. Magnani B, Magelli C: Captopril in mild heart failure: Preliminary observations of a long-term, double-blind, placebo-controlled multicentre trial. *Postgrad Med J* 1986;62(suppl 1):153-158.
59. Bayliss J, Canepa-Anson R, Norell MS, et al: Vasodilatation with captopril and prazosin in chronic heart failure: Double blind study at rest and on exercise. *Br Heart J* 1986;55:265-273.
60. Mettauer B, Rouleau JL, Bichet D, et al: Differential long-term intrarenal and neurohormonal effects of captopril and prazosin in patients with chronic congestive heart failure: Importance of initial plasma renin activity. *Circulation* 1986;73:492-502.

61. Packer M, Lee WH, Medina N, et al: Hemodynamic and clinical significance of the pulmonary vascular response to long-term captopril therapy in patients with severe chronic heart failure. *J Am Coll Cardiol* 1985;6:635-645.

62. Shaw TR, Duncan FM, Williams BC, et al: Plasma free captopril concentrations during short and long term treatment with oral captopril for heart failure. *Br Heart J* 1985;54:160-165.

63. Creager MA, Faxon DP, Weiner DA, et al: Hemodynamic and neurohumoral response to exercise in patients with congestive heart failure treated with captopril. *Br Heart J* 1985;53:431-435.

64. Cleland JG, Dargie HJ, Hodsman GP, et al: Captopril in heart failure: A double-blind controlled trial. *Br Heart J* 1984;52:530-535.

65. Packer M, Medina N, Yushak M: Correction of dilutional hyponatremia in severe chronic heart failure by converting-enzyme inhibition. *Ann Intern Med* 1984;199:782-789.

66. Packer M, Medina N, Yushak M: Efficacy of captopril in low-renin congestive heart failure: Importance of sustained reactive hyperreninemia in distinguishing responders from nonresponders. *Am J Cardiol* 1984;54:771-777.

67. Packer M, Medina N, Yushak M: Relation between serum sodium concentration and the hemodynamic and clinical responses to converting enzyme inhibition with captopril in severe heart failure. *J Am Coll Cardiol* 1984;3:1035-1043.

68. Massie BM, Kramer BL, Topic N: Long-term captopril therapy for chronic congestive heart failure. *Am J Cardiol* 1984;53:1316-1320.

69. Chatterjee K, Parmley WW, Cohn JN, et al: A cooperative multicenter study of captopril in congestive heart failure: Hemodynamic effects and long-term response. *Am Heart J* 1985;110(suppl 2):439-447.

70. Awan NA, Amsterdam EA, Hermanovich J, et al: Long-term hemodynamic and clinical efficacy of captopril therapy in ambulatory management of severe chronic congestive heart failure. *Am Heart J* 1982;103;474-479.

71. Kayanakis JG, Fauvel JM, Giraud P, et al: Long-term treatment of congestive heart failure by captopril: Hemodynamic, biological and clinical effects. *Eur Heart J* 1981;2:75-81.

72. Romankiewicz JA, Brogden RN, Heel RC, et al: Captopril: An update review of its pharmacological properties and therapeutic efficacy in congestive heart failure. *Drugs* 1983;25:6-40.

73. Fouad FM, Tarazi RC, Bravo EL: Successful management of heart failure with captopril: Relation to angiotensin II—aldosterone suppression. *World Conference on Clinical Pharmacology and Therapeutics*, London, August 3-9, 1980.

74. Maslowski AH, Nicholls MG, Ikram H, et al: Hemodynamic, hormonal and electrolyte responses to withdrawal of long-term captopril treatment for heart failure. *Lancet* 1981;2:959-961.

75. Fitzgerald DJ, O'Callaghan WG, O'Malley K, et al: Clinical and hemodynamic responses to captopril and hydralazine in chronic congestive heart failure: The importance of preload reduction. *Br J Clin Pharmacol* 1982;14:2175-2225.

76. Levine TB, Olivari MT, Cohn JN: Dissociation of the responses of the renin-angiotensin system and sympathetic nervous system to a vasodilator stimulus in congestive heart failure. *Int J Cardiol* 1986;12:165-173.

77. Froer RL, Hall D, Blasini R, et al: Prazosin versus captopril in patients with congestive heart failure. *Am J Cardiol* 1982;49:988.

78. Kluger J, Cody RJ, Laragh JH: The contribution of sympathetic tone and the renin-angiotensin system to severe chronic congestive heart failure: Response to specific inhibitors (prazosin and captopril). *Am J Cardiol* 1982;49:1667-1674.

79. Lee CL, Walsh WF: Comparison of captopril and prazosin in patients with refractory heart failure. *Aust NZ J Med* 1982;12:323.

80. Packer M, Medina N, Yushak M: Comparative hemodynamic and clinical effects of long-term treatment with prazosin and captopril for severe chronic congestive heart failure secondary to coronary heart disease or idiopathic dilated cardiomyopathy. *Am J Cardiol* 1986;57:1323-1327.

81. Packer M, Medina N, Yushak M: Role of the renin-angiotensin system in the development of hemodynamic and clinical tolerance to long-term prazosin therapy in patients with severe chronic heart failure. *J Am Coll Cardiol* 1986;7:671-680.

82. Awan NA, Garrett L, DeMaria AN, et al: Ambulatory prazosin treatment of chronic congestive heart failure: Development of late tolerance reversible by higher dosage and interrupted substitution therapy. *Am Heart J* 1981;101:541-547.

83. Colucci WS, Wynne J, Holman BL, et al: Long-term therapy of heart failure with prazosin: A randomized double-blind trial. *Am J Cardiol* 1980;45:337-344.

84. Packer M, Meller J, Medina N, et al: Hemodynamic characterization of tolerance to long-term hydralazine therapy in severe chronic heart failure. *N Engl J Med* 1982;306:57-62.

85. Rouleau JL, Warnica JW, Burgess JA: Prazosin and congestive heart failure: Short- and long-term therapy. *Am J Med* 1981;71:147-152.

86. Massie BM, Packer M, Hanlon JT, et al: Hemodynamic responses to combined therapy with captopril and hydralazine in patients with severe heart failure. *J Am Coll Cardiol* 1983;2:338-344.

87. Alicandri C, Fariello R, Boni E, et al: Comparison of captopril and digoxin in mild to moderate heart failure. *Postgrad Med J* 1986;62(suppl 1):170-175.

88. Cleland JGF, Dargie HJ, Pettigrew A, et al: The effects of captopril on serum digoxin and urinary urea and digoxin clearances in patients with congestive heart failure. *Am Heart J* 1986;112:130-135.

89. Walsh WF, Greenberg BH: Results of long-term vasodilator therapy in patients with refractory congestive heart failure. *Circulation* 1981;64:499-507.

90. Cohn JN, Archibald DG, Ziesche S, et al: Effect of vasodilator therapy on mortality in chronic congestive heart failure. *N Engl J Med* 1986;314:1547-1552.

91. Arnold SB, William RL, Ports TA, et al: Attenuation of prazosin effect on cardiac output in chronic heart failure. *Ann Intern Med* 1979;91:345-349.

92. Pitt B: Natural history of patients with congestive heart failure: Potential role of converting enzyme inhibitors in improving survival. *Am J Med* 1986;81(suppl 4C):32-35.

93. Lee WH, Packer M: Prognostic importance of serum sodium concentration and its modification by converting-enzyme inhibition in patients with severe chronic heart failure. *Circulation* 1986;73:257-267.

94. Furberg CD, Yusuf S: Effect of vasodilators on survival in chronic congestive heart failure. *Am J Cardiol* 1985;55:1110-1113

95. CONSENSUS Trial Study Group: Effects of enalapril on mortality in severe congestive heart failure. *N Engl J Med* 1987;316:1429-1435.

96. Packer M, Medina N, Yushak M, et al: Hemodynamic patterns of response during long-term captopril therapy for severe chronic heart failure. *Circulation* 1983;64:803-812.

97. Dzau VJ, Hollenberg NK: Renal response to captopril in severe heart failure: Role of furosemide in natriuresis and reversal of hyponatremia. *Ann Intern Med* 1984;100:777-782.

98. Pfeffer JM, Pfeffer MA, Braunwald E: Hemodynamic benefits and prolonged survival with long-term captopril therapy in rats with myocardial infarction and heart failure. *Circulation* 1987;75(suppl 1):149-155.

99. Cody RJ, Franklin KW, Laragh JH: Postural hypotension during tilt with chronic captopril and diuretic therapy of severe congestive heart failure. *Am Heart J* 1982;103:480-484.

100. Duchin KL, Singhvi SM, Willard DA, et al: Captopril kinetics. *Clin Pharmacol Ther* 1982;31:452-458.

101. Devlin RG, Fleiss PM: Captopril in human blood and breast milk. *J Clin Pharmacol* 1981;21:110-113.

102. Onoyama K, Hirakata H, Kunitoshi I, et al: Blood concentration and urinary excretion of captopril (SQ 14,225) in patients with chronic renal failure. *Hypertension* 1981;3:456-459.

103. Hirakata H, Onoyama K, Iseki K, et al: Captopril (SQ 14225) clearance during hemodialysis treatment. *Clin Nephrol* 1981;16:321-323.

104. Ikram H, Maslowski AH, Nicholls MG: Hemodynamic effects of dobutamine in patients with congestive heart failure receiving captopril. *Br Heart J* 1981;46:528-530.

105. Cody RJ, Schaer GL, Covit AB, et al: Captopril kinetics in chronic congestive heart failure. *Clin Pharmacol Ther* 1982;32:721-726.

106. Montgomery AJ, Shephard AN, Emslie-Smith D: Severe hyponatremia and cardiac failure successfully treated with captopril. *Br Med J* 1982;284:1085-1086.

107. Luderer JR, Lookingbill DP, Schneck DW, et al: Captopril-induced skin eruptions. *J Clin Pharmacol* 1982;22:151-154.

108. Wilkin JK, Kirkendall WM: Pityriasis rosea–like rash from captopril. *Arch Dermatol* 1982;118:186-187.

109. Cooper RA: Captopril-associated neutropenia: Who is at risk? *Arch Intern Med* 1983;143:659-660.

110. Nicholls MG, Maslowski AH, Ikram H, et al: Ulceration of the tongue: A complication of captopril therapy. *Ann Intern Med* 1981;94:659.

111. Hess B, Keusch G, Neftel K, et al: Severe electrolyte disorders during the therapy of heart failure with the ACE-inhibitor enalapril. *Schweiz Med Wochenschr* 1986;116:1331-1336.

BERTRAM PITT, MD

Evaluation and Treatment of Chronic Compensated and New-Onset Mild to Moderate Heart Failure

The major goals in the treatment of heart failure are to improve (1) patient well-being, (2) exercise performance, and (3) survival. While there is increasing evidence that the combination of a diuretic, digitalis, and a vasodilator such as the combination of hydralazine and isosorbide dinitrate[1] or a converting-enzyme inhibitor[2] is effective in improving survival in patients with moderate to severe heart failure, the situation in patients with stable chronic heart failure or those with early mild to moderate heart failure is less certain.

For the purposes of this discussion, *severe heart failure* is defined as systolic dysfunction and manifest decompensation. Systolic dysfunction is evidenced by a reduction in left ventricular ejection fraction. Decompensation is manifest by fluid retention associated with peripheral edema and/or pulmonary congestion; a severe limitation in exercise performance, usually New York Heart Association class III or IV; and symptoms such as dyspnea on exertion, orthopnea, paroxysmal nocturnal dyspnea, cough, and/or fatigue. *Compensated chronic heart failure* refers to that stage of heart failure during which treatment has relieved most of the symptoms, but ventricular dysfunction persists and exercise tolerance may still be reduced. *New-onset mild to moderate heart failure* refers to dyspnea on exertion, a decrease in exercise capacity, or fatigue developing in a patient with objective evidence of systolic cardiac dysfunction. Excluded from this discussion are patients with symptoms or signs of heart failure without systolic dysfunction, such as those with hypertensive heart disease in whom there is a primary abnormality of diastolic function, and those with potentially correctable forms of heart failure, such as those with valvular heart disease. The approach to the patient with underlying hypertensive or valvular heart disease must focus on the natural history and correction of the underlying heart disease and is not discussed in further detail in this chapter.

The initial evaluation of new-onset mild to moderate heart failure should attempt to document a cardiac cause for the patient's symptoms, exclude any correctable causes of heart failure, and determine functional capacity and long-term prognosis. Pulmonary disease as a cause for dyspnea, fatigue, and/or bibasilar rales should be excluded by history, chest x-ray, and, if in doubt, objective pulmonary function studies. Causes of noncardiac edema, such as hypoalbuminemia, drug-induced peripheral edema, or idiopathic lymphedema, should be sought. Significant valvular heart disease should be excluded by careful physical examination and, if in doubt, echocardiography. In patients with unexplained cardiac enlargement on physical examination or chest x-ray, care should be taken to exclude pericardial effusion caused by tumor or infarction or other causes of cardiac enlargement such as amyloidosis. Myocardial ischemia as a cause of intermittent pulmonary congestion should be excluded by history and, if necessary, objective exercise stress testing, ambulatory ECG monitoring, or both. The finding of a normal rest and exercise radionuclide ventriculogram is useful in excluding systolic dysfunction as a cause of a patient's symptoms of dyspnea or fatigue. Dyspnea or fatigue may, of course, occur in patients with normal systolic function, because of diastolic dysfunction secondary to left ventricular hypertrophy or restrictive heart disease. Patients with a recent onset of symptoms of heart failure with evidence of diffuse ventricular hypokinesis without a clear explanation of its cause should be suspected of having occult myocarditis, and biopsy evidence should be sought.

Once it is established that the patient's symptoms and/or signs are due to a primary cardiac abnormality and the cause (eg, ischemic heart disease or idiopathic cardiomyopathy) is determined, reversible factors such as electrolyte abnormalities or the use of a negative inotropic drug such as disopyramide should be eliminated. After the patient's condition has been evaluated and is stable, exercise testing should be considered. Objective exercise testing may detect occult ventricular arrhythmias and provides baseline data to judge the efficacy of therapy and disease progression. There is, however, currently no agreement as to the best method of measuring exercise performance in a patient with heart failure.

THERAPY Results from the Veterans Administration Vasodilator Heart Failure Trial (V-HeFT)[1] and from the Northern Scandinavian Study (CONSENSUS)[2] have provided evidence that vasodilator drugs added to conventional therapy with digoxin and diuretics can prolong survival in heart failure. The V-HeFT study was carried out in patients with ventricular dysfunction and exercise intolerance. Although this study included patients with mild, moderate, and moderately severe heart failure, an exercise protocol requirement excluded patients too sick to exercise and the persistence of symptoms despite digoxin and diuretic therapy tended to exclude the most mild form of this syndrome. The CONSENSUS study was confined to patients with class IV failure who were by definition symptomatic at rest.

Although these studies provide strong support for a role of vasoconstriction as a contributing factor to progression of heart failure in the patient population studied, application of this principle to the patient with mild heart failure must be considered speculative. Until the results of several ongoing, large, prospective randomized trials of vasodilators in heart failure, such as the study of left ventricular dysfunction (SOLVD) sponsored by the National Heart, Lung and Blood Institute, the second Veterans Administration Heart Failure Trial (V-HeFT-II), and the study of acute ventricular enlargement (SAVE), are available, any conclusions about therapy for chronic compensated or new-onset mild heart failure are premature. Current discussions of such therapy must be based on the effect of a given therapeutic strategy on patient well-being and long-term exercise performance. Earlier discussions based on acute hemodynamic evaluation and short-term exercise studies must be revised in view of the increasing recognition that there is a relatively poor correlation between the acute hemodynamic effects of a given agent and its long-term effects on exercise performance and patient well-being.[3-5] There are currently no convincing data to predict long-term improvement in exercise performance from acute hemodynamic measurements including left ventricular filling pressure, cardiac index, and peripheral vascular resistance.[3] Similarly, the short-term effects of a therapeutic agent on exercise performance may not be maintained over the long term.[4,5]

The recently completed prospective, double-blind, randomized trial of digitalis versus captopril in patients with mild to moderate heart failure[6] may be valuable in deciding on an interim strategy for the treatment of chronic compensated or new-onset heart failure. In this study, patients younger than 75 years of age with a left ventricular ejection fraction less than or equal to 40% and a treadmill exercise performance limited by dyspnea or fatigue of more than four minutes but less than the age-predicted maximum were randomized to receive either digoxin, captopril, or placebo while taking a diuretic if needed after withdrawal from baseline vasodilator therapy, digoxin, or both. Increased use of diuretic was allowed during the trial if necessitated by the patient's symptoms. Other entry criteria included the presence of sinus rhythm and either ischemic heart disease, primary myocardial disease, or heart failure without significant valvular regurgitation after valve replacement. Three hundred patients meeting these criteria were entered into the study protocol and followed for six months. The effect of the three therapeutic strategies (captopril, digoxin, or placebo), in conjunction with diuretic if needed, on the following outcomes was evaluated: exercise performance, change in New York Heart Association functional class, need for emergency room visits and hospitalization for heart failure, ventricular arrhythmias, left ventricular ejection fraction, and safety profile.

The mean age of the study population was 57 years; over 80% of the patients were male. Approximately two thirds of the patients had ischemic heart disease; one third, primary myocardial disease. The mean duration of heart failure at entry into the study was three years, with 87% of the patients in New York Heart Association class I or II. The mean exercise time on a modified Naughton protocol was approximately nine minutes. The mean left ventricular ejection fraction was 25%. Half of the patients had more than ten ventricular premature beats (VPBs) per hour at entry into the study.

In this study, patients maintained on a regimen of captopril and a diuretic if needed had a significantly improved exercise performance and New York Heart Association functional class compared with the placebo group (diuretic alone if needed). Patients taking digoxin and a diuretic if needed also had an improvement in exercise performance and functional class, but this was not significant compared with the placebo group nor as great as that found in the captopril group, although this difference was not statistically significant. Patients receiving captopril who had had ten or more VPBs an hour on the baseline ambulatory ECG had a significant reduction in the incidence of ventricular premature beats, compared to the digoxin-treated group. The patients in this study maintained on a regimen of placebo and a diuretic if needed had significantly more visits to the emergency room and admissions to the hospital for heart failure than either the captopril or the digoxin group, even though during the course of the study the placebo group had a significant increase in diuretic usage compared with the other two treatment groups. Patients taking digoxin did, however, have a significant increase in left ventricular ejection fraction, compared with both the placebo and captopril groups.

The captopril group had a greater incidence of side effects (dizziness or lightheadedness). These side effects were, however, usually transient, were alleviated by reducing the dose of diuretic, and did not result in any increase in patient dropout from the study. Because of the relatively small sample size, there were too few deaths to reach any conclusions as to the relative effect of the three treatment strategies on survival.

A recent survey of internists and cardiologists in the United States suggested that most physicians prescribe diuretics alone or in combination with digoxin for patients with chronic heart failure.[7] Vasodilator therapy was used only infrequently (<10%) and was reserved for those with more severe heart failure. The results of the captopril-digoxin study in patients with mild to moderate heart failure[6] and the encouraging data on the effects of vasodilators on mortality in patients with moderate to severe heart failure[1,2] suggest that vasodilators be used more frequently to treat patients with chronic compensated and mild to moderate heart failure. The reasoning for this recommendation is outlined briefly below.

Diuretics   Diuretics when used alone are effective in relieving peripheral edema and pulmonary congestion and in improving exercise performance. The results of the captopril-digoxin study in patients with mild to moderate heart failure[6] suggest, however, that a combination of a converting-enzyme inhibitor and a diuretic is more effective than a diuretic alone in improving exercise performance and New York Heart Association functional class. In a previous study the strategy of increasing diuretic dosage was suggested to be more effective than the addition of a converting-enzyme inhibitor in improving exercise performance in patients with mild to moderate heart failure.[8] This earlier study was, however, carried out in a relatively small number of patients, and exercise performance was determined after only a few weeks. The finding that the maximal effects of converting-enzyme inhibition may not be evident for several weeks[9] and the results of the longer multicenter captopril-digoxin study[6] suggest that converting-enzyme inhibition plus a diuretic may be more effective than a diuretic alone in the treatment of chronic compensated or mild to moderate heart failure. Use of a diuretic alone in a patient with heart failure tends to stimulate secondary neurohumoral mechanisms, including the renin-angiotensin system, vasopressin, and catecholamines.[10,11] Stimulation of the renin-angiotensin system results in an increase in both systemic and coronary vascular resistance.[12] In some instances use of a diuretic such as furosemide may actually precipitate pulmonary edema because of systemic vasoconstriction secondary to neurohumoral stimulation.[13] Diuretics also lead

to hypokalemia in 20% to 25% of patients treated for heart failur
hypokalemia associated with diuretic usage may occur despite conc
use of oral potassium replacement and often cannot be corrected unl
accompanying diuretic-induced magnesium deficiency is corrected.
pokalemia resulting from diuretic usage in patients with heart failure
have an important effect on patient survival. There is a clear relation: ..p
between the degree of hypokalemia and the incidence of ventricular tachycardia.[15] This is especially important in view of the recent study by Gottlieb
et al,[16] which showed that diuretic-induced hypokalemia and neurohumoral
activation were the most important factors associated with the occurrence
of ventricular arrhythmias in patients with heart failure, and the finding that
approximately half of the deaths in patients with heart failure are sudden,
presumably caused by a ventricular arrhythmia.[17] These considerations and
the findings in the captopril-digoxin trial[6] argue against the use of diuretics
as sole therapy in patients with heart failure. These considerations do not,
however, negate the effectiveness of diuretics as part of a more comprehensive
therapeutic regimen. In combination with a converting-enzyme inhibitor, the
risk of diuretic-induced hypokalemia and secondary neurohumoral activation
is reduced. The question as to whether this combination will reduce the
incidence of sudden cardiac death in patients with heart failure must await
further study. In contrast, in combination with digoxin, diuretic-induced hypokalemia and secondary neurohumoral activation persists. The occurrence
of hypokalemia and secondary neurohumoral activation including catecholamine release in a digitalized patient may further increase the risk of ventricular
arrhythmias and sudden cardiac death.

Digoxin   Digitalis has been the mainstay of therapy for heart failure
for over 200 years. In patients with moderate to severe
heart failure characterized by a dilated heart and a third
heart sound there is suggestive evidence that digoxin is
effective in improving ventricular performance, exercise
duration, and functional class.[18] The effect of digoxin in patients with chronic
compensated and new-onset mild to moderate heart failure is less certain.
In several studies of patients with chronic compensated heart failure in sinus
rhythm, digoxin has been withdrawn and the patients followed over several
months without adverse effect in the vast majority.[19-23] In a recent randomized
study of patients with chronic compensated heart failure, Fleg et al[24] found
that administration of digoxin resulted in a significant improvement in left
ventricular ejection fraction but no significant improvement in exercise performance. Similarly, the results of the captopril-digoxin trial[6] in patients with
mild to moderate heart failure show that digoxin significantly improves left
ventricular ejection fraction without a concomitant increase in exercise performance compared with placebo. Both digoxin and captopril were, however,
effective in protecting the patient from manifest heart failure, as evidenced
by a lower incidence of visits to the emergency room and hospitalization for
heart failure, compared with the placebo group. Nevertheless, even if digoxin
were as effective as a converting-enzyme inhibitor in improving exercise
performance and patient well-being in chronic compensated or early mild
to moderate heart failure, the potentially beneficial effects (discussed above)
of converting-enzyme inhibitors on serum potassium and secondary neurohumoral activation would favor the use of a converting-enzyme inhibitor
and a diuretic as an alternative to digoxin and a diuretic. Because digitalis
toxicity occurs in approximately 20% of digitalized patients[25] and in view of

the uncertain effect of digoxin on survival,[26] especially in patients with underlying ischemic heart disease, a prudent strategy for the management of chronic compensated or new-onset mild to moderate heart failure may be to attempt therapy with a converting-enzyme inhibitor and a diuretic. If symptoms or signs persist or the patient fails to tolerate the converting-enzyme inhibitor, digoxin should be added. The favorable effect of digoxin on ejection fraction in the captopril-digoxin trial could constitute in some physicians' views an indication for more routine digoxin usage. However, data to support a long-term benefit of digoxin are not available.

Vasodilators Converting-enzyme inhibitors in conjunction with a diuretic and digoxin have been found effective in improving survival in patients with class IV heart failure.[2] Similarly, the combination of hydralazine–isosorbide dinitrate with a diuretic and digoxin improves survival in patients with more moderate degrees of heart failure.[1] Although vasodilators are currently reserved for severe heart failure,[7] the evidence that they improve survival[1,2] and the results of the captopril-digoxin study[6] suggest that they will find increasing use in patients with chronic compensated and mild to moderate heart failure. Insight into the question as to whether vasodilator therapy with hydralazine–isosorbide dinitrate or converting-enzyme inhibitor is superior will come from the results of the ongoing V-HeFT-II study, in which the effect of these two vasodilator strategies on survival is being compared. Although final judgment as to the relative merits of the two vasodilator strategies will have to await further study, it should be pointed out that direct-acting vasodilators may stimulate secondary neurohumoral mechanisms and that tolerance to the effect of some of these drugs has been demonstrated in some studies.[4,5,27] It should also be emphasized that not all vasodilators are equally effective. For example, prazosin has been associated with tachyphylaxis[5] and did not improve survival in patients in the V-HeFT trial.[1] Converting-enzyme inhibitors, on the other hand, may be less likely to show tolerance[9,28-30] and cause secondary neurohumoral activation. In one study that directly compared captopril and hydralazine–isosorbide dinitrate, there was significantly greater neurohumoral activation with hydralazine–isosorbide dinitrate.[27] In a small single-blind study of captopril or hydralazine added to conventional therapy in patients with severe heart failure, there was significantly greater symptomatic improvement and symptom-limited exercise tolerance in patients treated with a converting-enzyme inhibitor.[30]

Calcium Channel Blockers The calcium channel blocking agents have had wide use in patients with angina pectoris and, because of their vasodilating properties, have also been evaluated in patients with heart failure.[31-33] Like other vasodilators, they tend to improve hemodynamics and exercise tolerance. However, unlike the direct-acting vasodilators and converting-enzyme inhibitors, the calcium channel blockers may have a negative inotropic action and in some instances have worsened heart failure.[34] Until a favorable risk-benefit ratio has been demonstrated for calcium channel blocking agents, they should not be used to treat heart failure. They may, however, have a role in cases in which coronary arterial spasm is a cause of ventricular dysfunction.

Positive Inotropic Agents   Several positive inotropic agents have been investigated over the past several years.[35] There is increasing evidence to suggest that phosphodiesterase inhibitors such as milrinone improve symptoms and exercise tolerance in patients with mild to moderate heart failure.[36] Their effect on survival is, however, questionable.[37] Until the results of further prospective randomized studies are available and the effect of phosphodiesterase inhibitors and other inotropic agents such as the β_1-agonists on survival is clearer, these agents must be considered of uncertain value in the treatment of mild to moderate heart failure.

β-Adrenergic Blockade   Although originally relatively contraindicated, β-blockers are finding increasing use in patients with heart failure. Patients in the Beta Blocker Heart Attack Trial (BHAT) with a history of heart failure before infarction or on entry into the hospital had a significantly greater improvement in survival than patients without a history of heart failure.[38] Studies in patients with idiopathic dilated cardiomyopathy treated with metoprolol[39] have suggested that long-term β-adrenergic receptor blockade may result in improved ventricular function, patient well-being, and survival. Some patients with heart failure, however, cannot tolerate even small doses of metoprolol. Until there is greater experience with β-blockers in patients with heart failure and clear benefit is demonstrated in prospective, randomized trials, β-blockers should be reserved for clinical investigation but not used in clinical practice for the treatment of heart failure.

CONCLUSION   After decades of little progress, therapy for patients with heart failure is in transition. There is increasing evidence that the natural history of severe heart failure may be favorably altered by vasodilator therapy.[1,2] While more definitive guidelines for the treatment of mild to moderate heart failure must await the results of the ongoing large, prospective, randomized trials, there is sufficient evidence, outlined above, to recommend that vasodilator therapy play an increasing role in the management of chronic compensated or mild to moderate heart failure. On the basis of the available data it seems reasonable to use a converting-enzyme inhibitor or direct-acting vasodilator and a diuretic in patients with chronic compensated or new-onset mild to moderate heart failure. Such patients probably should not be maintained on a regimen of diuretics alone. The precise role of digoxin in this patient population has not yet been defined, although it may appropriately be reserved for those who fail to respond adequately to the initial therapy.

REFERENCES

1. Cohn JN, Archibald DG, Ziesche S, et al: Effect of vasodilator therapy on mortality in chronic congestive heart failure. *N Engl J Med* 1986;314:1547-1552.
2. The CONSENSUS Trial Study Group: Effects of enalapril on mortality in severe congestive heart failure. *N Engl J Med* 1987;316:1429-1435.
3. Franciosa JA, Goldsmith SR, Cohn JV: Contrasting immediate and long term effects of isosorbide dinitrate on exercise capacity in congestive heart failure. *Am J Med* 1980;67:557-560.
4. Franciosa JA, Weber KT, Levine TB: Hydralazine in the long term treatment of chronic heart failure: Lack of difference from placebo. *Am Heart J* 1982;104:587-594.
5. Packer M, Meller J, Gorlin R, et al: Hemodynamic and clinical tachyphylaxis to prazosin-mediated afterload reduction in severe chronic congestive heart failure. *Circulation* 1979;59:531-539.
6. The Captopril-Digoxin Multicenter Research Group: Comparative effects of therapy with captopril and digoxin in patients with mild to moderate heart failure. *JAMA* 1988;259:539-544.
7. Hlatky MA, Fleg JL, Hinton PC, et al: Physician practice in the management of congestive heart failure. *J Am Coll Cardiol* 1986;8:966-970.
8. Cleland JGF, Dargie HJ, Ball SG: Effects of enalapril in heart failure: A double blind study of effects on exercise performance, renal function, hormones and metabolic state. *Br Heart J* 1985;54:305-312.
9. Topic N, Kramer B, Massie B: Acute and long-term effects of captopril on exercise cardiac performance and exercise capacity in congestive heart failure. *Am Heart J* 1982;104:1172-1179.
10. Ikram H, Chan W, Espiner EA, et al: Haemodynamic and hormone responses to acute and chronic furosemide therapy in congestive heart failure. *Clin Sci* 1980;59:443-449.
11. Bayliss J, Norell M, Canepa-Anson R, et al: Untreated heart failure: Clinical and lneuroendocrine effects of introducing diuretics. *Br Heart J* 1987;57:17-22.
12. Magrini F, Shimizu M, Roberts N, et al: Converting-enzyme inhibition and coronary blood flow. *Circulation* 1987;75(suppl 1):168-174.
13. Francis GS, Siegel RM, Goldsmith SR, et al: Acute vasodilator response to intravenous furosemide in patients with chronic congestive heart failure. *Ann Intern Med* 1985;103:1-6.
14. Johansson BW: Hypokalemia in cardiac decompensation. *Acta Pharmacol Toxicol* 1984;54(suppl 1):103-106.
15. Nordrehaug JE: Malignant arrhythmias in relation to serum potassium values in patients with an acute myocardial infarction. *Acta Med Scand* 1981;suppl 647: 101-107.
16. Gottlieb SS, Blum MA, Kukin ML, et al: Which patients with congestive heart failure have malignant ventricular tachyarrhythmias in high risk subsets (abstract)? *J Am Coll Cardiol* 1987;9(suppl A):33A.
17. Wilson JR, Schwartz JS, Sutton MSJ, et al: Prognosis in severe heart failure: Relation to hemodynamic measurements and ventricular ectopic activity. *J Am Coll Cardiol* 1983;2:403-410.
18. Lee DC, Johnson RA, Bingham JE, et al: Heart failure in outpatients: A randomized trial of digoxin versus placebo. *N Engl J Med* 1986;306:699-705.
19. Gheorghiade M, Beller GA: Effects of discontinuing maintenance digoxin therapy in patients with ischemic heart disease and congestive heart failure in sinus rhythm. *Am J Cardiol* 1983;51:1243-1250.
20. Johnston GD, McDevitt DG: Is maintenance digoxin necessary in patients with sinus rhythm? *Lancet* 1979;1:567-570.
21. Hull SM, Mackintosh A: Discontinuation of maintenance digoxin therapy in general practice. *Lancet* 1977;2:1054-1055.

22. Dall JL: Maintenance digoxin in elderly patients. *Br Med J* 1970;2:705-706.

23. Fleg JL, Gottlieb SH, Lakatta EG: Is digoxin really important in treatment of compensated heart failure? A placebo-controlled crossover trial in patients with sinus rhythm. *Am J Med* 1982;73:244-250.

24. Fleg JL, Rothfeld B, Wright J, et al: Does digoxin enhance exercise left ventricular function in patients with congestive heart failure (abstract)? *J Am Coll Cardiol* 1987;9(suppl A):132A.

25. Beller GA, Smith TW, Abelmann WH, et al: Digitalis intoxication: A prospective clinical study with serum level correlations. *N Engl J Med* 1971;284:989-997.

26. Yusuf S, Wittes J, Bailey K, et al: Digitalis—a new controversy regarding an old drug: The pitfalls of inappropriate methods. *Circulation* 1986;73:14-18.

27. Daly P, Rouleau JL, Cousineau D, et al: Effects of captopril and a combination of hydralazine and isosorbide dinitrate on myocardial sympathetic tone in patients with severe congestive heart failure. *Br Heart J* 1986;56:152-157.

28. Awan NA, Amsterdam EA, Hermanovich J, et al: Long-term hemodynamic and clinical efficacy of captopril therapy in ambulatory management of severe chronic congestive heart failure. *Am Heart J* 1982;103:474-479.

29. Fitzpatrick D, Ikram H, Nicholls MG: Double-blind placebo-controlled withdrawal of long-term captopril heart failure therapy (abstract). *Circulation* 1983;68(suppl 3):130.

30. Schofield PM, Lawrence G, Testa T, et al: A randomized comparison of hydralazine and captopril in the treatment of severe congestive heart failure (abstract). *J Am Coll Cardiol* 1987;9(suppl A):103A.

31. Leier CV, Patrick TJ, Hermiller J, et al: Nifedipine in congestive heart failure: Effects on resting and exercise hemodynamics and regional blood flow. *Am Heart J* 1984;108:1461-1468.

32. Ferlinz J, Citron PD: Hemodynamic and myocardial performance characteristics after verapamil use in congestive heart failure. *Am J Cardiol* 1983;51:1339-1345.

33. Walsh RW, Porter CB, Starling MR, et al: Beneficial hemodynamic effects of intravenous and oral diltiazem in severe congestive heart failure. *J Am Coll Cardiol* 1984;3:1044-1050.

34. Brooks N, Cattell M, Pidgeon J, et al: Unpredictable response to nifedipine in severe cardiac failure. *Br Med J* 1980;281:1324.

35. Colucci WS, Wright RF, Braunwald E: New positive inotropic agents in the treatment of congestive heart failure: Mechanisms of action and recent clinical developments. *N Engl J Med* 1986;314:349-358.

36. Baim DS, McDowell AV, Cherniles J, et al: Evaluation of a new bipyridine inotropic agent—milrinone—in patients with severe congestive heart failure. *N Engl J Med* 1983;309:748-756.

37. Packer M, Leier CV: Survival in congestive heart failure during treatment with drugs with positive inotropic actions. *Circulation* 1987;75(suppl 4):55-63.

38. Chadda K, Goldstein S, Byington R, et al: Effect of propranolol after acute myocardial infarction in patients with congestive heart failure. *Circulation* 1986;73:503-510.

39. Swedberg K, Hjalmarson A, Waagstein F, et al: Prolongation of survival in congestive cardiomyopathy by beta-receptor blockade. *Lancet* 1979;1:1374-1376.

12

Survival in Patients with Chronic Congestive Heart Failure and Its Potential Modification by Drug Therapy

---

During the last 20 years, a variety of inotropic, diuretic, and vasodilator drugs have been developed that can ameliorate the symptoms and enhance the functional capacity of patients with congestive heart failure.[1] Despite these advances, however, the mortality of patients with congestive heart failure remains very high (Fig. 12-1). The annual mortality rate ranges from 15% to 60%, depending on the severity of the underlying disease; nearly 200,000 patients die of congestive heart failure each year.[2]

Do the drugs that we have developed for the treatment of heart failure alter mortality? Are efforts directed at improving symptoms likely to prolong life? An affirmative response to these questions would suggest that the physiologic derangements that limit productivity also limit longevity, but this might not be true. Previous experience in the treatment of systemic hypertension has shown that drugs that correct physiologic abnormalities may not produce expected benefits with respect to morbidity and mortality.[3] It is important, therefore, to closely examine the issue of survival in patients with chronic congestive heart failure, to investigate whether therapeutic interventions can modify the long-term outcome of these patients, and to determine if these benefits are achieved independently of the ability of these agents to ameliorate symptoms or improve exercise tolerance.

For purposes of this chapter, we will restrict our review to those patients with congestive heart failure due to disorders of the left heart that are associated with poor left ventricular systolic function. We will not consider patients with surgically correctable lesions, hypertrophic states, or left ventricular diastolic abnormalities.

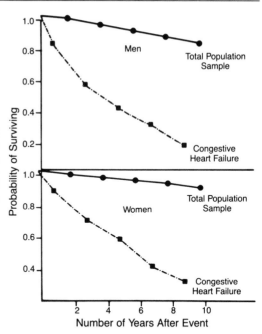

Fig. 12-1. Survival of patients with congestive heart failure in the Framingham study. (Adapted from McKee et al.[4] Reprinted, by permission of *The New England Journal of Medicine*, 285;1441-1446, 1971.)

MORTALITY IN CONGESTIVE HEART FAILURE

Although the issue of mortality in congestive heart failure has been evaluated in numerous reports, these studies differ substantially in a number of important aspects and therefore do not provide a coherent perspective of the problem. First, previous investigators examined patients with markedly different demographic, hemodynamic, and clinical characteristics. Some evaluated only ambulatory patients who could tolerate formal treadmill testing, whereas others enrolled only critically ill patients who could tolerate prolonged invasive hemodynamic monitoring. Second, previous reports defined the syndrome of congestive heart failure in different ways. In some mortality studies the diagnosis of congestive heart failure was made clinically and did not require confirmation of left ventricular dysfunction,[4] whereas other studies followed the long-term outcome of patients with left ventricular dysfunction, whether or not they had symptoms of heart failure.[5,6] Third, previous studies enrolled patients at different stages in the disease process. Early reports followed patients after their initial presentation to the physician,[4] whereas recent studies evaluated patients referred to tertiary care centers with refractory symptoms.[7] All of these analytical dilemmas considerably limit the ability to assess the risk of mortality in the individual patient with congestive heart failure and to determine if a proposed therapeutic intervention exerts a favorable effect on survival.

Mechanism of Death in Heart Failure

Death in congestive heart failure is a result of a progressive disorder of left ventricular function, which is accompanied by both mechanical and electrical sequelae, and is exacerbated by peripheral hemodynamic and neurohormonal factors. After an initial insult to the myocardium, a number of physiologic forces are triggered that lead to cardiac dilatation and loss of contractile function, as ventricular muscle is gradually replaced by noncon-

tractile fibrous tissue. At some stage in this progression to end-s
ventricular dysfunction, symptoms become apparent to the patient a
time become increasingly severe and resistant to treatment. Eventually, c
performance becomes insufficient to sustain the circulation, and death re
The precise pathophysiologic events that lead to this terminal inabili
maintain circulatory homeostasis remain poorly understood. However,
event is usually clinically sudden, although it is usually preceded by seve
symptoms and is almost always accompanied by a severe tachy- or brady-
arrhythmia, which occurs secondary to the rapidly deteriorating hemodynamic
state. Very few patients with heart failure actually die from refractory hypotension
and electromechanical dissociation without an intervening terminal arrhythmia.

This progressive deterioration in cardiac performance
leading to refractory symptoms and death is not the only mechanism of
death in patients with left ventricular disease. At any time after the onset of
cardiac dilatation and dysfunction, electrical automatic or reentry circuits
may emerge within the myocardium that predispose to the formation of
malignant ventricular arrhythmias.[8] If these are sustained and are not interrupted
by medical therapy, death in a patient with left ventricular dysfunction may
rapidly supervene, even though left ventricular mechanical function may be
only modestly compromised and would (in the absence of the arrhythmia)
be capable of supporting the circulation. Sudden death may occur early in
the course of the disease before any symptoms of heart failure have been
noted by the patient, but these arrhythmic events become increasingly frequent
as the left ventricle becomes progressively more compromised. During the
terminal stages of left ventricular dysfunction, malignant rhythm disturbances
may become so common that it may be nearly impossible to determine (with
certainty) if the terminal arrhythmia observed at the time of death played a
primary or secondary role in the demise of the patient.

Traditionally, clinicians have attempted to approach this
uncertainty by estimating the severity of circulatory impairment immediately
prior to death, based on the patient's symptoms. If the patient's clinical status
became worse in the days before his or her demise, physicians generally
assumed that significant hemodynamic deterioration had recently occurred,
and thus any terminal arrhythmia could be considered a secondary event
and attributable to the mechanical consequences of the left ventricular
dysfunction. On the other hand, if the patient did not note any exacerbation
of symptoms of heart failure prior to death, no preterminal hemodynamic
deterioration could be inferred, and the fatal arrhythmia was presumed to
be primary. On the basis of this classification, previous reports suggested
that 30% to 45% of deaths in chronic heart failure were sudden, whereas
50% of deaths could be ascribed to mechanical progression of the underlying
disease.[9] Unfortunately, symptoms are not a reliable reflection of the occurrence
of preterminal hemodynamic events. Consequently, the hemodynamic deterioration that occurs before death may remain clinically silent, and if so,
the patient's death may be incorrectly categorized as a sudden arrhythmic
demise (because of the lack of symptoms) even though it resulted from
mechanical failure of the left ventricle.

Can we then ever be certain about the mode of death in
patients with congestive heart failure? At first, we might believe that our
dilemma would be easier if we were able to observe patients closely in the
hours and days before their terminal event. Ironically, such close attention

might merely exacerbate our confusion. As patients with heart failure approach the time of death, they usually manifest multiple deficits of cardiac function. Many have *both* arrhythmias and heart failure in the last few weeks of life, and it may be impossible to determine (with confidence) how these multiple factors interact pathophysiologically to lead to the patient's demise. As Bigger has emphasized,[10] a single cause of death usually cannot be satisfactorily identified even when a patient with heart failure dies in the intensive care unit during continuous electrocardiographic and hemodynamic monitoring. Even under the closest scrutiny, we cannot determine if the terminal arrhythmia played a primary or secondary role in the demise of the patient. Any mechanism of death that is assigned under these conditions is highly judgmental and is strongly subject to the biases of the investigator; the designation "sudden death" cannot be considered to be a reliable indicator of an arrhythmic mechanism of death. Except for a few extreme examples, the final event in most patients with congestive heart failure is a multifactorial death.

This realization—that most deaths in heart failure are multifactorial—should not, however, dissuade physicians from attempting to minimize the various contributory mechanical and electrical factors that interact to determine the patient's demise. Should interventions that selectively address the hemodynamic or electrophysiologic abnormalities be developed in the future, logic would suggest that these approaches be applied in concert in an effort to reduce *total* cardiovascular mortality in this disease.

DETERMINANTS OF MORTALITY IN HEART FAILURE

Congestive heart failure represents a complex clinical syndrome characterized by abnormalities of left ventricular function and neurohormonal regulation, which are accompanied by effort intolerance, fluid retention, and reduced longevity. Since in most patients the pathophysiologic components of the disease become increasingly abnormal over time, any assessment of disease severity (based on one pathophysiologic factor) is likely to be reasonably correlated with long-term prognosis. The finding of such a statistical association, however, does not imply a cause-and-effect relationship. Conversely, the lack of a statistical relationship between a specific pathophysiologic variable and mortality does not preclude an important role for such a factor in determining survival.

Why should statistical significance be so poorly correlated with biologic significance in these patients? Any potentially useful prognostic variable can be shown to accurately presage long-term outcome only if the patient cohort being evaluated includes patients with a wide range of values for that variable. Conversely, an important prognostic factor cannot be shown to have any predictive value if it is present in all of the patients enrolled in the study. Hence, when assessing the value of any report concerning mortality in heart failure, it is important to pay close attention to the demographic, hemodynamic, clinical, and neurohormonal characteristics of the patients who were enrolled in the study. Unfortunately, many reports have confined their attention to patients with advanced disease who are able to undergo intensive (and frequently invasive) testing; this restricted view has limited the ability of some reports to discern a prognostic role for some variables of pathophysiologic importance.

Etiology of Disease

In most patients with congestive heart failure, left ventricular dysfunction is the result of coronary artery disease or a primary (usually idiopathic) myocardial disorder. Does the etiology of left ventricular dysfunction influence survival?

In studies in which coronary artery disease has been the principal etiologic factor (those derived from tertiary referral centers), the cause of heart failure was not usually an important determinant of mortality.[11-13] In contrast, in studies in which the fraction of patients with an idiopathic dilated cardiomyopathy has been large (those conducted at Veterans Administration hospitals), patients with coronary artery disease had a worse long-term prognosis than patients with a dilated cardiomyopathy.[14,15]

Why should the presence of coronary artery disease alter the prognosis of patients with congestive heart failure? There are two possible explanations. First, the difference in the risk of mortality between patients with an idiopathic and ischemic cardiomyopathy may not be related to the etiology of the disease but to the timing of the diagnosis. Because of the slowly advancing nature of the disorder, patients with an idiopathic dilated cardiomyopathy may be detected earlier in the course of the disease at a time when left ventricular performance is only moderately compromised. In contrast, patients with coronary artery disease commonly experience a sudden and large loss of viable myocardium, such that the magnitude of left ventricular dysfunction may already be severe at the time when symptoms first appear. Second, the difference in the prognosis of etiology-based subgroups may be related to *true* differences in the rate of progression of these two disorders. Patients with coronary artery disease may experience additional ischemic events that may further compromise myocardial function[16]; in contrast, patients with an idiopathic dilated cardiomyopathy may undergo spontaneous remission of their disorder.[5,17] Such spontaneous remissions may be unlikely to occur in patients with far advanced disease with disabling symptoms at rest, who are likely to be referred to tertiary care centers.

Symptoms and Functional Capacity

The clinical assessment is widely used by clinicians to judge the severity of heart failure, but its prognostic utility has not been clearly defined. At first glance, it would seem that symptoms should be strongly predictive of long-term outcome, since exercise tolerance becomes more limited as the heart failure state progresses. Patients with disabling symptoms do fare worse than those with asymptomatic left ventricular dysfunction (Fig. 12-2)[18]; the prognosis may be particularly poor in patients exhibiting progressive clinical deterioration.[13] Yet, symptoms remain highly subjective, are subject to considerable patient and physician bias, and can be rapidly improved by drugs that have no apparent effect on mortality. Since nearly all patients with heart failure who are seen by physicians are already receiving some treatment in an attempt to modify their clinical status, can we still use symptoms to predict survival in these patients?

As in the case of other prognostic factors, the ability of symptoms to predict mortality depends on the patient cohort being evaluated. In studies of patients with a wide range of symptoms, exercise tolerance was an important predictor of long-term outcome, whether this was assessed subjectively (by New York Heart Association functional class)[11,13,18,19] or objectively (by measurement of maximum oxygen consumption)[16,20]; this was not true in studies that restricted their analysis to severely ill patients.[12,21] It is noteworthy

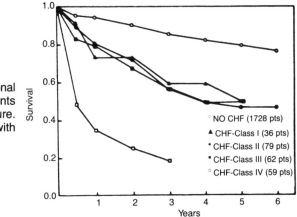

Fig. 12-2. Relation of functional status and survival in patients with congestive heart failure. (Adapted from Califf et al[18] with permission.)

that the principal utility of this functional assessment appeared to be in the identification of patients with extreme exercise intolerance—those with symptoms at rest (functional class IV) or with a maximum oxygen consumption less than 10 mL/kg/min—both of whom have an extremely poor prognosis. When such individuals are omitted from the analysis, the assessment of symptoms and functional capacity in the patient with congestive heart failure appears to provide little prognostic information.[21,22]

Ventricular Dimensions and Ejection Fraction
Nearly all patients with congestive heart failure have dilated hearts; therefore the measurement of cardiac dimensions (either radiographically or echocardiographically) does not predict the long-term outcome of these patients,[23] except if patients with heart failure are compared with individuals who have minimal disease.[5]

The left ventricular ejection fraction is the measure of cardiac performance most commonly used to predict mortality in patients with congestive heart failure. This variable is a powerful prognostic indicator in patients recovering from an acute myocardial infarction as well as in those with clinically stable coronary artery disease.[6,24] Its value in these settings, however, derives primarily from the fact that comparisons are made between patients with normal and abnormal cardiac performance.[22] In the setting of congestive heart failure, in which nearly all patients have an abnormal left ventricular ejection fraction, is the measurement of left ventricular ejection fraction still useful in predicting survival? Again, the answer seems to depend on the patient cohort being evaluated. In reports that include patients with a wide spectrum of disease severity, the left ventricular ejection fraction remains a powerful prognostic factor (Fig. 12-3),[15,18,25,26] whereas it has provided little prognostic information in the studies of patients with refractory symptoms, in which nearly all patients had severe left ventricular dysfunction (ejection fraction < 30%).[11,12,27]

Should we then avoid using noninvasive imaging to predict long-term outcome in the patient with severe congestive heart failure? Although the assessment of left ventricular ejection fraction may provide little information in such cases, the measurement of right ventricular function may be of considerable prognostic value. Concomitant right ventricular dysfunction in patients with left heart failure appears to indicate an advanced severity or

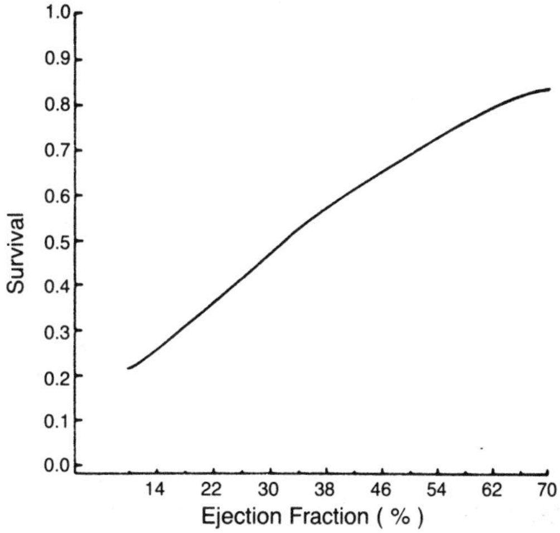

Fig. 12-3. Relation of left ventricular ejection fraction and survival in congestive heart failure. (Adapted from Califf et al[18] with permission.)

chronicity of the underlying disease, and therefore it can be used to identify those patients with the most dismal long-term outcome among those with a very low left ventricular ejection fraction.[28-31] In patients with only moderate left ventricular dysfunction, however, right ventricular ejection fraction is usually well preserved and thus has little discriminant value in predicting survival.[22]

Central Hemodynamic Variables

The severity of hemodynamic abnormalities predicts mortality in patients with acute heart failure secondary to a myocardial infarction[32]; therefore we might expect that a similar relationship exists between hemodynamic variables and survival in patients with chronic heart failure. Support for this hypothesis comes from studies that have evaluated patients with a wide range of hemodynamic abnormalities. In these reports, patients with a markedly depressed cardiac output and stroke work index and a markedly elevated left ventricular filling pressure and systemic vascular resistance had a significantly worse prognosis than patients with near normal values for these hemodynamic variables (Fig. 12-4).[5,13,25-27,30,33-35] However, in studies in which all patients showed severe hemodynamic abnormalities, values for cardiac output and left ventricular filling pressure provided little independent prognostic information.[11,12]

Fig. 12-4. Relation of central hemodynamic variables and survival in congestive heart failure. (Adapted from BM Massie, T Ports, K Chatterjee, et al, Long-term vasodilator therapy for heart failure: Clinical response and its relationship to hemodynamic measurements, *Circulation* 1981;63:269-278, by permission of the American Heart Association, Inc.)

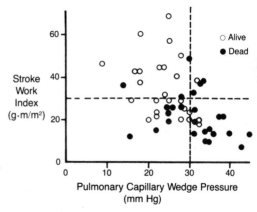

Can we then conclude that invasive hemodynamic measurements should not be used to predict mortality in such severely ill patients? Hemodynamic measurements performed *at rest* may tell us little about the ability of the myocardium to respond to circulatory stress. If such hemodynamic variables were assessed during exercise, however, such information might prove more useful, but no study has yet investigated the relation between exercise hemodynamics and survival in chronic heart failure. Alternatively, if we could measure the ability of the heart to respond favorably to a positive inotropic stimulus or to show deleterious effects following the administration of a negative inotropic agent, such information could prove to be more valuable in predicting long-term outcome than hemodynamic measurements during unstressed conditions.[27,36] For example, in 63 patients with severe heart failure, Tan showed that hemodynamic variables assessed during the infusion of dobutamine were a better predictor of mortality than these same hemodynamic variables measured in the absence of the inotropic stimulus.[27] Similarly, in 29 patients with severe heart failure, we showed that the change in hemodynamic variables noted following the short-term administration of the cardiodepressant drug nifedipine was an accurate predictor of long-term prognosis.[36] Patients who showed a negative inotropic effect with nifedipine had a worse long-term outcome than patients who tolerated the drug well. This pharmacologic challenge provided more powerful predictive information concerning the risk of subsequent death than the hemodynamic state at rest.

Ventricular Arrhythmias
As left ventricular performance deteriorates in patients with congestive heart failure, ventricular arrhythmias become an increasingly frequent occurrence. As the left ventricular ejection fraction declines to less than 30% and symptoms become resistant to medical therapy, frequent and complex ventricular ectopic beats are found in 80% to 95% of patients with heart failure; 40% to 60% of these patients have nonsustained ventricular tachycardia (Table 12-I).[9,11,25,37-46] Because sudden death occurs so frequently in patients with heart failure, we might surmise that patients with the most frequent or most serious arrhythmias are at greatest risk of a fatal arrhythmia. Unfortunately, this does not seem to be the case. The finding of a malignant ventricular arrhythmia during ambulatory monitoring is a strong predictor of *total* mortality, but it does not presage which patients will die suddenly (Table 12-I).[9,11,19,25,30,37-46] Furthermore, neither ventricular stimulation during invasive electrophysiologic testing nor the finding of late diastolic potentials on signal-averaged electrocardiograms provides additional discriminant information in predicting sudden death.[9,44,47,48] Hence, complex ventricular arrhythmias may be more a reflection of the severity of hemodynamic and functional abnormalities than a specific pathophysiologic event. This concept may explain why antiarrhythmic drug therapy may suppress ventricular arrhythmias but may not prolong life in these severely ill patients[43,45,49]; however, this issue remains a source of considerable controversy.[46,50]

Neurohormonal Variables
The sympathetic nervous system is activated in patients with congestive heart failure in proportion to the clinical severity of their illness.[51,52] Thus it is not surprising that there is a relation between plasma norepinephrine and survival in this disorder.[28,53] As with other factors discussed above, the prognostic importance of this measurement appears to depend

Table 12-1. Ventricular arrhythmias in congestive heart failure

Study*	Number of Patients	% Mortality/ Avg Follow-up (months)	% Patients with VT	Relation of VT to Total Mortality	Relation of VT to Sudden Death
Huang et al[40]	35	11/34	60	No	No
Constanzo-Nordin et al[41]	55	16/14	40	No	No
von Olshausen et al[39]	60	12/12	42	Yes	No
Neri et al[45]	62	29/30	47	—	—
Meinertz et al[44]	42	17/16	36	Yes	No
Meinertz et al[37]	74	26/11	49	Yes	Yes
Unverferth et al[25]	69	35/12	41	Yes	—
Chakko et al[43]	43	37/16	48	Yes	No
Holmes et al[38]	31	45/14	39	Yes	No
Dargie et al[46]	84	58/31	61	Yes	—
Baim et al[30]	100	63/12	59	Yes	No
Wilson et al[11]	77	65/12	51	Yes	No
Maskin et al[42]	35	71/?	71	—	—

*Studies listed in order of increasing severity of heart failure.
Avg = average; VT = ventricular tachycardia.

on the patient cohort being studied. In patients with mild to moderate heart failure, plasma catecholamines seem to reflect the evolution of hemodynamic and functional abnormalities, and hence provide much of the same prognostic information as the assessment of left ventricular ejection fraction or exercise tolerance.[54] On the other hand, in the patient with severe chronic heart failure (in whom conventional hemodynamic variables may no longer be an accurate estimate of the severity of the underlying disease process), plasma norepinephrine appears to accurately predict long-term mortality (Fig. 12-5).[28,53]

Similarly, the renin-angiotensin system is activated in patients with congestive heart failure in proportion to the clinical severity of the disease, and hence there is a relation between plasma renin activity and mortality in this disorder.[55] Insofar as an inverse relationship exists between plasma renin activity and serum sodium concentration in these patients,[56-59] it is expected that there would be a relation between serum sodium concen-

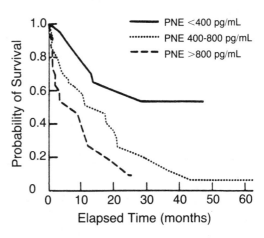

Fig. 12-5. Relation of plasma catecholamines (plasma norepinephrine, PNE) and survival in congestive heart failure. (Adapted from Cohn et al.[53] Reprinted, by permission of *The New England Journal of Medicine*, 311;819-823, 1984.)

survival in this disorder.[12,53] As in the case of plasma catecholamines, he prognostic importance of this measurement depends on the hort being studied. In patients with mild to moderate heart failure, yponatremia is uncommon, assessment of the activity of the renin-in system is unlikely to provide useful prognostic information. On ιιе ω.... hand, in patients with severe heart failure in whom hyponatremia is a common occurrence, serum sodium concentration is a powerful predictor of long-term outcome.[12]

In 142 patients with severe (class IV) chronic heart failure whom we treated with direct-acting vasodilator drugs, five variables were found to contribute independently to the prediction of survival: serum sodium concentration, serum bilirubin, serum creatinine concentration, age, and left ventricular stroke work index.[60] Among these five variables, serum sodium concentration was the most powerful predictor of long-term prognosis (Fig. 12-6). When patients were divided into three groups based on their pretreatment serum sodium concentration, patients with a normal serum sodium concentration (> 137 mEq/L) fared significantly better than did patients with mild hyponatremia (133 to 137 mEq/L) or patients with moderate to severe hyponatremia (< 133 mEq/L). Further analysis showed that the patients whose serum sodium concentration ranged from 138 to 140 mEq/L fared similarly to the patients with a serum sodium concentration greater than 140 mEq/L. This observation confirms our hypothesis that serum sodium concentration is unlikely to be of prognostic significance in a cohort consisting only of those patients with normal values for this variable (ie, those with mild to moderate heart failure).

Fig. 12-6. Relation of serum sodium concentration and survival in congestive heart failure. (Adapted from WH Lee, M Packer, Prognostic importance of serum sodium concentration and its modification by converting-enzyme inhibition in patients with severe chronic heart failure, *Circulation* 1986;73:257-267, by permission of the American Heart Association, Inc.)

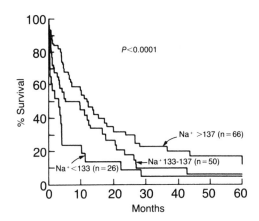

Conclusions   Based on the data cited above, we can conclude that a number of hemodynamic, structural, functional, and neurohormonal variables can predict survival in patients with chronic heart failure. The predictive value for each variable, however, depends largely on the patient cohort being examined. In patients with mild to moderate heart failure who demonstrate a wide range of abnormalities of left ventricular function, the measurement of left ventricular systolic performance (by invasive or noninvasive measures)

is likely to provide the most powerful prognostic information. In contrast, in patients with severe heart failure with symptoms at rest or upon minimal exertion, the measurement of neurohormonal variables (plasma catecholamines and serum sodium concentration), ventricular arrhythmias, and right ventricular function will be the most useful in predicting long-term outcome. These observations suggest that different variables should be utilized at different stages in the disease process in order to gauge its severity and to measure its progression.

EFFECT OF TREATMENT ON MORTALITY   Having elucidated the primary determinants of survival in chronic heart failure, we should ask the following questions: Does modification of these prognostic factors alter the long-term outcome of these severely ill patients? Does an improvement of symptoms and functional capacity lead to a prolongation of life? Are efforts directed at increasing the left ventricular ejection fraction and improving the hemodynamic state associated with a favorable impact on mortality? Unfortunately, most of the interventions that have been developed for the treatment of heart failure do not *selectively* address these determinant factors. Rather, they act to simultaneously modify several factors. Occasionally, drug treatment may favorably influence some factors, while adversely affecting others.

Digitalis   Although the role of digitalis in the treatment of heart failure has been controversial, the preliminary analyses of two large multicenter placebo-controlled trials indicate that digitalis therapy improves symptoms, enhances exercise tolerance, and increases left ventricular performance in patients with chronic heart failure.[61,62] Is this improvement in symptoms and ejection fraction associated with prolonged survival? Neither of the two multicenter trials was large enough to detect any impact of digitalis therapy on mortality, but both studies showed that treatment with digitalis was associated with a slight but significant increase in the frequency and complexity of ventricular arrhythmias on ambulatory electrocardiographic monitoring, even in the presence of nontoxic serum concentrations of the drug. This finding underscores concerns that digitalis may adversely affect the survival of patients with congestive heart failure who have experienced a recent myocardial infarction.

     In retrospective analyses of data collected during large-scale intervention trials in patients recovering from an acute myocardial infarction, patients treated with digitalis experienced a higher mortality than those not treated with the drug.[63-68] However, none of these studies was designed to specifically examine the impact of digitalis on survival, and patients were not randomly assigned to treatment with the drug but were selected for therapy by their primary physicians based on the usual clinical indications.[67] Accordingly, patients treated with digitalis were older, had a more frequent history of prior infarction, had more frequent cardiomegaly and cardiac arrhythmias, had worse left ventricular function, and were more frequently given diuretics and antiarrhythmic drugs than patients who did not receive the drug.[69] To what extent was the excess mortality seen in patients treated with digitalis the result of conditions that led physicians to prescribe the drug? In five of the six studies, the mortality in digitalis-treated patients no longer appeared to be enhanced, once attempts were made to correct for baseline differences in pretreatment variables between the treatment groups. One study,[63] however, noted a persistent excess mortality in a retrospectively defined subset of patients with congestive heart failure and complex ventricular arrhythmias, and all studies noted a persistent trend toward enhanced mortality, even when baseline differences were considered. When the data from four of these studies were pooled, Bigger et al[66] concluded that there was a persistent risk associated with digitalis use that could not be explained by baseline differences between the treatment groups.

Despite these concerns, we cannot conclude that digitalis exerts a detrimental effect on the mortality of patients with congestive heart failure. The statistical techniques used to correct for baseline differences among treatment groups in the six multicenter trials cited above assume that all factors that determine mortality are known and can be accounted for in evaluating the interaction of treatment and mortality.[69] Unfortunately, these patients were incompletely characterized; in many cases, left ventricular function was not assessed and coronary anatomy remained undefined. Because these variables are unknown and cannot be incorporated into a statistical model, they may contribute to observed differences in mortality that may otherwise be ascribed to an effect of treatment. This is especially true if these unrecorded variables were apparent to the prescribing physician and thus influenced his or her decision to administer digitalis.

The influence of digitalis on the survival of patients with chronic heart failure can be assessed only by randomly assigning therapy with the drug to patients in whom there is no clear therapeutic mandate for the drug (ie, those without atrial tachyarrhythmias). The National Institutes of Health is presently considering such a trial, yet such a study may be extremely difficult to carry out once it becomes clear that digitalis is of benefit in patients with normal sinus rhythm. The true impact of digitalis on the survival of patients with chronic heart failure may never be known.

Diuretics   Because diuretics have become indispensable for the treatment of fluid retention in patients with chronic heart failure, there have been no large-scale placebo-controlled trials to evaluate the impact of this class of drugs on symptoms or survival in patients with heart failure. The limited data from objectively performed studies confirm the widespread clinical impression that diuretics improve symptoms and prolong exercise tolerance in patients with the disease.[70-72] Short-term therapy with these drugs is associated with amelioration of many of the hemodynamic and neurohormonal abnormalities seen in patients with heart failure,[72,73] but vigorous intravenous or long-term oral therapy may be associated with neurohormonal activation and depletion of intracellular electrolytes (potassium and magnesium).[72-76] Diuretics deplete potassium and magnesium by promoting the renal excretion of these cations; such excretion is potentiated by diuretic-induced hyperaldosteronism and metabolic alkalosis.[77-79] The high circulating levels of catecholamines in patients with chronic heart failure may exacerbate the occurrence and severity of hypokalemia (by enhancing the movement of potassium into cells by a β_2-receptor-mediated mechanism) and may directly potentiate the arrhythmogenic effects of the hypokalemic state.[80-83] This proarrhythmic interaction between serum potassium concentration and circulating catecholamines (Fig. 12-7) has been convincingly demonstrated in diuretic-treated patients suffering from an acute myocardial infarction.[84-86]

Can the electrolyte deficits caused by diuretic therapy be detrimental to the survival of patients with chronic heart failure? This question cannot be answered with certainty, but we do know that electrolyte deficits may provoke or exacerbate the occurrence of malignant (and fatal) ventricular arrhythmias in these patients,[87] and this may occur as a result of a number of interactive mechanisms. Hypokalemia may directly predispose patients with heart failure to lethal ventricular arrhythmias,[88,89] it may potentiate the arrhythmias secondary to digitalis and catecholamines,[90] it may interfere with the efficacy of antiarrhythmic drugs,[91] and it may enhance the proarrhythmic potential of antiarrhythmic drug therapy.[92] Magnesium depletion may exacerbate ventricular arrhythmias by similar pathogenetic mechanisms.[93-95]

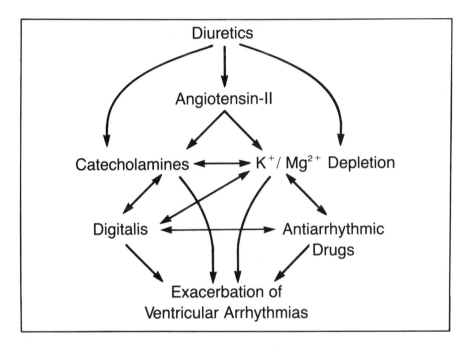

Fig. 12-7. Mechanisms of diuretic-induced ventricular arrhythmias in congestive heart failure. (Adapted from M Packer, SS Gottlieb, PD Kessler, *Am J Med* 1986;80[suppl 4A]:23-29.)

Can ventricular arrhythmias in patients with congestive heart failure be treated by interventions that restore normal levels of electrolytes? Several clinical studies have shown that in patients with arrhythmias associated with hypokalemia and hypomagnesemia, administration of potassium and magnesium salts reduces the frequency and complexity of these rhythm disturbances and prevents the subsequent occurrence of sudden death without long-term antiarrhythmic drug therapy.[87,96,97] The therapeutic approach is more complicated, however, when potassium and magnesium deficits coexist, as is so commonly the case. Under such circumstances, repletion of magnesium appears to be critical to the success of treatment. Administration of potassium salts alone frequently fails to restore normal circulating levels of potassium or normal sinus rhythm, whereas magnesium therapy corrects the hypomagnesemia *and* the hypokalemia as well as the accompanying tachyarrhythmias.[97,98] Once corrected, combined electrolyte deficits are best prevented by the use of potassium-sparing diuretics and by converting-enzyme inhibitors, which not only replete potassium but act to preserve magnesium as well.[99-101]

Diuretics may also provoke the occurrence of ventricular arrhythmias in patients with heart failure by increasing the activity of the renin-angiotensin system. Angiotensin-II may exacerbate electrolyte-related ventricular ectopy by promoting aldosterone-mediated losses of potassium and magnesium by the kidney[77,79] or may be directly proarrhythmic through its ability to potentiate the central and peripheral actions of the sympathetic nervous system.[102,103] This may explain why in three double-blind, placebo-controlled trials of diuretic-treated patients with heart failure, treatment with converting-enzyme inhibitors reduced the frequency and complexity of ventricular arrhythmias, and this improvement was associated with an increase in total body and circulating levels of potassium and a decrease in circulating catecholamines.[104-106] Of the two factors identified in these studies, the restoration of normal potassium homeostasis appeared to be the more important, because the rise in serum potassium concentration correlated better with the reduction in ventricular arrhythmias.[107] This concept is consistent with the data of Cleland et al, who showed that the greatest depletion of potassium was seen in patients whose heart failure was accompanied by the highest circulating levels of angiotensin-II.[106-108] Accordingly, the most pronounced antiarrhythmic effects of converting-enzyme inhibition were seen in diuretic-treated patients with the highest plasma renin activity.[106,107]

Catecholamines Short-term therapy with intravenous or oral catecholamines produces marked hemodynamic and clinical improvement in patients with chronic heart failure[109-112]; therefore we might be encouraged to consider these agents as a means of prolonging life in patients with chronic heart failure. Because the myocardium becomes depleted of catecholamines as the heart failure state progresses,[113] it is possible that such depletion contributes to the progressive loss of contractile function that occurs over time. If this is true, catecholamine therapy might retard progression of the underlying disease. Unfortunately, long-term treatment with β-receptor agonists has not produced sustained hemodynamic and clinical benefits in patients with heart failure,[114-116] in part because prolonged exposure to these drugs results in a decrease in the density of active β-receptors ("down regulation") and loss of the drugs' hemodynamic and clinical efficacy.[117-119] In addition, long-term therapy with catecholamines may exacerbate myocardial ischemia and ventricular arrhythmias.[120]

Should these results raise concerns about a deleterious effect of oral or intravenous catecholamines on the survival of patients with chronic heart failure? Three lines of circumstantial evidence underscore this concern. First, a single long-term follow-up study reported a disturbing 32% mortality after three months in 63 patients treated with the oral β-agonist pirbuterol[121]; this event rate was considerably higher than that expected in this patient population. Second, trials with a number of oral and intravenous β-agonists have been halted, in part because of reports of worsening arrhythmias during treatment with these drugs.[112,122,123] Third, the benefits of β-blockers in patients with an acute myocardial infarction (especially with a history of congestive heart failure) appear to be lost when β-agonist properties are incorporated into the pharmacologic profile of the drug.[124] In fact, when patients with a remote myocardial infarction receive long-term treatment with β-blockers with intrinsic sympathomimetic activity, their mortality appears to be increased when compared with a control group treated with placebo.[125]

Can we conclude from these reports that catecholamines are directly detrimental to the survival of patients with congestive heart failure? As in the case of digitalis, we cannot be certain about the influence of these drugs on mortality in the absence of a randomized, placebo-controlled trial specifically designed to address this question. It is therefore noteworthy that such a placebo-controlled trial has recently been completed in the United States.[126] Sixty patients with severe (class IV) chronic heart failure were randomly assigned to treatment with intermittent dobutamine or placebo: 31 patients received dobutamine intravenously (48 h/wk), and 29 patients received a weekly infusion of placebo. The trial was halted prematurely when 15 of the 20 deaths that occurred in the study were seen in patients assigned to or crossed over to treatment with dobutamine. These findings are of particular interest in view of the unfavorable prognosis associated with high circulating levels of catecholamines when these are observed to occur spontaneously in patients with chronic heart failure.[53]

Phospho-diesterase Inhibitors
A third class of positive inotropic agent, the phosphodiesterase inhibitor, has undergone extensive clinical evaluation during the last nine years. These agents include amrinone, milrinone, enoximone, piroximone, and CI-914.

All of these agents produce both positive inotropic and systemic vasodilator effects by their ability to increase intracellular cyclic adenosine monophosphate (AMP) (by inhibiting its degradation).[127] As such, these agents share a similar biochemical mechanism of action with the catecholamines, which also increase intracellular cyclic AMP (by stimulating its synthesis).

Should we then be concerned about a potential detrimental effect of these drugs on survival, just as we were with the oral and intravenous catecholamines? There may be many reasons to be concerned about a detrimental effect on survival following the use of drugs that increase the inotropic state of the myocardium by increasing intracellular cyclic AMP. Insofar as the decrease in contractility seen in heart failure is a compensatory mechanism that acts to lower energy utilization by the failing heart,[128] any drug-induced augmentation of the inotropic state could increase myocardial energy consumption and accelerate the death of the myocardial cell. This acceleration may be particularly likely to occur in patients with coronary artery disease, in whom the balance between energy production and energy consumption is precarious. There is special concern about agents that increase the inotropic state by increasing intracellular cyclic AMP. This nucleotide may be directly toxic to myocardial cells by setting into motion a number of energy-consuming reactions that lead to an increase in cytosolic calcium; such toxicity may be enhanced by agents that stimulate cyclic AMP synthesis (such as catecholamines) or retard its degradation (such as phosphodiesterase inhibitors).[129-131] Reports of accelerated progression of disease and provocation of ventricular tachyarrhythmias have appeared from uncontrolled trials in patients with chronic heart failure treated with amrinone and milrinone.[132-137]

Have these concerns (raised on the basis of theoretical considerations) been confirmed in patients with chronic heart failure treated with phosphodiesterase inhibitors? Uncontrolled studies in 301 patients with heart failure treated with amrinone, milrinone, enoximone, piroximone, and CI-914 have reported a very high one-year mortality rate (approximately 74%).[30,120,134-146] This mortality rate appears to be higher than similarly uncontrolled data from follow-up studies of patients treated with oral vasodilators (captopril, hydralazine, nitrates, and prazosin), in which the observed one-year mortality rate is only 45%.[120] Yet we cannot reach any conclusions from a direct comparison of mortality rates, because we cannot be certain that patients entered into the vasodilator trials were comparable to those treated with positive inotropic agents. Even though both groups of patients had severe symptoms (class IV) and severe hemodynamic abnormalities before treatment, and both groups had been unresponsive to previous therapy with available inotropic and vasodilator drugs, the two groups may still differ in several significant respects. The dilemma here is not dissimilar to that discussed earlier in this chapter with respect to the effect of digitalis on mortality. It is possible that unmeasured variables were present before therapy in patients treated with positive inotropic agents that contributed significantly both to the decision to refer such patients for therapy and to their extremely poor prognosis.

These questions about the effect of phosphodiesterase inhibitors on mortality in chronic heart failure cannot be resolved without a prospectively designed double-blind, placebo-controlled trial. The single published trial for which data are available (a three-month multicenter study) did not observe a higher mortality rate in patients treated with amrinone than in patients treated with placebo.[147] Yet this trial also did not demonstrate that amrinone was effective in the treatment of congestive heart failure, possibly because patients could not be treated with therapeutic doses of the study drug because of severe drug toxicity. This study leads us to conclude that subtherapeutic doses of amrinone do not exert an adverse effect on survival, but it provides little information about the potential impact of therapeutically effective doses of phosphodiesterase inhibitors on long-term prognosis. A more recently completed (and as yet unpublished) multicenter placebo-controlled trial, however, did demonstrate that patients treated with another phosphodiesterase inhibitor, CI-914, had a significantly higher mortality than patients treated with placebo. Because of this finding, CI-914 has been withdrawn from further clinical investigation by its manufacturer.

Direct-Acting Vasodilators

Direct-acting vasodilators (hydralazine, isosorbide dinitrate, and minoxidil) and the α-adrenergic antagonists (prazosin and trimazosin) were the first oral vasodilators used to improve left ventricular performance in patients with chronic heart failure, and thus were considered ideal candidates for a trial to test the impact of vasodilator therapy on the survival of patients with chronic heart failure.[148] Enthusiasm for these drugs waned, however, when it became clear that most were unable to improve the clinical status of patients with chronic heart failure when administered for long periods of time.[1]

Treatment with hydralazine was complicated by an unpredictable hemodynamic response and a high frequency of adverse reactions,[149,150] minoxidil therapy was associated with severe fluid retention and tachycardia,[151] and the administration of prazosin and trimazosin was frequently accompanied by loss of hemodynamic and clinical efficacy during long-term treatment.[152,153] For these reasons, none of these drugs proved to be superior to placebo therapy in double-blind, controlled clinical trials.[1,151,154,155] The only direct-acting vasodilator drug that was shown to be effective in the symptomatic treatment of chronic heart failure was isosorbide dinitrate,[156,157] but therapy with this agent was complicated by the need for frequent daily dosing and the potential for pharmacologic tolerance to its hemodynamic and clinical effects.[158,159] Because of these disappointing results, many investigators no longer expected that direct-acting vasodilator drugs could favorably influence the long-term survival of patients with chronic heart failure.

Nevertheless, the Veterans Administration Cooperative Study on Vasodilator Therapy of Heart Failure (V-HeFT) did demonstrate (in a large-scale multicenter placebo-controlled trial) that some direct-acting vasodilators can reduce mortality in patients with chronic heart failure (Fig. 12-8).[15] A total of 642 ambulatory middle-aged men with mild to moderate failure were enrolled in 11 participating hospitals; all patients had cardiac enlargement or left ventricular dysfunction and reduced exercise capacity. Of these patients, 273 patients were randomly assigned to receive placebo in addition to digitalis and diuretics; 186 were assigned to a combination of hydralazine and isosorbide dinitrate (300 mg and 160 mg daily, respectively); and 183 were assigned to treatment with prazosin (20 mg daily). At the end of 0.5 to 5.7 years of follow-up (mean 2.3 years), 44% of the placebo group, 39% of the hydralazine-nitrate group, and 50% of the prazosin group had died. Based on the Cox life-table regression model, there was a 28% reduction in mortality risk in the hydralazine-nitrate group compared with the placebo group, whereas there was no reduction in mortality in the prazosin group. The benefits of hydralazine-nitrate were apparent in all subgroups of patients in the study and were not influenced by prerandomization variables.[160] The study did not attempt to distinguish between sudden death and death secondary to congestive heart failure.

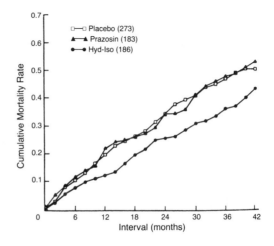

Fig. 12-8. Influence of direct-acting vasodilator drugs on mortality in congestive heart failure: the Veterans Administration Cooperative Study on Vasodilator Therapy of Heart Failure. (Hyd-Iso = hydralazine and isosorbide dinitrate.) (From Cohn et al.[15] Reprinted, by permission of *The New England Journal of Medicine*, 314;1547-1552, 1986.)

How did the combination of hydralazine and isosorbide dinitrate improve survival in these patients with mild to moderate heart failure? Additional analyses indicated that an improved survival was closely related to an improved left ventricular ejection fraction in this study[161]; this was seen more frequently in patients treated with hydralazine and nitrates than in patients treated with placebo. Yet, despite a persistent reduction in systemic blood pressure, left ventricular performance and long-term survival were not improved by prazosin, presumably because its vasodilator effects were not accompanied by a favorable change in left ventricular function.[15,153] We cannot conclude from these results, however, that the left ventricular ejection fraction can be used as a surrogate endpoint for mortality in patients with chronic heart failure, because a variety of interventions such as minoxidil and dobutamine may increase left ventricular ejection fraction but adversely affect long-term outcome.[126,151]

Unfortunately, the combination of hydralazine and isosorbide dinitrate was not well tolerated in this multicenter trial. More patients required the withdrawal of either hydralazine or nitrate therapy (or both) than required the discontinuation of placebo (38% vs 22%); in addition, there was no evidence presented that the hydralazine-nitrate combination ameliorated the symptoms of patients with heart failure or enhanced their exercise capacity.[162] Although converting-enzyme inhibitors appear to be better tolerated than direct-acting vasodilators and consistently improve the clinical state of treated patients,[1,163] the impact of converting-enzyme inhibitors on mortality was not examined in the Veterans Administration study. A direct comparison of hydralazine-nitrate and a converting-enzyme inhibitor (enalapril) is now being carried out in a second Veterans Administration trial in a similar patient population (V-HeFT-II).[15,160]

Converting-Enzyme Inhibitors

Because converting-enzyme inhibitors produce consistent short- and long-term hemodynamic and clinical benefits in chronic heart failure, there has been enormous interest in the possibility that these drugs can prolong life in patients with this disease, especially in view of the reduction in mortality noted with a combination of hydralazine and isosorbide dinitrate in the Veterans Administration trial.

Preliminary evidence that converting-enzyme inhibitors may enhance survival in congestive heart failure was first derived from studies of their use in experimental models of the disease. In dogs with tachycardia-induced heart failure, captopril attenuated the progressive increase in systemic vascular resistance that was noted to accompany the onset of left ventricular dysfunction.[164] In rats with left ventricular dysfunction induced by an experimental myocardial infarction, captopril reduced the progressive increase in left ventricular dimensions and diastolic pressures that followed the initial insult to the myocardium, and prolonged survival; this appeared to be particularly true in rats with moderate-sized infarcts.[165,166] Finally, captopril reduced the frequency of ventricular arrhythmias induced by experimental coronary reperfusion, in part because of the drug's ability to decrease the outpouring of myocardial catecholamines that accompanied the arrhythmogenic state.[103]

These encouraging experimental data were subsequently supported by clinical reports of improved survival in patients enrolled in long-term vasodilator studies. After pooling the short-term mortality data from prospectively conducted double-blind placebo-controlled trials, Furberg and Yusuf[167] concluded that only converting-enzyme inhibitors seemed to reduce the mortality of patients with severe chronic heart failure; no favorable trend was apparent in trials using direct-acting vasodilator drugs (but this analysis was performed before the release of the V-HeFT results). In a retrospective analysis of patients treated with a variety of vasodilator interventions, Lee and I[12] observed a significant interaction between activation of the renin-angiotensin system, serum sodium concentration, and mortality in patients with congestive heart failure. Patients with hyponatremia had the most marked activation of the renin-angiotensin system and the highest cardiovascular mortality—a fact that could not be explained by the degree of left ventricular dysfunction. Was their poor prognosis related then to activation of the renin-angiotensin system? When hyponatremic patients were treated with converting-enzyme inhibitors, serum sodium concentration increased towards normal values,[168] and the mortality rate in these patients was reduced to that expected in patients without activation of the renin-angiotensin system.[12] In contrast, there appeared to be no selective benefit on survival (when compared with direct-acting vasodilators) when converting-enzyme inhibitors were administered to patients with a normal serum sodium concentration, who did not show marked increases in plasma renin activity. These data suggested a deleterious role for angiotensin-II in the long-term outcome of patients with chronic heart failure—a role that could be neutralized by treatment with converting-enzyme inhibitors.

Definitive evidence to support a favorable effect of converting-enzyme inhibitors on the survival of patients with chronic heart failure was finally forthcoming with the publication of the Cooperative North Scandinavian Enalapril Survival Study (CONSENSUS).[169] This trial randomly assigned 253 elderly men and women with severe (class IV) heart failure to treatment with a converting-enzyme inhibitor (enalapril, target dose 20 to 40 mg daily) or placebo, in addition to treatment with digitalis, diuretics, and direct-acting vasodilators. Treatment with enalapril reduced mortality by 31% at the end of one year (Fig. 12-9). It is noteworthy that this favorable effect on mortality was associated with correction of the hyponatremic state and was observed even in patients treated with direct-acting vasodilators; this observation confirms the predictions Lee and I made in our retrospective analysis.[12,162] Furthermore, unlike V-HeFT, the beneficial effect of therapy on survival in CONSENSUS was associated with substantial clinical improvement,[169] even though symptomatic hypotension, renal insufficiency, and potassium retention occurred more frequently in patients treated with enalapril than those treated with placebo.[162]

Can the result of the CONSENSUS trial be extrapolated to all patients with chronic heart failure? In some ways, the patient cohort studied in the CONSENSUS trial was unusual. These patients were older (mean age 71), had higher systemic blood pressures, and had a higher incidence of atrial fibrillation than patients enrolled in previous heart failure studies.[169] Moreover, all patients in CONSENSUS had class IV symptoms; the vast majority of patients with chronic heart failure (who are ambulatory) were not entered into this trial. It is therefore reassuring that the results of CONSENSUS have been confirmed in a second multicenter trial of 105 patients with moderately severe chronic heart failure (functional class II or

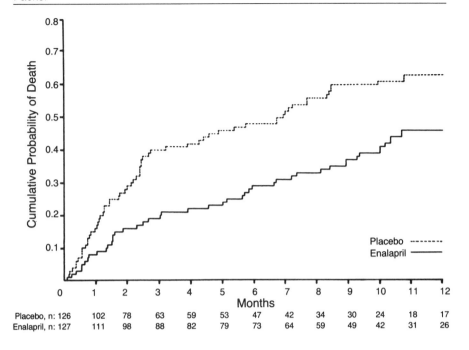

Fig. 12-9. Influence of converting-enzyme inhibition with enalapril on mortality in severe chronic congestive heart failure: the CONSENSUS Trial. (Adapted from the CONSENSUS Trial Study Group.[169] Reprinted, by permission of *The New England Journal of Medicine*, 316;1429-1435, 1987.)

III) who participated in a three-month double-blind comparison of captopril (300 mg daily) and placebo (Captopril Multicenter Heart Failure Trial).[170,171] During the trial, 11 of 52 patients (21%) assigned to placebo died, compared with only 2 of 53 patients (4%) assigned to treatment with captopril ($P < 0.01$; Fig. 12-10). This study also demonstrated a favorable effect of captopril in ameliorating the symptoms and increasing the exercise capacity of patients with chronic heart failure. The preliminary results from two other randomized clinical trials[172,173] provide further support for the concept that converting-enzyme inhibition improves the long-term outcome of patients with chronic heart failure.

How do converting-enzyme inhibitors exert their favorable effects on mortality in chronic heart failure? The mortality reduction noted in the CONSENSUS trial was attributed entirely to a reduction in death from progressive heart failure[169]; the investigators could not discern any decrease in the incidence of sudden death in these patients. Although the determination of the cause of death was made prospectively, it is difficult to determine how the CONSENSUS investigators could reach this conclusion with confidence. As noted earlier in this chapter, it is very difficult to determine the mode of death in patients with class IV heart failure.[10] All death is sudden; therefore, the traditional classification of mortality relies heavily on the symptomatic status of the patient immediately prior to his or her demise. In a patient with symptoms of dyspnea at rest, all death will be considered to be secondary to progressive congestive heart failure. A mortal event may be classified as

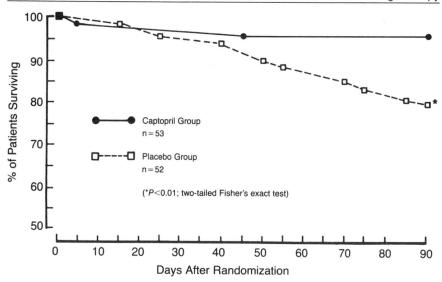

Fig. 12-10. Influence of converting-enzyme inhibition (with captopril) on mortality in moderately severe chronic congestive heart failure: the Captopril Multicenter Heart Failure Trial. (Adapted from Dennick et al,[171] based on reanalysis of results of a study reported by Captopril Multicenter Research Group.[170] Reprinted, by permission of *The New England Journal of Medicine* 317;1350, 1987.)

sudden only if the highly symptomatic patient improves during therapy and remains clinically improved at the time of death. Because converting-enzyme inhibition produced symptomatic improvement more frequently than placebo therapy,[169,170] deaths among those treated with enalapril would be more likely to be classified as sudden deaths (when compared with placebo), regardless of the true pathogenesis of these events. The uncertainty of the findings of CONSENSUS (with respect to the mode of death) is underscored by the mode of death in the Captopril Multicenter Heart Failure Trial, in which eight patients died suddenly during placebo administration, whereas only one patient died suddenly while taking captopril (ie, the improvement in survival was primarily related to a reduction in sudden death and not death from progressive heart failure). Given this confusion, it is not surprising that the V-HeFT investigators did not classify the mode of death in their study.[15]

Can these beneficial effects of converting-enzyme inhibition on mortality be extrapolated to patients with asymptomatic left ventricular dysfunction? This exciting possibility is now the focus of two separate studies. The prevention arm of the SOLVD trial (Studies of Left Ventricular Dysfunction), sponsored by the National Institutes of Health, will evaluate the impact of converting-enzyme inhibition (with enalapril) on mortality in 4,600 patients with a left ventricular ejection fraction less than 35% but without symptoms of heart failure.[148] The SAVE trial (Survival and Ventricular Enlargement) will examine the effect of converting-enzyme inhibition (with captopril) on mortality in 4,000 minimally symptomatic patients who have recently experienced an acute myocardial infarction and who have a left ventricular ejection fraction less than 40%.[174] Both studies are expected to be completed and analyzed by 1991.

β-Adrenergic Blocking Drugs

If neurohormonal activation is detrimental to survival in chronic heart failure, we might expect that neurohormonal antagonists other than converting-enzyme inhibitors might exert favorable effects on long-term outcome in these patients. The results of controlled and uncontrolled trials suggest that long-term β-blockade improves exercise capacity and left ventricular ejection fraction in patients with an idiopathic dilated cardiomyopathy.[175-178] Of note, the most marked improvement during β-blockade has been observed in patients with the most advanced heart failure (ie, lowest left ventricular ejection fraction and highest heart rates) before therapy,[175] who presumably had the most markedly increased levels of plasma catecholamines.

Do these elevated levels of catecholamines increase the mortality of patients with chronic heart failure? No definitive data are available to adequately address this question, but two clinical studies of β-blockers in patients with an idiopathic dilated cardiomyopathy suggest that this may be the case. Swedberg et al[179] treated 24 patients with congestive heart failure with metoprolol and compared their long-term outcome with 13 matched historical control subjects; survival at one and two years was 83% and 69%, respectively, in the treated group, compared with 49% and 19% in the control group ($P < 0.01$). Anderson et al[180] randomly assigned 50 patients to treatment with metoprolol (in addition to standard therapy) or to standard therapy alone. By intention to treat, no difference was noted between the two groups during long-term follow-up; by actual treatment received, however, a favorable trend ($P = 0.12$) was noted after 24 months in metoprolol-treated patients.

Further support for a beneficial effect of β-blockade on the survival of patients with congestive heart failure comes from the subanalyses of the long-term outcome of patients with ischemic heart disease who were enrolled into randomized clinical trials of β-blockers shortly after an acute myocardial infarction. A number of large-scale, long-term, double-blind, placebo-controlled trials have shown that β-blockers decrease the mortality rate of post-myocardial-infarction patients when initiated between one and three weeks after the event.[124] In the Beta Blocker Heart Attack Trial, this beneficial effect of β-blockade (with propranolol) was particularly noteworthy in patients with a history of congestive heart failure or whose index infarction was complicated by congestive heart failure.[181,182] The most remarkable therapeutic effect of propranolol in this high-risk cohort was a 47% reduction in the incidence of sudden death (compared with placebo-treated patients); in contrast, β-blockade produced no significant reduction in sudden death in randomized patients who did not have a history of congestive heart failure. Similar results have been noted in the subanalysis of other β-blocker trials.[183,184]

Definitive evidence that β-blockade prolongs life in patients with congestive heart failure awaits the completion of large-scale multicenter trials of patients randomly assigned to treatment with a β-blocker or placebo. One such study (Metoprolol in Dilated Cardiomyopathy) has already been initiated with an intent to enroll and randomly assign 520 patients with an idiopathic dilated cardiomyopathy to treatment with metoprolol or placebo. Other trials using other β-blockers are also being planned.

CONCLUSION Convincing data are now available that some drugs developed to treat the symptoms of patients with chronic congestive heart failure can also modify the natural history of the disorder. Because ventricular wall stress is an important factor that accelerates disease progression,[165] it is logical to assume that any agent that produces sustained amelioration of loading conditions in the left ventricle is potentially capable of prolonging life.[15] All presently available inotropic, diuretic, and vasodilator drugs can improve left ventricular performance, but the mechanisms by which such benefits are achieved differ substantially, and such differences may greatly modify the expected impact of treatment on long-term outcome. In this regard, pharmacologic interventions that improve left ventricular function by reducing neurohormonal activation may exert a more favorable long-term effect on survival than agents that increase (or mimic an increase in) neurohormonal activity.[162] If the latter effect is sufficiently marked, treatment could adversely affect morbidity and mortality. Confirmation of this hypothesis awaits the completion of ongoing randomized clinical trials.

REFERENCES

1. Packer M: Vasodilator and inotropic therapy for severe chronic heart failure: Passion and skepticism. *J Am Coll Cardiol* 1983;2:841-852.
2. Packer M: Prolonging life in patients with congestive heart failure: The next frontier. *Circulation* 1987;75(suppl 4):1-3.
3. Multiple Risk Factor Intervention Trial Research Group: Multiple risk factor intervention trial: Risk factor changes and mortality results. *JAMA* 1982;248:1465-1477.
4. McKee PA, Castelli WP, McNamara PM, et al: The natural history of congestive heart failure: The Framingham Study. *N Engl J Med* 1971;285:1441-1446.
5. Fuster V, Gersh BJ, Giuliani ER, et al: The natural history of idiopathic dilated cardiomyopathy. *Am J Cardiol* 1981;47:525-531.
6. Brushke AVG, Proudfit WL, Sones FM Jr: Progress study of 590 consecutive nonsurgical cases of coronary disease followed 5-9 years: II. Ventriculographic and other correlations. *Circulation* 1973;47:1154-1163.
7. Massie BM, Conway M: Survival of patients with congestive heart failure: Past, present, and future prospects. *Circulation* 1987;75(suppl 4):11-19.
8. White CW, Mirro MJ, Lund DD, et al: Alterations in ventricular excitability in conscious dogs during development of chronic heart failure. *Am J Cardiol* 1986;250:H1022-H1029.
9. Packer M: Sudden unexpected death in patients with congestive heart failure: A second frontier. *Circulation* 1985;72:681-685.
10. Bigger JT Jr: Why patients with congestive heart failure die: Arrhythmias and sudden cardiac death. *Circulation* 1987;75(suppl 4):29-35.
11. Wilson JR, Schwartz JS, St. John Sutton M, et al: Prognosis in severe heart failure: Relation to hemodynamic measurements and ventricular ectopic activity. *J Am Coll Cardiol* 1983;2:403-410.
12. Lee WH, Packer M: Prognostic importance of serum sodium concentration and its modification by converting-enzyme inhibition in patients with severe chronic heart failure. *Circulation* 1986;73:257-267.
13. Massie BM, Ports T, Chatterjee K, et al: Long-term vasodilator therapy for heart failure: Clinical response and its relationship to hemodynamic measurements. *Circulation* 1981;63:269-278.

14. Franciosa JA, Wilen M, Ziesche S, et al: Survival in men with severe chronic heart failure due to either coronary heart disease or idiopathic dilated cardiomyopathy. *Am J Cardiol* 1983;51:831-836.
15. Cohn JN, Archibald DG, Ziesche S, et al: Effect of vasodilator therapy on mortality in chronic congestive heart failure: Results of a Veterans Administration Cooperative Study. *N Engl J Med* 1986;314:1547-1552.
16. Likoff MJ, Chandler SL, Kay HR: Clinical determinants of mortality in chronic congestive heart failure secondary to idiopathic dilated or to ischemic cardiomyopathy. *Am J Cardiol* 1987;59:634-638.
17. Figulla HR, Rahlf G, Nieger M, et al: Spontaneous hemodynamic improvement or stabilization and associated biopsy findings in patients with congestive cardiomyopathy. *Circulation* 1985;71:1095-1104.
18. Califf RM, Bounous P, Harrell FE, et al: The prognosis in the presence of coronary artery disease, in Braunwald E, Mock MB, Watson JT (eds): *Congestive Heart Failure*. New York, Grune & Stratton, 1982, pp 31-40.
19. Glover DR, Littler WA: Factors influencing survival and mode of death in severe ischemic heart failure. *Br Heart J* 1987;57:125-132.
20. Szlachcic J, Massie BM, Kramer BL, et al: Correlates and prognostic implication of exercise capacity in chronic congestive heart failure. *Am J Cardiol* 1985;55:1037-1042.
21. Franciosa JA, Wilen MM, Baker BJ: Functional capacity and long-term survival in chronic left ventricular failure (abstract). *Circulation* 1983;69(suppl 3):149.
22. Franciosa JA: Why patients with heart failure die: Hemodynamic and functional determinants of survival. *Circulation* 1987;75(suppl 4):20-27.
23. Baker BJ, Leddy C, Galie N, et al: Predictive value of M-mode echocardiography in patients with congestive heart failure. *Am Heart J* 1986;111:697-702.
24. Taylor GJ, Humphries JO, Mellits ED, et al: Predictors of clinical course, coronary anatomy and left ventricular function after recovery from acute myocardial infarction. *Circulation* 1980;62:960-970.
25. Unverferth DV, Magorien DR, Moeschberger ML, et al: Factors influencing the one year mortality of dilated cardiomyopathy. *Am J Cardiol* 1984;54:147-152.
26. Schwartz F, Mall G, Zebe H, et al: Determinants of survival in congestive cardiomyopathy: Quantitative morphologic findings and left ventricular hemodynamics. *Circulation* 1984;70:923-928.
27. Tan LB: Cardiac pumping capability and prognosis in heart failure. *Lancet* 1986;2:1360-1363.
28. Creager MA, Faxon DP, Halperin JL, et al: Determinants of clinical response and survival in patients with congestive heart failure treated with captopril. *Am Heart J* 1982;104:1147-1154.
29. Polak JF, Holman L, Wynne J, et al: Right ventricular ejection fraction: An indicator of increased mortality in patients with congestive heart failure associated with coronary artery disease. *J Am Coll Cardiol* 1983;2:217-224.
30. Baim DS, Colucci WS, Monrad ES, et al: Survival of patients with severe congestive heart failure treated with oral milrinone. *J Am Coll Cardiol* 1986;7:661-670.
31. Lee WH, Packer M: Importance of right ventricular function as the primary determinant of clinical response and long-term survival in patients with severe heart failure treated with converting-enzyme inhibitors (abstract). *J Am Coll Cardiol* 1985;5:461.
32. Forrester J, Diamond G, Swan HJC: Correlative classification of clinical and hemodynamic function after myocardial infarction. *Am J Cardiol* 1977;39:137-145.
33. Hamby RI: Primary myocardial disease: A prospective clinical and hemodynamic evaluation in 100 patients. *Medicine* 1970;49:55-78.
34. Yatteau RF, Peter RH, Behar VS, et al: Ischemic cardiomyopathy: The myopathy of coronary artery disease. *Am J Cardiol* 1974;34:520-525.

35. Hatle L, Stake G, Storstein O: Chronic myocardial disease: II. Haemodynamic findings related to long-term prognosis. *Acta Med Scand* 1976;199:407-411.
36. Packer M, Lee WH, Medina N, et al: Prognostic importance of the immediate hemodynamic response to nifedipine in patients with severe left ventricular dysfunction. *J Am Coll Cardiol* 1987;10:1303-1311.
37. Meinertz T, Hofmann F, Kasper W, et al: Significance of ventricular arrhythmias in idiopathic dilated cardiomyopathy. *Am J Cardiol* 1984;53:902-907.
38. Holmes J, Kubo SH, Cody RJ, et al: Arrhythmias in ischemic and nonischemic dilated cardiomyopathy: Prediction of mortality by ambulatory electrocardiography. *Am J Cardiol* 1985;55:146-151.
39. von Olshausen K, Schafer A, Mehmel HC, et al: Ventricular arrhythmias in idiopathic dilated cardiomyopathy. *Br Heart J* 1984;51:195-201.
40. Huang SK, Messer JV, Denes P: Significance of ventricular arrhythmias in idiopathic dilated cardiomyopathy: Observations in 35 patients. *Am J Cardiol* 1983;51:507-512.
41. Constanzo-Nordin MR, O'Connell JB, Englemeier RS, et al: Dilated cardiomyopathy: Functional status, hemodynamics, arrhythmias, and prognosis. *Cathet Cardiovasc Diagn* 1985;11:445-453.
42. Maskin CS, Siskind SJ, LeJemtel TH: High prevalence of nonsustained ventricular tachycardia in severe congestive heart failure. *Am Heart J* 1984;107:896-901.
43. Chakko CS, Gheorghiade M: Ventricular arrhythmias in severe heart failure: Incidence, significance, and effectiveness of antiarrhythmic therapy. *Am Heart J* 1985;109:497-504.
44. Meinertz T, Tresse N, Kasper W, et al: Determinants of prognosis in idiopathic dilated cardiomyopathy as determined by programmed electrical stimulation. *Am J Cardiol* 1985;56:337-341.
45. Neri R, Mestroni L, Salvi A, et al: Ventricular arrhythmias in dilated cardiomyopathy: Efficacy of amiodarone. *Am Heart J* 1987;113:707-715.
46. Dargie HJ, Cleland JGF, Leckie BJ, et al: Relation of arrhythmias and electrolyte abnormalities to survival in patients with severe chronic heart failure. *Circulation* 1987;75(suppl 4):98-107.
47. Stamato NJ, O'Connell JB, Murdock DK, et al: The response of patients to dilated cardiomyopathy to programmed electrical stimulation. *Am Heart J* 1986;112:505-508.
48. Das SK, Morady F, DiCarlo L, et al: Prognostic usefulness of programmed ventricular stimulation in idiopathic dilated cardiomyopathy without symptomatic ventricular arrhythmias. *Am J Cardiol* 1986;58:998-1000.
49. Wilson JR: Use of antiarrhythmic drugs in patients with heart failure: Clinical efficacy, hemodynamic results, and relation to survival. *Circulation* 1987;75(suppl 4):64-73.
50. Parmley WW, Chatterjee K: Congestive heart failure and arrhythmias: An overview. *Am J Cardiol* 1986;57:34B-37B.
51. Thomas JA, Marks BH: Plasma norepinephrine in congestive heart failure. *Am J Cardiol* 1978;41:233-243.
52. Francis GS, Goldsmith SR, Cohn JN: Relationship of exercise capacity to resting left ventricular performance and basal plasma norepinephrine levels in patients with congestive heart failure. *Am Heart J* 1982;104:725-731.
53. Cohn JN, Levine TB, Olivari MT, et al: Plasma norepinephrine as a guide to prognosis in patients with chronic congestive heart failure. *N Engl J Med* 1984;311:819-823.
54. Cohn JN, Rector T, Olivari MT, et al: Plasma norepinephrine, ejection fraction and maximal oxygen consumption as prognostic variables in congestive heart failure (abstract). *Circulation* 1985;72(suppl 3):285.
55. Dzau VJ, Colucci WS, Hollenberg NK, et al: Relation of the renin-angiotensin-aldosterone system to clinical state in congestive heart failure. *Circulation* 1981;63:645-651.

56. Dzau VJ, Packer M, Lilly LS, et al: Prostaglandins in severe heart failure: Relation to activation of the renin-angiotensin system and hyponatremia. *N Engl J Med* 1984;310:347-352.
57. Levine TB, Franciosa JA, Vrobel T, et al: Hyponatremia as a marker for high renin heart failure. *Br Heart J* 1982;47:161-166.
58. Brown JJ, Davies DL, Johnson VW, et al: Renin relationships in congestive cardiac failure, treated and untreated. *Am Heart J* 1970;80:329-342.
59. Packer M, Medina N, Yushak M: Relation between serum sodium concentration and the hemodynamic and clinical responses to converting enzyme inhibition with captopril in severe heart failure. *J Am Coll Cardiol* 1984;3:1035-1043.
60. Packer M, Lee WH, Kessler PD, et al: Role of neurohormonal mechanisms in determining survival in patients with severe chronic heart failure. *Circulation* 1987;75(suppl 4):80-92.
61. The Captopril-Digitalis Research Group: Comparison of effects of captopril and digoxin on ejection fraction, exercise tolerance, clinical status, and arrhythmias in patients with mild-to-moderate heart failure (abstract). *J Am Coll Cardiol* 1987;9:203A.
62. DiBianco R, Shabetai R, Kostuk W, et al: Oral milrinone and digoxin in heart failure: Results of a placebo-controlled, prospective trial of each agent and the combination (abstract). *Circulation* 1987;76(suppl 4):256.
63. Moss AJ, Davis HT, Conrad DL, et al: Digitalis-associated cardiac mortality after myocardial infarction. *Circulation* 1981;65:1150-1156.
64. Ryan TJ, Bailey KR, McCabe CH, et al: The effects of digitalis on survival in high-risk patients with coronary artery disease: The Coronary Artery Surgery Study (CASS). *Circulation* 1983;67:735-742.
65. Madsen EB, Gilpin E, Menning H, et al: Prognostic importance of digitalis after acute myocardial infarction. *J Am Coll Cardiol* 1984;3:681-689.
66. Bigger JT, Fleiss JL, Rolnitzky LM, et al: Effect of digitalis treatment on survival after acute myocardial infarction. *Am J Cardiol* 1985;55:623-630.
67. Muller JE, Turi ZG, Stone PH, et al: Digoxin therapy and mortality after myocardial infarction. *N Engl J Med* 1986;314:265-271.
68. Byington R, Goldstein S: Association of digitalis therapy with mortality in survivors of acute myocardial infarction: Observations in the Beta-Blocker Heart Attack Trial. *J Am Coll Cardiol* 1985;6:976-982.
69. Yusuf S, Wittes J, Bailey K, et al: Digitalis—a new controversy regarding an old drug: The pitfalls of inappropriate methods. *Circulation* 1986;73:14-18.
70. Stampfer M, Epstein SE, Beiser GD, et al: Hemodynamic effects of diuretics at rest and during upright exercise in patients with impaired cardiac function. *Circulation* 1968;37:900-911.
71. Cowley AJ, Stainer K, Wynne RD, et al: Symptomatic assessment of patients with heart failure: Double-blind comparison of increasing doses of diuretics and captopril in moderate heart failure. *Lancet* 1986;2:770-772.
72. Bayliss J, Norell M, Canepa-Anson R, et al: Untreated heart failure: Clinical and neuroendocrine effects of introducing diuretics. *Br Heart J* 1987;57:17-22.
73. Nicholls MG, Espiner EA, Donald RA, et al: Aldosterone and its regulation during diuresis in patients with gross congestive heart failure. *Clin Sci Mol Med* 1974;47:301-315.
74. Ikram H, Chan W, Espiner EA, et al: Haemodynamic and hormone responses to acute and chronic frusemide therapy in congestive heart failure. *Clin Sci* 1980;59:443-449.
75. Francis GS, Siegel RM, Goldsmith SR, et al: Acute vasoconstrictor response to intravenous furosemide in patients with chronic congestive heart failure: Activation of the neurohumoral axis. *Ann Intern Med* 1985;103:1-6.
76. Packer M, Gottlieb SS, Kessler PD: Hormone-electrolyte interactions in the pathogenesis of lethal cardiac arrhythmias in patients with congestive heart failure: Basis of a new physiologic approach to control of arrhythmia. *Am J Med* 1986;80(suppl 4A):23-29.

77. Knochel JP: Diuretic-induced hypokalemia. *Am J Med* 1984;77(suppl 5A):18-27.
78. Hollifield JW: Potassium and magnesium abnormalities: Diuretics and arrhythmias in hypertension. *Am J Med* 1984;77(suppl 5A):28-32.
79. Horton R, Biglieri EG: Effect of aldosterone on the metabolism of magnesium. *Clin Endocrinol Metab* 1962;22:1187-1192.
80. Rosa RM, Silva P, Young BJ, et al: Adrenergic modulation of extrarenal potassium disposal. *N Engl J Med* 1980;302:431-434.
81. Brown MJ, Brown DC, Murphy MB: Hypokalemia from beta$_2$-receptor stimulation by circulating epinephrine. *N Engl J Med* 1983;309:1414-1419.
82. Struthers AD, Whitesmith R, Reid JL: Prior thiazide diuretic treatment increases adrenaline-induced hypokalemia. *Lancet* 1983;1:1358-1361.
83. Vincent HH, Boomsma F, Man in't Veld AJ, et al: Effects of selective and nonselective beta-agonists on plasma potassium and norepinephrine. *J Cardiovasc Pharmacol* 1984;6:107-114.
84. Nordrehaug JE, von der Lippe G: Hypokalemia and ventricular fibrillation in acute myocardial infarction. *Br Heart J* 1983;50:525-529.
85. Dyckner T, Helmers C, Lundman T, et al: Initial potassium level in relation to early complications and prognosis in patients with an acute myocardial infarction. *Acta Med Scand* 1975;197:207-210.
86. Solomon RJ, Cole AG: Importance of potassium in patients with acute myocardial infarction. *Acta Med Scand* 1981;647(suppl):87-93.
87. Packer M, Lee WH: Provocation of hyper- and hypokalemic sudden death during treatment with and withdrawal of converting-enzyme inhibition in severe chronic congestive heart failure. *Am J Cardiol* 1986;57:347-348.
88. Wilkoff BL, Schaal SF, Muir WW, et al: Diuretic effects on rhythm in chronic ischemic canine model (abstract). *Clin Res* 1985;33:821A.
89. Fisch C: Relation of electrolyte disturbances to cardiac arrhythmias. *Circulation* 1973;47:408-419.
90. Steiness E, Olesen KH: Cardiac arrhythmias induced by hypokalemia and potassium loss during maintenance digoxin therapy. *Br Heart J* 1976;38:167-172.
91. Watanabe Y, Dreifus LS, Likoff W: Electrophysiologic antagonism and synergism of potassium and antiarrhythmic agents. *Am J Cardiol* 1963;12:702-710.
92. Winkle RA, Mason JW, Griffin JC, et al: Malignant ventricular tachyarrhythmias associated with the use of encainide. *Am Heart J* 1981;102:857-864.
93. Dyckner T, Wester PO: Relation between potassium, magnesium and cardiac arrhythmias. *Acta Med Scand* 1981;suppl 647:163-169.
94. Camara EJ, Cruz TR, Massri JM, et al: Muscle magnesium content and cardiac arrhythmias during treatment of congestive heart failure due to chronic chagasic cardiomyopathy. *Braz J Med Biol Res* 1986;19:49-58.
95. Sheehan JP, Seelig MS: Interactions of magnesium and potassium in the pathogenesis of cardiovascular disease. *Magnesium* 1984;3:301-314.
96. Bertuso JR, Flaker GC, Ruder MA, et al: Do patients with cardiac arrest and hypokalemia require antiarrhythmic drug therapy (abstract)? *Circulation* 1984;70(suppl 2):443.
97. Chadda K, Ballas M, Bodenheimer MM: Efficacy of magnesium replacement in patients with hypomagnesemia and cardiac arrhythmia (abstract). *Circulation* 1984;70(suppl 2):444.
98. Whang R, Aikawa JK: Magnesium deficiency and refractoriness to potassium repletion. *J Chronic Dis* 1977;30:65-68.
99. Ryan MP, Ryan MF, Counihan TB: The effect of diuretics on lymphocyte magnesium and potassium. *Acta Med Scand* 1981;suppl 647:153-161.
100. Devane J, Ryan MP: Urinary magnesium excretion during amiloride administration in saline-loaded rats (abstract). *Br J Pharmacol* 1979;67:493P.
101. Ryan MP, Phillips O: Diuretic-induced calcium and magnesium excretion in the rat. *Ir J Med Sci* 1977;146:303.

102. Francis GS: Neurohumoral mechanisms involved in congestive heart failure. *Am J Cardiol* 1985;55:15A-21A.
103. van Gilst WH, de Graeff PA, Wesseling H, et al: Reduction in reperfusion arrhythmias in the ischemic isolated rat heart by angiotensin converting enzyme inhibitors: A comparison of captopril, enalapril, and HOE 498. *J Cardiovasc Pharmacol* 1986;8:722-728.
104. Cleland JGF, Dargie HJ, Hodsman GP, et al: Captopril in heart failure: A double-blind controlled trial. *Br Heart J* 1984;52:530-535.
105. Webster MWL, Fitzpatrick A, Nicholls MG, et al: Effect of enalapril on ventricular arrhythmias in congestive heart failure. *Am J Cardiol* 1985;56:566-569.
106. Cleland JGF, Dargie HJ, Ball SG, et al: Effects of enalapril in heart failure: A double-blind study of effects on exercise performance, renal function, hormones, and metabolic state. *Br Heart J* 1985;54:305-312.
107. Cleland JG, Dargie HJ, Robertson JL, et al: Heart failure, renin, potassium and arrhythmias (abstract). *Circulation* 1985;72(suppl 3):283.
108. Cleland JGF, Dargie HJ, East BW, et al: Total body and serum electrolyte composition in heart failure: The effects of captopril. *Eur Heart J* 1985;6:681-688.
109. Unverferth DV, Magorien RD, Lewis RP, et al: Long-term benefit of dobutamine in patients with congestive cardiomyopathy. *Am Heart J* 1980;100:622-630.
110. Liang C-S, Sherman LG, Doherty JU, et al: Sustained improvement in patients with congestive heart failure after short-term infusion of dobutamine. *Circulation* 1984;69:113-119.
111. Awan NA, Meedham KE, Evenson MK, et al: Hemodynamic actions of prenalterol in severe congestive heart failure due to chronic coronary artery disease. *Am Heart J* 1981;101:158-161.
112. Sharma B, Hoback J, Francis GS, et al: Pirbuterol: A new oral sympathomimetic amine for the treatment of congestive heart failure. *Am Heart J* 1981;102:533-541.
113. Chidsey CA, Braunwald E, Morrow AG: Catecholamine excretion and cardiac stores of norepinephrine in congestive heart failure. *Am J Med* 1966;39:442-451.
114. Weber KT, Andrews V, Janicki JS, et al: Pirbuterol, an oral beta-adrenergic receptor agonist, in the treatment of chronic cardiac failure. *Circulation* 1982;66:1262-1267.
115. Lambertz H, Meyer J, Erbel R: Long-term hemodynamic effects of prenalterol in patients with severe congestive heart failure. *Circulation* 1984;69:298-305.
116. Roubin GS, Choong CVP, Devenish-Meares S, et al: β-Adrenergic stimulation of the failing ventricle: A double-blind randomized trial of sustained oral therapy with prenalterol. *Circulation* 1984;69:955-962.
117. Unverferth DV, Blaunford H, Kates RE, et al: Tolerance to dobutamine after a 72-hour infusion. *Am J Med* 1980;69:262-266.
118. Klein NA, Siskind SJ, Frishman WH, et al: Hemodynamic comparison of intravenous amrinone and dobutamine in patients with chronic congestive heart failure. *Am J Cardiol* 1981;48:170-175.
119. Colucci WS, Alexander RW, Williams GH, et al: Decreased lymphocyte beta-adrenergic receptor density in patients with heart failure and tolerance to the beta-adrenergic agonist pirbuterol. *N Engl J Med* 1981;305:185-190.
120. Packer M, Leier CV: Survival in congestive heart failure during treatment with drugs with positive inotropic actions. *Circulation* 1987;75(suppl 4):55-59.
121. Dawson JR, Canepa-Anson R, Kuan P, et al: Symptoms, haemodynamics, and exercise capacity during long term treatment of chronic heart failure: Experience with pirbuterol. *Br Heart J* 1983;50:282-289.
122. Mettauer B, Rouleau JL, Burgess JH: Detrimental arrhythmogenic and sustained beneficial hemodynamic effects of oral salbutamol in patients with chronic congestive heart failure. *Am Heart J* 1985;109:840-847.
123. David S, Zaks JM: Arrhythmias associated with intermittent outpatient dobutamine infusion. *Angiology* 1986;37:86-91.

124. Yusuf S, Peto R, Lewis J, et al: Beta blockade during and after myocardial infarction: An overview of the randomized trials. *Prog Cardiovasc Dis* 1985;27:335-371.

125. Taylor SH, Silke B, Ebbutt A, et al: A long-term prevention study with oxprenolol in coronary heart disease. *N Engl J Med* 1982;307:1293-1301.

126. Dies F, Krell MJ, Whitlow P, et al: Intermittent dobutamine in ambulatory outpatients with chronic cardiac failure (abstract). *Circulation* 1986;74(suppl 2):39.

127. Endoh M, Yamashita S, Taira N: Positive inotropic effect of amrinone in relation to cyclic nucleotide metabolism in the canine ventricular muscle. *J Pharmacol Exp Ther* 1982;221:775-783.

128. Katz AM: Biochemical "defect" in the hypertrophied and failing heart: Deleterious or compensatory? *Circulation* 1973;47:1076-1079.

129. Lee JC, Downing SE: Cyclic AMP and the pathogenesis of myocardial injury. *Res Commun Chem Pathol Pharmacol* 1980;27:305-318.

130. Mantorana PA: The role of cyclic AMP in isoprenaline-induced cardiac necrosis in the rat. *J Pharm Pharmacol* 1971;23:200-203.

131. Ebbesen P: Myocardial degeneration in mice treated with dibutyryl cyclic AMP and/or theophylline. *Virchows Arch Pathol Anat Histol* 1976;372:89-95.

132. Maskin CS, Forman R, Klein NA, et al: Long-term amrinone therapy in patients with severe heart failure: Drug-dependent hemodynamic benefits despite progression of the disease. *Am J Med* 1982;72:113-118.

133. Sinoway LS, Maskin CS, Chadwick B, et al: Long-term therapy with a new cardiotonic agent, WIN 47203: Drug-dependent improvement in cardiac performance and progression of the underlying disease. *J Am Coll Cardiol* 1983;2:327-331.

134. Packer M, Medina N, Yushak M: Hemodynamic and clinical limitations of long-term inotropic therapy with amrinone in patients with severe chronic heart failure. *Circulation* 1984;70:1038-1047.

135. Leier CV, Dalpiaz K, Huss P, et al: Amrinone therapy for congestive heart failure in outpatients with idiopathic dilated cardiomyopathy. *Am J Cardiol* 1983;52:304-308.

136. Askins JC, Anderson JL, Gilbert EM, et al: Arrhythmogenic potential of prolonged intravenous milrinone (abstract). *Circulation* 1985;72(suppl 3):405.

137. Ferrick KJ, Fein SA, Ferrick AM, et al: Effect of milrinone on ventricular arrhythmias in patients with congestive heart failure (abstract). *Circulation* 1986;74(suppl 2):508.

138. Petein M, Levine TB, Cohn JN: Persistent hemodynamic effects without long-term clinical benefits in response to oral piroximone (MDL 19,205) in patients with congestive heart failure. *Circulation* 1986;73(suppl 3):230-236.

139. Rubin SA, Tabak L: MDL 17,043: Short- and long-term cardiopulmonary and clinical effects in patients with heart failure. *J Am Coll Cardiol* 1985;5:1422-1427.

140. Shah PK, Amin DK, Hulse S, et al: Inotropic therapy for refractory congestive heart failure with oral fenoximone (MDL-17,043): Poor long-term results despite early hemodynamic and clinical improvement. *Circulation* 1985;71:326-331.

141. Simonton C, Chatterjee K, Cody R, et al: Milrinone in congestive heart failure: Acute and chronic hemodynamic and clinical evaluation. *J Am Coll Cardiol* 1985;6:453-459.

142. Maskin CS, Mancini D, Chadwick B, et al: Clinical response to long-term milrinone therapy in severe chronic heart failure: Two-year experience (abstract). *Circulation* 1984;70(suppl 2):168.

143. Lee WH, Packer M: Does inotropic therapy shorten survival in patients with severe chronic heart failure (abstract)? *Circulation* 1985;72(suppl 2):283.

144. Uretsky BF, Generalovich T, Verbalis JG, et al: MDL 17,043 therapy in severe congestive heart failure: Characterization of the acute and chronic hemodynamic, pharmacokinetic, hormonal, and clinical response. *J Am Coll Cardiol* 1985;5:1414-1421.

145. Jafri SM, Burlew BS, Goldberg AD, et al: Hemodynamic effects of a new type III phosphodiesterase inhibitor (CI-914) for congestive heart failure. *Am J Cardiol* 1986;57:254-259.

146. Kinney EL, Carlin B, Ballard JO, et al: Clinical experience with amrinone in patients with advanced congestive heart failure. *J Clin Pharmacol* 1982;22:433-440.

147. Massie B, Bourassa M, DiBianco R, et al: Long-term oral administration of amrinone for congestive heart failure: Lack of efficacy in a multicenter controlled trial. *Circulation* 1985;71:963-971.

148. Francis GS: The survival hypothesis: How small uncontrolled studies should influence the design of large-scale clinical trials. *Circulation* 1987;75(suppl 4):74-79.

149. Packer M, Meller J, Medina N, et al: Provocation of myocardial ischemic events during initiation of vasodilatory therapy for severe chronic heart failure: Clinical and hemodynamic evaluation of 52 consecutive patients with ischemic cardiomyopathy. *Am J Cardiol* 1981;48:939-946.

150. Packer M, Meller J, Medina N, et al: Importance of left ventricular chamber size in determining the response to hydralazine in severe chronic heart failure. *N Engl J Med* 1980;303:250-255.

151. Franciosa JA, Jordan RA, Wilen MM, et al: Minoxidil in patients with chronic left heart failure: Contrasting hemodynamic and clinical effects in a controlled trial. *Circulation* 1984;70:63-68.

152. Packer M, Meller J, Gorlin R, et al: Hemodynamic and clinical tachyphylaxis to prazosin-mediated afterload reduction in severe chronic congestive heart failure. *Circulation* 1979;59:531-539.

153. Packer M, Medina N, Yushak M: Role of the renin-angiotensin system in the development of hemodynamic and clinical tolerance to long-term prazosin therapy in patients with severe chronic heart failure. *J Am Coll Cardiol* 1986;7:671-680.

154. Markham RV, Corbett JR, Gilmore A, et al: Efficacy of prazosin in the management of chronic congestive heart failure: A 6-month randomized double-blind placebo-controlled study. *Am J Cardiol* 1983;51:1346-1352.

155. Franciosa JA, Weber KT, Levine TB, et al: Hydralazine in the long-term treatment of chronic heart failure: Lack of difference from placebo. *Am Heart J* 1982;104:587-594.

156. Franciosa JA, Nordstrom LA, Cohn JN: Nitrate therapy for congestive heart failure. *JAMA* 1978;240:443-446.

157. Leier CV, Huss P, Magorien RD, et al: Improved exercise capacity and differing arterial and venous tolerance during chronic isosorbide dinitrate therapy for congestive heart failure. *Circulation* 1983;67:817-822.

158. Thadani U, Manyari D, Parker JO, et al: Tolerance to the circulatory effects of oral isosorbide dinitrate: Rate of development and cross-tolerance to glyceryl trinitrate. *Circulation* 1980;61:526-535.

159. Parker JO, Farrell B, Lahey KA, et al: Effect of intervals between doses on the development of tolerance to isosorbide dinitrate. *N Engl J Med* 1987;316:1440-1444.

160. Cohn JN, Archibald DG, Francis GS, et al: Veterans Administration Cooperative Study on Vasodilator Therapy of Heart Failure: Influence of prerandomization variables on the reduction of mortality by treatment with hydralazine and isosorbide dinitrate. *Circulation* 1987;75(suppl 4):49-54.

161. Archibald DG, Cohn JN, and VA Cooperative Study Group: A treatment-associated increase in ejection fraction predicts long-term survival in congestive heart failure: The V-HeFT Study (abstract). *Circulation* 1986;74(suppl 2):309.

162. Packer M: Do vasodilators prolong life in heart failure? *N Engl J Med* 1987;316:1471-1473.

163. Packer M, Lee WH, Bair J, et al: Does vasodilator therapy alter prognosis in patients with severe chronic heart failure? Comparative effects of hydralazine and captopril on clinical outcome and survival in 175 patients treated over a 6-year period (abstract). *J Am Coll Cardiol* 1984;3:561.

164. Riegger GAJ, Liebau G, Holzschuh M, et al: Role of the renin-angiotensin system in the development of congestive heart failure in the dog as assessed by chronic converting-enzyme blockage. *Am J Cardiol* 1984;53:614-618.

165. Pfeffer JM, Pfeffer MA, Braunwald E: Influence of chronic captopril therapy on the infarcted left ventricle of the rat. *Circ Res* 1985;57:84-95.

166. Pfeffer MA, Pfeffer JM, Steinberg C, et al: Survival after an experimental myocardial infarction: Beneficial effects of long-term therapy with captopril. *Circulation* 1985;72:406-412.

167. Furberg CD, Yusuf S: Effect of vasodilators on survival in chronic congestive heart failure. *Am J Cardiol* 1985;55:1110-1113.

168. Packer M, Medina N, Yushak M: Correction of dilutional hyponatremia in severe chronic heart failure by converting-enzyme inhibition. *Ann Intern Med* 1984;100:782-789.

169. The CONSENSUS Trial Study Group: Effects of enalapril on·mortality in severe congestive heart failure: Results of the Cooperative North Scandinavian Enalapril Survival Study (CONSENSUS). *N Engl J Med* 1987;316:1429-1435.

170. Captopril Multicenter Research Group: A placebo-controlled trial of captopril in refractory chronic congestive heart failure. *J Am Coll Cardiol* 1983;2:755-763.

171. Dennick LG, Maskin CS, Meyer JH, et al: Enalapril for congestive heart failure (letter). *N Engl J Med* 1987;317:1350.

172. Kleber FX, Laube A, Osterkorn K, et al: Captopril in mild to moderate heart failure over 18 months: Effects on morbidity and mortality (abstract). *J Am Coll Cardiol* 1987;9:42A.

173. Lilly L, Dzau VJ, Williams GH, et al: Captopril vs hydralazine in advanced congestive heart failure: Comparison of one year survival (abstract). *Circulation* 1985;72(suppl 3):408.

174. Pfeffer MA, Pfeffer JM: Ventricular enlargement and reduced survival after myocardial infarction. *Circulation* 1987;75(suppl 4):93-97.

175. Engelmeier RS, O'Connell JB, Walsh R, et al: Improvement in symptoms and exercise tolerance by metoprolol in patients with dilated cardiomyopathy: A double-blind, randomized, placebo-controlled trial. *Circulation* 1985;72:536-546.

176. Waagstein F, Hjalmarson A, Varnauskas E, et al: Effect of chronic beta-adrenergic receptor blockade in congestive cardiomyopathy. *Br Heart J* 1975;37:1022-1036.

177. Swedberg K, Hjalmarson A, Waagstein F, et al: Beneficial effects of long-term beta-blockade in congestive cardiomyopathy. *Br Heart J* 1980;44:117-133.

178. Swedberg K, Hjalmarson A, Waagstein F, et al: Adverse effects of beta-blockade withdrawal in patients with congestive cardiomyopathy. *Br Heart J* 1980;44:134-142.

179. Swedberg K, Hjalmarson A, Waagstein F, et al: Prolongation of survival in congestive cardiomyopathy by beta-receptor blockade. *Lancet* 1979;1:1374-1376.

180. Anderson J, Lutz JR, Gilbert EM, et al: A randomized trial of low-dose beta-blockade therapy for idiopathic dilated cardiomyopathy. *Am J Cardiol* 1985;55:471-475.

181. Chadda K, Goldstein S, Byington R, et al: Effect of propranolol after acute myocardial infarction in patients with congestive heart failure. *Circulation* 1986;73:503-510.

182. Furberg CD, Hawkins CM, Lichstein E, for the Beta-Blocker Heart Attack Trial Study Group: Effect of propranolol in postinfarction patients with mechanical or electrical complications. *Circulation* 1984;69:761-765.

183. Hansteen V, Moinchen E, Lorentsen E, et al: One year's treatment with propranolol after myocardial infarction: Preliminary report of Norwegian multicentre trial. *Br Med J* 1982;284:155-160.
184. Olsson G, Rehnquist N: Effect of metoprolol in postinfarction patients with increased heart size. *Eur Heart J* 1986;7:468-474.

JAY N. COHN, MD

13

A Comprehensive Approach to the Treatment of Congestive Heart Failure

In order to pursue a rational and comprehensive approach to the therapy of congestive heart failure, it is essential to establish appropriate goals of therapy and understand the use of diuretics, vasodilators, and inotropic drugs, which form the cornerstone of the pharmacologic management of the disease.

GOALS OF THERAPY There are two goals of therapy. The first is to improve the quality of life for the patient; the second is to prolong life. Quantitation of the quality of a patient's life has been an elusive measurement, and a number of questionnaires are now being specifically designed for use in patients with heart failure. It is clear that exercise tolerance alone does not serve as a surrogate for overall quality of life analysis, although reduced exercise tolerance is one of the factors that affect the life-style of the patient with heart failure.

Most clinical trials have been designed with an exercise tolerance endpoint, because it can be quantitated and should be improved by effective therapy. Although congestive heart failure has in the past been regarded as a contraindication to exercise testing, it is now apparent that progressive exercise testing to maximal tolerated levels is a safe procedure and can provide quantitation of the severity of functional disability and of the response to therapy. Exercise testing can be carried out either on a bicycle ergometer or on a treadmill. The exercise protocol used for this purpose is usually different from that used in patients with angina and often necessitates beginning at a lower work load and increasing in more gradual steps. In many laboratories, it has become customary to monitor oxygen consumption during exercise testing to approximate the maximal oxygen consumption that the patient can achieve during progressive exercise loading. The equipment required for this purpose is somewhat complex and moderately expensive, but it is gaining popularity in many exercise laboratories dedicated to quantitative assessment.

Most patients will have started initial therapy for heart failure before consideration is given to more aggressive pharmacologic approaches; therefore, the usual reason for carrying out a quantitative exercise test is to determine whether the patient's present therapy is adequate to restore normal functional capacity. If the patient is capable of carrying out all of his or her normal life activities without symptoms and is willing to forgo strenuous exertion, of which he or she is no longer capable, then it may be that the therapy has achieved its desired goal in terms of quality of life. If, on the other hand, the patient's life-style is significantly impaired because of the cardiac disability, especially if exercise testing confirms considerable reduction in maximum capability, then more aggressive attempts to improve symptoms are indicated. When oxygen consumption measurements are utilized, a peak of greater than 25 mL/kg/min may be assumed to represent an essentially normal level that should not be a deterrent to an active life-style. Elderly or sedentary individuals may be comfortable with oxygen consumption of greater than 15 mL/kg/min; levels less than 15 mL/kg/min are usually associated with considerable impairment in life-style.

The goal of prolonging life in heart failure is now a rational expectation of therapy. This is due to the results of two recent controlled trials, one in patients with mild to moderate heart failure treated with hydralazine and isosorbide dinitrate, and one in class IV heart failure patients treated with enalapril. The reported efficacy of these two vasodilator regimens in reducing mortality provides support for the concept that vasodilator therapy should be employed in all patients with heart failure, regardless of their symptoms.

The other consideration to be kept in mind during treatment of patients with heart failure is that sudden death is a common cause of their demise. Because ventricular arrhythmias are common in patients with heart failure, they may represent a harbinger of the sudden death syndrome. Assessment of the effect of therapeutic efforts on premature ventricular depolarizations may be an appropriate concern. Unfortunately, the relationship between these ventricular premature depolarizations and sudden death, and the impact of therapeutic suppression of these ventricular arrhythmias have not been established. Holter monitoring is the most effective means of quantitating the frequency of ventricular premature beats and asymptomatic episodes of ventricular tachycardia.

NONPHARMA-COLOGIC MEASURES Although the emphasis in this book has been on pharmacologic therapy, simple adjustments in life-style that may influence cardiac and peripheral vascular function should not be disregarded. These measures include weight reduction to decrease the burden on the cardiovascular system, salt restriction to decrease the renal tubular burden of sodium, and a regular dynamic exercise program to avoid the deconditioning that may aggravate the exercise disability in patients with heart failure. In the overall management of the patient, avoidance of stresses that may produce a sustained increase in left ventricular wall tension, such as prolonged isometric exercise, and avoidance of drugs that may reduce myocardial contractility should also be considered.

Surgical intervention and catheterization procedures have an important therapeutic role in certain patients with heart failure. Improved surgical techniques and better pre- and postoperative care now make it possible to perform operations with remarkable safety on patients with severe ventricular dysfunction. Furthermore, catheter angioplasty and valvuloplasty have made it possible to perform corrective procedures without the operative risk in selected patients. Therefore, it is imperative to examine patients with heart failure carefully for epicardial coronary stenoses and valve deformities, which may have an important role in the etiology of the heart failure syndrome. Recognition of the prevalence of silent myocardial ischemia has increased the complexity of this evaluation, because the absence of angina pectoris no longer excludes significant ischemia as a contributing factor to ventricular dysfunction.

DIURETICS   The use of diuretics in patients with advanced heart failure is still necessary. This is because impairment of renal sodium excretion appears to be an early manifestation of cardiac dysfunction and because none of the therapeutic approaches studied to date have been generally effective in completely reversing this renal manifestation of heart failure. Diuretics not only relieve the symptoms of congestion that result from excess sodium retention; they also reduce ventricular volume and thus reduce left ventricular wall stress. Reduction of left ventricular wall stress reduces myocardial oxygen consumption and appears to result in an improvement of the functional capacity of the left ventricle. In view of the fact that cardiac performance is also dependent on filling pressure by virtue of the Frank-Starling relationship, excessive reduction of the filling pressure by overly aggressive use of diuretics may reduce cardiac output and further impair functional capacity, renal perfusion, and sodium excretion. Therefore, the use of diuretics to adjust volume in patients with heart failure involves careful titration aimed at reducing cardiac filling pressure to the lowest level compatible with stable forward output.

Because of their potency and relative ease of administration, loop diuretics such as furosemide have become the mainstay of diuretic therapy for patients with congestive heart failure. In milder forms of heart failure, however, use of the less potent thiazide diuretics may be sufficient to maintain normal fluid balance. If patients are able to adhere to restricting their sodium intake, mild, intermittently administered diuretic treatment may be all that is necessary. Some patients may require only one or two doses of a diuretic per week in order to maintain dry weight, and sometimes diuretics are not necessary in patients who can restrict their sodium intake. In more severe degrees of heart failure when use of loop diuretics is necessary, dosage adjustments should be made on the basis of close monitoring of the fluid volume status. The most effective means of monitoring are visual inspection of the jugular venous pressure and daily recording of the patient's weight. The goal of diuretic therapy is to maintain intravascular volume at the lowest well-tolerated level, and the venous pressure provides a useful guide to that level. Visual inspection of the height of the venous pressure by observing the deep venous pulse in the neck provides a very valuable guide. The response of this central venous pressure to right upper quadrant abdominal compression yields additional insight into the adequacy of intravascular volume. A positive hepatojugular reflux test always implies the presence of

295

an expanded volume that is best reduced. A negative hepatojugular reflux test is consistent with a nonexpanded volume. If the physician is able to identify the body weight that matches normal central venous pressure and is associated with a negative response to the hepatojugular reflux test and good peripheral perfusion, then that body weight may subsequently serve as a guideline for the patient who is monitoring his or her own requirement for diuretics. Indeed, in the management of diuretic therapy for heart failure it is often best to enlist the participation of the patient. Thus, when there is increased body weight and especially if this increase in weight is associated with any recurrence of symptoms, an increase in diuretic dose should be administered. If body weight is decreased, especially if it is accompanied by weakness or dizziness compatible with a falling cardiac output, then reduction of diuretic dose may be indicated.

Furosemide may be administered to patients with congestive heart failure either once daily or in multiple daily doses. Many patients prefer to complete the entire diuretic response early in the day, within the course of a few hours. Others prefer more gentle diuresis during the day, in which case the dose may be given on two or three occasions. In more severe congestive states when the furosemide dose must be increased to high levels in order to achieve an adequate diuresis, the addition of a second diuretic to modest doses of furosemide is usually more effective than further increases in furosemide dosage. I have found the addition of metolazone to furosemide to be a particularly useful combination. A single dose of 2.5 mg or 5 mg of metolazone given approximately 30 minutes before the morning dose of furosemide usually produces a considerable augmentation of diuresis. A similar response may be achieved with the addition of thiazide diuretics.

Maintenance of normal serum potassium is, of course, an important consideration during diuretic therapy. This can be accomplished either with administration of supplemental potassium or the addition of a potassium-retaining diuretic such as amiloride, triamterene, or spironolactone. In patients receiving a converting-enzyme inhibitor, potassium supplementation or potassium-retaining drugs are required less often. Frequent monitoring of serum potassium as well as monitoring of blood urea nitrogen concentrations provides useful guides to the efficacy and safety of these potassium-supporting measures.

VASODILATOR DRUGS   The decision to initiate vasodilator therapy is based upon the desire to improve functional capacity in the patient with congestive heart failure or to favorably influence survival. There is probably no absolute contraindication to administering vasodilator drugs in the patient with heart failure except the presence of severe hypotension associated with symptoms of inadequate perfusion. Even when arterial pressure is in the lower range of normal, cautious administration of vasodilator drugs may be appropriate. Certain findings may particularly encourage the early use of vasodilators. If arterial pressure is elevated or in the upper range of normal, aggressive vasodilator therapy as a means to lower impedance may be indicated. If mitral regurgitation or aortic regurgitation complicates the myocardial dysfunction, vasodilator drugs may be especially useful in augmenting forward output at the expense of the regurgitant flow. Initiation of vasodilator therapy does presuppose that the patient has documented left ventricular failure and the physician is certain that the left ventricle is dilated and has poor systolic function. This documentation is best quantitated with an echocardiogram or measurement of the radionuclide ejection fraction. Chest x-ray alone may often provide misleading information regarding the severity of left ventricular disease.

Therapy may be initiated with any of the available vaso-dilator regimens. If symptoms are predominantly related to shortness of breath on exertion and if the venous pressure is elevated, then a drug that increases venous capacitance and reduces cardiac filling pressures should be an important component of therapy. If, on the other hand, the patient complains predominantly of fatigue on exertion yet venous pressures are normal, then consideration should be given to the use of agents that act on the arterial circulation to reduce impedance and improve cardiac output. Many of the drug regimens accomplish both an increase in venous capacitance and decrease in arterial resistance; therefore, this distinction between backward symptoms and forward symptoms is not always necessary.

Hydralazine has served as an effective arterial dilator in many individuals and may be initiated in doses of 50 to 100 mg twice daily. In some patients it may be necessary to increase the dose to 400 or even 600 mg daily. Because of the high incidence of side effects as the dose is increased to high levels, many physicians turn to other agents rather than use higher doses of hydralazine. For example, hydralazine is often given in combination with a nitrate, which has a predominant venous effect, thus complementing hydralazine's predominant effect on the arterial circulation and its comparatively minor effect on the venous circulation. Isosorbide dinitrate given orally in doses from 20 to 80 mg four times daily may be an effective means of increasing venous capacitance and lowering the filling pressure of the heart. Newer transdermal nitroglycerin preparations may also be effective, but they usually require daily use of patches of 40 to 80 cm^2, which probably should be removed at night to inhibit the development of drug tolerance.

Captopril and other angiotensin converting-enzyme in-hibitors are gaining widespread popularity as vasodilators in heart failure because they have been demonstrated to improve exercise capacity and quality of life in patients with heart failure that is unresponsive to conventional therapy. This therapy must be initiated with somewhat more care than the other vasodilator therapy, because the initial response to the drug may result in a profound fall in blood pressure. In patients with low serum sodium, which serves as a marker for a high plasma renin activity, therapy should be initiated with a very low dose such as 6.25 mg of captopril. Close observation of the patient for the first hour and a half after dosage administration is necessary to document the extent of the fall in blood pressure. If the fall in blood pressure has been only modest and is not associated with any adverse symptoms, then therapy may be initiated at doses of 12.5 mg three times daily. This dose may then be increased after several days to 25 or 50 mg three times daily. If the patient does not show evidence of a low serum sodium level or severe decompensation, then the initial dose may be 25 mg and the same subsequent regimen can be followed. Doses as high as 100 mg three times daily may occasionally be necessary to achieve the desired therapeutic goal. Enalapril is a converting-enzyme inhibitor with a slower onset and longer duration of effect. Doses of from 5 to 40 mg in two divided doses daily may be effective. In all cases the response to converting-enzyme inhibitors should be monitored by frequent assessment of venous pressure, symptoms, blood chemistry values including renal function and electrolytes, and blood count and urinalysis, because of the rare occurrence of neutropenia.

Prazosin was employed as a vasodilator, but tolerance to its hemodynamic effect in several studies and the failure to prolong life in the Veterans Administration Cooperative Study of Vasodilatory Therapy of Heart Failure (V-HeFT) has now rendered this agent nearly obsolete as a vasodilator for heart failure.

Minoxidil is an alternate arterial vasodilator that may be employed in patients who are intolerant or unresponsive to hydralazine or converting-enzyme inhibitors. Minoxidil 10 to 20 mg twice daily may produce a sustained vasodilator effect that may be associated with considerable improvement in cardiac output. Unwanted side effects of minoxidil, especially abnormal hair growth, limit its use in women. Sodium retention may also become more prominent during minoxidil therapy and may require adjustment of the diuretic dosage. This drug should probably always be used in conjunction with a nitrate or a converting-enzyme inhibitor.

INOTROPIC DRUGS Digitalis has been widely used for the treatment of congestive heart failure for generations and is still employed by most physicians in the United States. Its use in other countries around the world, particularly the United Kingdom, has decreased in recent years because of questionable efficacy and the possibility of adverse effects. The benefit-risk ratio for digitalis therapy in patients with congestive heart failure who have normal sinus rhythm remains controversial. It is clear that low-dose digoxin is safer than previously used higher doses, and it is likely that digoxin produces a slight but measurable improvement in left ventricular performance and a slight but measurable reduction of heart rate in many patients with heart failure. This evidence for modest efficacy has been thought by some to be outweighed by the arrhythmogenic potential of the drug. Although concern about an increased mortality in digoxin-treated patients was raised in a few retrospective studies, recent data do not support the idea that digoxin therapy increases the risk of sudden death.

Because of the modest efficacy of digitalis and its possible risk, considerable effort has been dedicated in recent years to the development of new orally effective inotropic drugs that may replace or supplement digitalis for inotropic support in patients with heart failure. None of these drugs is currently marketed for chronic use, and clinical studies of their efficacy and safety are still under way. These agents form at least two separate classes: drugs that work through β-adrenergic receptors, and drugs that are nonadrenergic.

The β-adrenergic agonists that have been employed include pirbuterol, prenalterol, terbutaline, salbutamol, and xamoterol. Some of these agents are predominantly β_2-agonists and therefore have their primary effect on the bronchi and the peripheral vasculature, whereas others have a predominantly β_1-agonistic effect with relatively little action on the β_2-receptor. It is likely that their effect on left ventricular function results from the summation of varying degrees of direct inotropism and varying degrees of vasodilation. The concern with these β-agonists is that the β-receptor may down regulate during chronic stimulation and that the pharmacologic effect may wane with time. Studies are under way to determine whether these drugs maintain efficacy during chronic administration.

The nonadrenergic drugs are a heterogeneous group of compounds with poorly established modes of action. Many of them have an inhibiting effect on phosphodiesterase and may lead to increased cardiac levels of cyclic adenosine monophosphate (AMP). Others may increase the permeability of the myocardial cell to calcium for excitation-contraction coupling or may actually increase the sensitivity of the contractile apparatus to calcium. Some of these drugs have rather potent acute effects, increasing contractility, but as yet the proof of efficacy during chronic administration has not been established, nor is their safety during chronic administration entirely established. Agents currently undergoing clinical trials include milrinone, enoximone, pimobendan, and OPC-8212.

The appropriate time for intervening with an inotropic drug versus a vasodilator drug remains controversial. Studies to date have focused primarily on patients with end-stage heart disease who often require combinations of vasodilators, inotropic drugs, and diuretics to obtain optimal therapeutic response. In less severe degrees of heart failure many patients continue to thrive while receiving only digitalis and diuretics. The addition of vasodilators to some of these patients' regimens improves functional capacity, but as yet inotropic drugs have not been carefully evaluated in this modestly impaired group of patients. What remains to be established is whether early recognition of signs of left ventricular dysfunction at a time when functional capacity is only modestly impaired will identify a group of patients in whom aggressive therapeutic interventions with either vasodilator or inotropic drugs will alter the natural history of the disease. A study in this patient population (Study of Left Ventricular Dysfunction, or SOLVD) is currently being carried out under the auspices of the National Heart, Lung and Blood Institute.

INDEX

A

ACE. See Angiotensin converting-enzyme inhibitors
Acetazolamide, 165, 168–172
  complications, 171
Acetylcholine, 52
Acidosis, as diuretic complication, 168–172
Acquired valvular regurgitation, digitalis treatment, 163
Activated charcoal, digitalis intoxication treatment, 158
Acute hypoxemia, digitalis and, 149
ADH. See Antidiuretic hormone
Adrenergic receptors, "down regulation," 52
Afterload, 19–33, 128–142. See also Ventricular performance
Aldosterone, 79–99, 109–111, 167, 228–229. See also Renin-angiotensin-aldosterone system
  angiotensin-II, 229
  atrial natriuretic factor, 82–86
  hyperaldosteronism, 165
  plasma renin activity and, 84–87
  potassium levels and, 80, 229
  renin-angiotensin-aldosterone system interactions and heart effects, 79–99
  sodium and, 80
    reabsorption, 89–90
  spironolactone and, 92, 170–171
  suppression of, 95
Alkalosis, as diuretic complication, 168–172
α-Adrenergic receptor blockers, 189, 201
α$_1$-Adrenergic agonists, 182–185
α$_1$-Adrenergic receptors, 182–185
Ambulatory ECG monitoring, 138
Amiloride, 168–172
  diuretic effects, 170
  serum potassium level and, 296
Amiodarone, digitalis intoxication and, 161
AMP. See Cyclic adenosine monophosphate
Amrinone, 180–183, 186–187
Angina pectoris, 256
  digitalis and, 162–163
Angiotensin. See also Angiotensin converting-enzyme inhibitors; Converting-enzyme inhibitors; Renin-angiotensin-aldosterone system
  angiotensin converting-enzyme inhibitors and, 118–120, 227–244
  atrial natriuretic factor, 82–86
  congestive heart failure and, 116
  heart failure and, 22, 116–117, 142
  hemorrhage, 110–112
  renin-angiotensin-aldosterone system interactions and heart effects, 51–52, 79–99

vascular tone, 87–89
  vasoconstriction and, 90–96
Angiotensin converting-enzyme inhibitors. See also Renin-angiotensin-aldosterone system
  acute hemodynamic effects, 229–232
  adverse effects, 240–243
  captopril, 87–89, 92–96, 117–121, 200–201, 219–220, 297
  comparison of different types, 237–238
  guidelines for clinical use, 239–244
  ischemic heart disease and, 232–233
  long-acting versus short-acting, 235
  mortality findings, 238–239
  well-being, feeling of, 237
Angiotensinogen, 167. See also Renin-angiotensin-aldosterone system
Angiotensin-I, 167. See also Renin-angiotensin-aldosterone system
  renin-angiotensin-aldosterone system interactions and heart effects, 79–99
  vasodilation effects, 201
Angiotensin-II, 59–60, 80, 91–92, 167. See also Renin-angiotensin-aldosterone system
  potassium levels and, 229
  renin levels and, 92
  renin-angiotensin-aldosterone system interactions and heart effects, 79–99
  vasoconstriction effects, 229
  vasodilation effects, 201
  well-being, feeling of, 237
Anorexia, digitalis intoxication and, 154–155
Antiarrhythmic agents, 157
Anticoagulants, in heart failure treatment, 141
Antidiuretic hormone, 228
  water handling in kidney and, 109
Aortic impedance, 5–6
Arginine vasopressin
  heart failure and, 8–9, 58–61
  vasoconstriction effects, 229
ARL 115 BS (sulmazole), 180, 189
Arrhythmias
  as diagnostic guidelines in heart failure, 57, 264
  digitalis actions on, 148
  digitalis intoxication and, 155–161
  electrolyte abnormalities and, 118
  inotropic therapy and, 192
  renal functioning and, 115
  sudden death, 294
  Wolff-Parkinson-White (WPW) tachyarrhythmias, 162
Arteriovenous fistulae, heart failure and, 113
Artificial heart, 10
Atrial fibrillation, 162
Atrial flutter, digitalis treatment, 162
Atrial natriuretic factor (ANF), 218. See also Atrial natriuretic peptide

INDEX

INDEX

INDEX

Sodium-potassium-adenosine
triphosphatase
digitalis and, 147–148
inhibitors, 111
Spironolactone, 165, 168–172
aldosterone inhibition, 92
serum potassium level and, 296
Splanchnic nerve, 52
Steroid-binding resins, digitalis
intoxication treatment, 158
Stress testing, 3–4. See also Exercise
testing
Strophanthidin, 25–26
Sulmazole (ARL 115 BS), 180, 189
Surgery, for heart failure, 10, 295
Sympathetic nervous system
abnormalities and heart failure, 56–57
central command, 53
heart failure and, 38–40, 52–57
norepinephrine and heart failure, 8–9
physiology of, 52–57
renal functioning and, 115–116
renal vascular response and, 112
renin release, 81–82
Systemic congestion, as symptom of
heart failure, 131–134
Systemic lupus erythematosus, captopril
and, 242

T

Tachycardia, 143, 146, 162
antiarrhythmic agents and, 157
digitalis and, 149
inotropic therapy and, 192
minoxidil effects and, 212–213
Tachyphylaxis, 256
prazosin side effect, 238–239
Tachypnea, 132
Taste alteration, as captopril side effect,
241–242
Teprotide, vasodilation effects, 201
Terbutaline, 298
Thiazides, 165, 295
furosemide and, 165–170
Thiocyanate toxicity, 206
Thyroid disease, digoxin and, 153
Treadmill exercise test, 137–138
Triamterene, 168–172
diuretic effects, 170
serum potassium level and, 296
Trimazosin, 215
Trimethaphan, 201, 206–207

U

Urinary tract calculi, as diuretic
complication, 168–172
Urination
antidiuretic hormone and, 109
glomerular filtration and, 107
kidney structure and processes of,
106–109
renal functioning and, 106–121

V

Vagus nerve, 52
Valvuloplasty, 295

Vascular response, in kidney, 112
Vascular tone, renin-angiotensin-
aldosterone system effects, 87–89
Vasoconstriction, 51–57. See also Renin-
angiotensin-aldosterone system;
Vasodilator therapy
captopril effects, 92–96
reversal of, 92–96
Vasodilator therapy, 144–145, 252–255,
269–270. See also specific
vasodilators by name
atrial natriuretic factor and, 64–65 (see
also Atrial natriuretic factor)
clinical guidelines, 190, 203–221
dopamine and, 70–71
for heart failure, 199–221, 256, 276–278,
296–298
hemodynamic effects, 202–220
mechanisms of action, 201–203
mortality findings, 238–239
myocardial ischemia, 200–201
rationale for, 199–200
recent advances in, 51
sodium nitroprusside, 203–206
ventricular diastolic compliance, 201
Vasopressin, 228
heart failure and, 8–9, 58–61
Venoconstriction, catecholamines and, 235
Ventricular arrhythmias. See Arrhythmias
Ventricular diastolic compliance,
vasodilators, 201
Ventricular function
captopril and, 236–240
evaluation procedures, 252–255
and filling pressure, 203
left ventricle, 33–35
pathophysiology, 49–71, 144–145
sodium nitroprusside and, 190, 204
Ventricular performance, 13–42
afterload, 20–33
aortic impedance, 5–6
contractility and, 22–37
determinants of, 14–33
digitalis and, 149, 156–161
ejection fraction, 266–267
preload, 7, 14–20
Verapamil, 216–217
digitalis and drug interactions, 160–161
vasodilation effects, 201
ventricular response and, 162
Visual disturbances, digitalis intoxication
and, 154–155
Vitamin B_{12} deficiency, 206

W

Water handling, kidney's defense of
extracellular fluid and plasma volume,
109–119
Weight reduction, captopril effects, 236
Well-being, captopril effects, 237
Wolff-Parkinson-White (WPW)
tachyarrhythmias, 162

X

Xamoterol, 298
Xenon activity, 115–116

CAPOTEN® TABLETS

Captopril Tablets

DESCRIPTION

CAPOTEN (captopril) is the first of a new class of antihypertensive agents, a specific competitive inhibitor of angiotensin I-converting enzyme (ACE), the enzyme responsible for the conversion of angiotensin I to angiotensin II. Captopril is also effective in the management of heart failure.

CAPOTEN (captopril) is designated chemically as 1-[(2S)-3-mercapto-2-methylpropionyl]-L-proline [MW 217.29].

Captopril is a white to off-white crystalline powder that may have a slight sulfurous odor; it is soluble in water (approx. 160 mg/mL), methanol, and ethanol and sparingly soluble in chloroform and ethyl acetate.

CAPOTEN (captopril) is available in potencies of 12.5 mg, 25 mg, 50 mg, and 100 mg as scored tablets for oral administration. Inactive ingredients: microcrystalline cellulose, corn starch, lactose, and stearic acid.

CLINICAL PHARMACOLOGY

Mechanism of Action

The mechanism of action of CAPOTEN (captopril) has not yet been fully elucidated. Its beneficial effects in hypertension and heart failure appear to result primarily from suppression of the renin-angiotensin-aldosterone system. However, there is no consistent correlation between renin levels and response to the drug. Renin, an enzyme synthesized by the kidneys, is released into the circulation where it acts on a plasma globulin substrate to produce angiotensin I, a relatively inactive decapeptide. Angiotensin I is then converted by angiotensin converting enzyme (ACE) to angiotensin II, a potent endogenous vasoconstrictor substance. Angiotensin II also stimulates aldosterone secretion from the adrenal cortex, thereby contributing to sodium and fluid retention.

CAPOTEN (captopril) prevents the conversion of angiotensin I to angiotensin II by inhibition of ACE, a peptidyldipeptide carboxy hydrolase. This inhibition has been demonstrated in both healthy human subjects and in animals by showing that the elevation of blood pressure caused by exogenously administered angiotensin I was attenuated or abolished by captopril. In animal studies, captopril did not alter the pressor responses to a number of other agents, including angiotensin II and norepinephrine, indicating specificity of action.

ACE is identical to "bradykininase," and CAPOTEN (captopril) may also interfere with the degradation of the vasodepressor peptide, bradykinin. Increased concentrations of bradykinin or prostaglandin E_2 may also have a role in the therapeutic effect of CAPOTEN.

Inhibition of ACE results in decreased plasma angiotensin II and increased plasma renin activity (PRA), the latter resulting from loss of negative feedback on renin release caused by reduction in angiotensin II. The reduction of angiotensin II leads to decreased aldosterone secretion, and, as a result, small increases in serum potassium may occur along with sodium and fluid loss.

The antihypertensive effects persist for a longer period of time than does demonstrable inhibition of circulating ACE. It is not known whether the ACE present in vascular endothelium is inhibited longer than the ACE in circulating blood.

Pharmacokinetics

After oral administration of therapeutic doses of CAPOTEN (captopril), rapid absorption occurs with peak blood levels at about one hour. The presence of food in the gastrointestinal tract reduces absorption by about 30 to 40 percent; captopril therefore should be given one hour before meals. Based on carbon-14 labeling, average minimal absorption is approximately 75 percent. In a 24-hour period, over 95 percent of the absorbed dose is eliminated in the urine; 40 to 50 percent is unchanged drug; most of the remainder is the disulfide dimer of captopril and captopril-cysteine disulfide.

Approximately 25 to 30 percent of the circulating drug is bound to plasma proteins. The apparent elimination half-life for total radioactivity in blood is probably less than 3 hours. An accurate determination of half-life of unchanged captopril is not, at present, possible, but it is probably less than 2 hours. In patients with renal impairment, however, retention of captopril occurs (see DOSAGE AND ADMINISTRATION).

Pharmacodynamics

Administration of CAPOTEN (captopril) results in a reduction of peripheral arterial resistance in hypertensive patients with either no change, or an increase, in cardiac output. There is an increase in renal blood flow following administration of CAPOTEN (captopril) and glomerular filtration rate is usually unchanged.

Reductions of blood pressure are usually maximal 60 to 90 minutes after oral administration of an individual dose of CAPOTEN (captopril). The duration of effect is dose related. The reduction in blood pressure may be progressive, so to achieve maximal therapeutic effects, several weeks of therapy may be required. The blood pressure lowering effects of captopril and thiazide-type diuretics are additive. In contrast, captopril and beta-blockers have a less than additive effect.

Blood pressure is lowered to about the same extent in both standing and supine positions. Orthostatic effects and tachycardia are infrequent but may occur in volume-depleted patients. Abrupt withdrawal of CAPOTEN has not been associated with a rapid increase in blood pressure.

In patients with heart failure, significantly decreased peripheral (systemic vascular) resistance and blood pressure (afterload), reduced pulmonary capillary wedge pressure (preload) and pulmonary vascular resistance, increased cardiac output, and increased exercise tolerance time (ETT) have been demonstrated. These hemodynamic and clinical effects occur after the first dose and appear to persist for the duration of therapy. Placebo controlled studies of 12 weeks duration in patients who did not respond adequately to diuretics and digitalis show no tolerance to beneficial effects on ETT; open studies, with exposure up to 18 months in some cases, also indicate that ETT benefit is maintained. Clinical improvement has been observed in some patients where acute hemodynamic effects were minimal.

Studies in rats and cats indicate that CAPOTEN (captopril) does not cross the blood-brain barrier to any significant extent.

INDICATIONS AND USAGE

Hypertension: CAPOTEN (captopril) is indicated for the treatment of hypertension.

In using CAPOTEN, consideration should be given to the risk of neutropenia/agranulocytosis (see WARNINGS).

CAPOTEN may be used as initial therapy for patients with normal renal function, in whom the risk is relatively low. In patients with impaired renal function, particularly those with collagen vascular disease, captopril should be reserved for hypertensives who have either developed unacceptable side effects on other drugs, or have failed to respond satisfactorily to drug combinations.

CAPOTEN is effective alone and in combination with other antihypertensive agents, especially thiazide-type diuretics. The blood pressure lowering effects of captopril and thiazides are approximately additive.

Heart Failure: CAPOTEN is indicated in the treatment of congestive heart failure in patients who have not responded adequately to treatment with diuretics and digitalis. Although the beneficial effect of captopril in heart failure does not require the presence of digitalis, most controlled clinical trial experience with captopril has been in patients receiving digitalis, as well as diuretic treatment. Consequently, CAPOTEN should generally be added to both of these agents except when digitalis use is poorly tolerated or otherwise not feasible.

CONTRAINDICATIONS

CAPOTEN is contraindicated in patients who are hypersensitive to this product.

WARNINGS

Neutropenia/Agranulocytosis

Neutropenia ($<1000/mm^3$) with myeloid hypoplasia has resulted from use of captopril. About half of the neutropenic patients developed systemic or oral cavity infections or other features of the syndrome of agranulocytosis.

The risk of neutropenia is dependent on the clinical status of the patient:

In clinical trials in patients with hypertension who have normal renal function (serum creatinine less than 1.6 mg/dL and no collagen vascular disease), neutropenia has been seen in one patient out of over 8,600 exposed.

In patients with some degree of renal failure (serum creatinine at least 1.6 mg/dL) but no collagen vascular disease, the risk of neutropenia in clinical trials was about 1 per 500, a frequency over 15 times that for uncomplicated hypertension. Daily doses of captopril were relatively high in these patients, particularly in view of their diminished renal function. In foreign marketing experience in patients with renal failure, use of allopurinol concomitantly with captopril has been associated with neutropenia but this association has not appeared in U.S. reports.

In patients with collagen vascular diseases (e.g., systemic lupus erythematosus, scleroderma) and impaired renal function, neutropenia occurred in 3.7 percent of patients in clinical trials.

While none of the over 750 patients in formal clinical trials of heart failure developed neutropenia, it has occurred during the subsequent clinical experience. About half of the reported cases had serum creatinine ≥ 1.6 mg/dL and more than 75 percent were in patients also receiving procainamide. In heart failure, it appears that the same risk factors for neutropenia are present.

The neutropenia has usually been detected within three months after captopril was started. Bone marrow examinations in patients with neutropenia consistently showed myeloid hypoplasia, frequently accompanied by erythroid hypoplasia and decreased numbers of megakaryocytes (e.g., hypoplastic bone marrow and pancytopenia); anemia and thrombocytopenia were sometimes seen.

In general, neutrophils returned to normal in about two weeks after captopril was discontinued, and serious infections were limited to clinically complex patients. About 13 percent of the cases of neutropenia have ended fatally, but almost all fatalities were in patients with serious illness, having collagen vascular disease, renal failure, heart failure or immunosuppressant therapy, or a combination of these complicating factors.

Evaluation of the hypertensive or heart failure patient should always include assessment of renal function.

If captopril is used in patients with impaired renal function, white blood cell and differential counts should be evaluated prior to starting treatment and at approximately two-week intervals for about three months, then periodically.

In patients with collagen vascular disease or who are exposed to other drugs known to affect the white cells or immune response, particularly when there is impaired renal function, captopril should be used only after an assessment of benefit and risk, and then with caution.

All patients treated with captopril should be told to report any signs of infection (e.g., sore throat, fever). If infection is suspected, white cell counts should be performed without delay.

Since discontinuation of captopril and other drugs has generally led to prompt return of the white count to normal, upon confirmation of neutropenia (neutrophil count $<1000/mm^3$) the physician should withdraw captopril and closely follow the patient's course.

Proteinuria

Total urinary proteins greater than 1 g per day were seen in about 0.7 percent of patients receiving captopril. About 90 percent of affected patients had evidence of prior renal disease or received relatively high doses of captopril (in excess of 150 mg/day), or both. The nephrotic syndrome occurred in about one-fifth of proteinuric patients. In most cases, proteinuria subsided or cleared within six months whether or not captopril was continued. Parameters of renal function, such as BUN and creatinine, were seldom altered in the patients with proteinuria.

Since most cases of proteinuria occurred by the eighth month of therapy with captopril, patients with prior renal disease or those receiving captopril at doses greater than 150 mg per day, should have urinary protein estimations (dip-stick on first morning urine) prior to treatment, and periodically thereafter.

Hypotension
Excessive hypotension was rarely seen in hypertensive patients but is a possible consequence of captopril use in severely salt/volume depleted persons such as those treated vigorously with diuretics, for example, patients with severe congestive heart failure (see PRECAUTIONS [Drug Interactions]).

In heart failure, where the blood pressure was either normal or low, transient decreases in mean blood pressure greater than 20 percent were recorded in about half of the patients. This transient hypotension may occur after any of the first several doses and is usually well tolerated, producing either no symptoms or brief mild lightheadedness, although in rare instances it has been associated with arrhythmia or conduction defects. Hypotension was the reason for discontinuation of drug in 3.6 percent of patients with heart failure.

BECAUSE OF THE POTENTIAL FALL IN BLOOD PRESSURE IN THESE PATIENTS, THERAPY SHOULD BE STARTED UNDER VERY CLOSE MEDICAL SUPERVISION. A starting dose of 6.25 or 12.5 mg tid may minimize the hypotensive effect. Patients should be followed closely for the first two weeks of treatment and whenever the dose of captopril and/or diuretic is increased.

Hypotension is not *per se* a reason to discontinue captopril. Some decrease of systemic blood pressure is a common and desirable observation upon initiation of CAPOTEN (captopril) treatment in heart failure. The magnitude of the decrease is greatest early in the course of treatment; this effect stabilizes within a week or two, and generally returns to pretreatment levels, without a decrease in therapeutic efficacy, within two months.

PRECAUTIONS
General
Impaired Renal Function
Hypertension—Some patients with renal disease, particularly those with severe renal artery stenosis, have developed increases in BUN and serum creatinine after reduction of blood pressure with captopril. Captopril dosage reduction and/or discontinuation of diuretic may be required. For some of these patients, it may not be possible to normalize blood pressure and maintain adequate renal perfusion.

Heart Failure—About 20 percent of patients develop stable elevations of BUN and serum creatinine greater than 20 percent above normal or baseline upon long-term treatment with captopril. Less than 5 percent of patients, generally those with severe preexisting renal disease, required discontinuation of treatment due to progressively increasing creatinine; subsequent improvement probably depends upon the severity of the underlying renal disease.

See CLINICAL PHARMACOLOGY, DOSAGE AND ADMINISTRATION, ADVERSE REACTIONS [Altered Laboratory Findings].

Valvular Stenosis: There is concern, on theoretical grounds, that patients with aortic stenosis might be at particular risk of decreased coronary perfusion when treated with vasodilators because they do not develop as much afterload reduction as others.

Surgery/Anesthesia: In patients undergoing major surgery or during anesthesia with agents that produce hypotension, captopril will block angiotensin II formation secondary to compensatory renin release. If hypotension occurs and is considered to be due to this mechanism, it can be corrected by volume expansion.

Information for Patients
Patients should be told to report promptly any indication of infection (e.g., sore throat, fever), which may be a sign of neutropenia, or of progressive edema which might be related to proteinuria and nephrotic syndrome.

All patients should be cautioned that excessive perspiration and dehydration may lead to an excessive fall in blood pressure because of reduction in fluid volume. Other causes of volume depletion such as vomiting or diarrhea may also lead to a fall in blood pressure; patients should be advised to consult with the physician.

Patients should be warned against interruption or discontinuation of medication unless instructed by the physician.

Heart failure patients on captopril therapy should be cautioned against rapid increases in physical activity.

Patients should be informed that CAPOTEN (captopril) should be taken one hour before meals (see DOSAGE AND ADMINISTRATION).

Drug Interactions
Hypotension—Patients on Diuretic Therapy: Patients on diuretics and especially those in whom diuretic therapy was recently instituted, as well as those on severe dietary salt restriction or dialysis, may occasionally experience a precipitous reduction of blood pressure usually within the first hour after receiving the initial dose of captopril.

The possibility of hypotensive effects with captopril can be minimized by either discontinuing the diuretic or increasing the salt intake approximately one week prior to initiation of treatment with CAPOTEN (captopril) or initiating therapy with small doses (6.25 or 12.5 mg). Alternatively, provide medical supervision for at least one hour after the initial dose. If hypotension occurs, the patient should be placed in a supine position and, if necessary, receive an intravenous infusion of normal saline. This transient hypotensive response is not a contraindication to further doses which can be given without difficulty once the blood pressure has increased after volume expansion.

Agents Having Vasodilator Activity: Data on the effect of concomitant use of other vasodilators in patients receiving CAPOTEN (captopril) for heart failure are not available; therefore, nitroglycerin or other nitrates (as used for management of angina) or other drugs having vasodilator activity should, if possible, be discontinued before starting CAPOTEN. If resumed during CAPOTEN therapy, such agents should be administered cautiously, and perhaps at lower dosage.

Agents Causing Renin Release: Captopril's effect will be augmented by antihypertensive agents that cause renin release. For example, diuretics (e.g., thiazides) may activate the renin-angiotensin-aldosterone system.

Agents Affecting Sympathetic Activity: The sympathetic nervous system may be especially important in supporting blood pressure in patients receiving captopril alone or with diuretics. Therefore, agents affecting sympathetic activity (e.g., ganglionic blocking agents or adrenergic neuron blocking agents) should be used with caution. Beta-adrenergic blocking drugs add some further antihypertensive effect to captopril, but the overall response is less than additive.

Agents Increasing Serum Potassium: Since captopril decreases aldosterone production, elevation of serum potassium may occur. Potassium-sparing diuretics such as spironolactone, triamterene, or amiloride, or potassium supplements should be given only for documented hypokalemia, and then with caution, since they may lead to a significant increase of serum potassium. Salt substitutes containing potassium should also be used with caution.

Inhibitors Of Endogenous Prostaglandin Synthesis: It has been reported that indomethacin may reduce the antihypertensive effect of captopril, especially in cases of low renin hypertension. Other nonsteroidal anti-inflammatory agents (e.g., aspirin) may also have this effect.

Drug/Laboratory Test Interaction
Captopril may cause a false-positive urine test for acetone.

Carcinogenesis, Mutagenesis and Impairment of Fertility
Two-year studies with doses of 50 to 1350 mg/kg/day in mice and rats failed to show any evidence of carcinogenic potential.

Studies in rats have revealed no impairment of fertility.

Animal Toxicology
Chronic oral toxicity studies were conducted in rats (2 years), dogs (47 weeks; 1 year), mice (2 years), and monkeys (1 year). Significant drug related toxicity included effects on hematopoiesis, renal toxicity, erosion/ulceration of the stomach, and variation of retinal blood vessels.

Reductions in hemoglobin and/or hematocrit values were seen in mice, rats, and monkeys at doses 50 to 150 times the maximum recommended human dose (MRHD). Anemia, leukopenia, thrombocytopenia, and bone marrow suppression occurred in dogs at doses 8 to 30 times MRHD. The reductions in hemoglobin and hematocrit values in rats and mice were only significant at 1 year and returned to normal with continued dosing by the end of the study. Marked anemia was seen at all dose levels (8 to 30 times MRHD) in dogs, whereas moderate to marked leukopenia was noted only at 15 and 30 times MRHD and thrombocytopenia at 30 times MRHD. The anemia could be reversed upon discontinuation of dosing. Bone marrow suppression occurred to a varying degree, being associated only with dogs that died or were sacrificed in a moribund condition in the 1 year study. However, in the 47-week study at a dose 30 times MRHD, bone marrow suppression was found to be reversible upon continued drug administration.

Captopril caused hyperplasia of the juxtaglomerular apparatus of the kidneys at doses 7 to 200 times the MRHD in rats and mice, at 20 to 60 times MRHD in monkeys, and at 30 times the MRHD in dogs.

Gastric erosions/ulcerations were increased in incidence at 20 and 200 times MRHD in male rats and at 30 and 65 times MRHD in dogs and monkeys, respectively. Rabbits developed gastric and intestinal ulcers when given oral doses approximately 30 times MRHD for only 5 to 7 days.

In the two-year rat study, irreversible and progressive variations in the caliber of retinal vessels (focal sacculations and constrictions) occurred at all dose levels (7 to 200 times MRHD) in a dose-related fashion. The effect was first observed in the 88th week of dosing, with a progressively increased incidence thereafter, even after cessation of dosing.

Pregnancy: Category C
Captopril was embryocidal in rabbits when given in doses about 2 to 70 times (on a mg/kg basis) the maximum recommended human dose, and low incidences of craniofacial malformations were seen. These effects in rabbits were most probably due to the particularly marked decrease in blood pressure caused by the drug in this species.

Captopril given to pregnant rats at 400 times the recommended human dose continuously during gestation and lactation caused a reduction in neonatal survival.

No teratogenic effects (malformations) have been observed after large doses of captopril in hamsters and rats.

Captopril crosses the human placenta.

There are no adequate and well-controlled studies in pregnant women. Captopril should be used during pregnancy, or for patients likely to become pregnant, only if the potential benefit justifies a potential risk to the fetus.

Nursing Mothers
Concentrations of captopril in human milk are approximately one percent of those in maternal blood. The effect of low levels of captopril on the nursing infant has not been determined. Caution should be exercised when captopril is administered to a nursing woman, and, in general, nursing should be interrupted.

Pediatric Use
Safety and effectiveness in children have not been established although there is limited experience with the use of captopril in children from 2 months to 15 years of age with secondary hypertension and varying degrees of

renal insufficiency. Dosage, on a weight basis, was comparable to that used in adults. CAPOTEN (captopril) should be used in children only if other measures for controlling blood pressure have not been effective.

ADVERSE REACTIONS

Reported incidences are based on clinical trials involving approximately 7000 patients.

Renal—About one of 100 patients developed proteinuria (see WARNINGS).

Each of the following has been reported in approximately 1 to 2 of 1000 patients and are of uncertain relationship to drug use: renal insufficiency, renal failure, polyuria, oliguria, and urinary frequency.

Hematologic—Neutropenia/agranulocytosis has occurred (see WARNINGS). Cases of anemia, thrombo-cytopenia, and pancytopenia have been reported.

Dermatologic—Rash, often with pruritus, and sometimes with fever, arthralgia, and eosinophilia, occurred in about 4 to 7 (depending on renal status and dose) of 100 patients, usually during the first four weeks of therapy. It is usually maculopapular, and rarely urticarial. The rash is usually mild and disappears within a few days of dosage reduction, short-term treatment with an antihistaminic agent, and/or discontinuing therapy; remission may occur even if captopril is continued. Pruritus, without rash, occurs in about 2 of 100 patients. Between 7 and 10 percent of patients with skin rash have shown an eosinophilia and/or positive ANA titers. A reversible associated pemphigoid-like lesion, and photosensitivity, have also been reported.

Angioedema of the face, mucous membranes of the mouth, or of the extremities has been observed in approximately 1 of 1000 patients and is reversible on discontinuance of captopril therapy. One case of laryngeal edema has been reported.

Flushing or pallor has been reported in 2 to 5 of 1000 patients.

Cardiovascular—Hypotension may occur; see WARNINGS and PRECAUTIONS [Drug Interactions] for discussion of hypotension on initiation of captopril therapy.

Tachycardia, chest pain, and palpitations have each been observed in approximately 1 of 100 patients.

Angina pectoris, myocardial infarction, Raynaud's syndrome, and congestive heart failure have each occurred in 2 to 3 of 1000 patients.

Dysgeusia—Approximately 2 to 4 (depending on renal status and dose) of 100 patients developed a diminution or loss of taste perception. Taste impairment is reversible and usually self-limited (2 to 3 months) even with continued drug administration. Weight loss may be associated with the loss of taste.

The following have been reported in about 0.5 to 2 percent of patients but did not appear at increased frequency compared to placebo or other treatments used in controlled trials: gastric irritation, abdominal pain, nausea, vomiting, diarrhea, anorexia, constipation, aphthous ulcers, peptic ulcer, dizziness, headache, malaise, fatigue, insomnia, dry mouth, dyspnea, cough, alopecia, paresthesias.

Altered Laboratory Findings

Elevations of liver enzymes have been noted in a few patients but no causal relationship to captopril use has been established. Rare cases of cholestatic jaundice, and of hepatocellular injury with or without secondary cholestasis, have been reported in association with captopril administration.

A transient elevation of BUN and serum creatinine may occur, especially in patients who are volume-depleted or who have renovascular hypertension. In instances of rapid reduction of longstanding or severely elevated blood pressure, the glomerular filtration rate may decrease transiently, also resulting in transient rises in serum creatinine and BUN.

Small increases in the serum potassium concentration frequently occur, especially in patients with renal impairment (see PRECAUTIONS).

OVERDOSAGE

Correction of hypotension would be of primary concern. Volume expansion with an intravenous infusion of normal saline is the treatment of choice for restoration of blood pressure.

Captopril may be removed from the general circulation by hemodialysis.

DOSAGE AND ADMINISTRATION

CAPOTEN (captopril) should be taken one hour before meals. Dosage must be individualized.

Hypertension—Initiation of therapy requires consideration of recent antihypertensive drug treatment, the extent of blood pressure elevation, salt restriction, and other clinical circumstances. If possible, discontinue the patient's previous antihypertensive drug regimen for one week before starting CAPOTEN.

The initial dose of CAPOTEN (captopril) is 25 mg bid or tid. If satisfactory reduction of blood pressure has not been achieved after one or two weeks, the dose may be increased to 50 mg bid or tid. Concomitant sodium restriction may be beneficial when CAPOTEN is used alone.

The dose of CAPOTEN in hypertension usually does not exceed 50 mg tid. Therefore, if the blood pressure has not been satisfactorily controlled after one to two weeks at this dose, (and the patient is not already receiving a diuretic), a modest dose of a thiazide-type diuretic (e.g., hydrochlorothiazide, 25 mg daily), should be added. The diuretic dose may be increased at one- to two-week intervals until its highest usual antihypertensive dose is reached.

If CAPOTEN (captopril) is being started in a patient already receiving a diuretic, CAPOTEN therapy should be initiated under close medical supervision (see WARNINGS and PRECAUTIONS [Drug Interactions] regarding hypotension), with dosage and titration of CAPOTEN as noted above.

If further blood pressure reduction is required, the dose of CAPOTEN may be increased to 100 mg bid or tid and then, if necessary, to 150 mg bid or tid (while continuing the diuretic). The usual dose range is 25 to 150 mg bid or tid. A maximum daily dose of 450 mg CAPOTEN should not be exceeded.

For patients with severe hypertension (e.g., accelerated or malignant hypertension), when temporary discontinuation of current antihypertensive therapy is not practical or desirable, or when prompt titration to more normotensive blood pressure levels is indicated, diuretic should be continued but other current antihypertensive medication stopped and CAPOTEN dosage promptly initiated at 25 mg bid or tid, under close medical supervision.

When necessitated by the patient's clinical condition, the daily dose of CAPOTEN may be increased every 24 hours or less under continuous medical supervision until a satisfactory blood pressure response is obtained or the maximum dose of CAPOTEN (captopril) is reached. In this regimen, addition of a more potent diuretic, e.g., furosemide, may also be indicated.

Beta-blockers may also be used in conjunction with CAPOTEN therapy (see PRECAUTIONS [Drug Interactions]), but the effects of the two drugs are less than additive.

Heart Failure—Initiation of therapy requires consideration of recent diuretic therapy and the possibility of severe salt/volume depletion. In patients with either normal or low blood pressure, who have been vigorously treated with diuretics and who may be hyponatremic and/or hypovolemic, a starting dose of 6.25 or 12.5 mg tid may minimize the magnitude or duration of the hypotensive effect (see WARNINGS, [Hypotension]); for these patients, titration to the usual daily dosage can then occur within the next several days.

For most patients the usual initial daily dosage is 25 mg tid. After a dose of 50 mg tid is reached, further increases in dosage should be delayed, where possible, for at least two weeks to determine if a satisfactory response occurs. Most patients studied have had a satisfactory clinical improvement at 50 or 100 mg tid. A maximum daily dose of 450 mg of CAPOTEN (captopril) should not be exceeded.

CAPOTEN is to be used in conjunction with a diuretic and digitalis. CAPOTEN therapy must be initiated under very close medical supervision.

Dosage Adjustment in Renal Impairment—Because CAPOTEN (captopril) is excreted primarily by the kidneys, excretion rates are reduced in patients with impaired renal function. These patients will take longer to reach steady-state captopril levels and will reach higher steady-state levels for a given daily dose than patients with normal renal function. Therefore, these patients may respond to smaller or less frequent doses.

Accordingly, for patients with significant renal impairment, initial daily dosage of CAPOTEN (captopril) should be reduced, and smaller increments utilized for titration, which should be quite slow (one- to two-week intervals). After the desired therapeutic effect has been achieved, the dose should be slowly back-titrated to determine the minimal effective dose. When concomitant diuretic therapy is required, a loop diuretic (e.g., furosemide), rather than a thiazide diuretic, is preferred in patients with severe renal impairment.

HOW SUPPLIED

12.5 mg tablets in bottles of 100 and 1000, **25 mg tablets** in bottles of 100 and 1000, **50 mg tablets** in bottles of 100 and 1000, and **100 mg tablets** in bottles of 100. Bottles contain a desiccant-charcoal canister.

Unimatic® unit-dose packs containing 100 tablets are also available for each potency: **12.5 mg, 25 mg, 50 mg,** and **100 mg.**

The **12.5 mg tablet** is a flat oval with a partial bisect bar; the **25 mg tablet** is a biconvex rounded square with a quadrisect bar; the **50 and 100 mg tablets** are biconvex ovals with a bisect bar.

All captopril tablets are white and may exhibit a slight sulfurous odor. Tablet identification numbers: 12.5 mg, **450**; 25 mg, **452**; 50 mg, **482**; and 100 mg, **485**.

Storage

Do not store above 86° F.   Keep bottles tightly closed (protect from moisture).   (J3-658L)

NOTES

NOTES

NOTES

NOTES